Comprehensive Virology 7

Comprehensive Virology

Edited by Heinz Fraenkel-Conrat
University of California at Berkeley

and Robert R. Wagner
University of Virginia

Editorial Board

Reproduction

Structure and Assembly

Regulation and Genetics

Interaction of Viruses and Their Hosts

Effects of Physical and Chemical Agents

Comprehensive

Edited by

Heinz Fraenkel-Conrat

Department of Molecular Biology and Virus Laboratory
University of California, Berkeley, California

and

Robert R. Wagner

Department of Microbiology
University of Virginia, Charlottesville, Virginia

Virology

7

Reproduction

Bacterial DNA Viruses

PLENUM PRESS · NEW YORK AND LONDON

Library of Congress Cataloging in Publication Data

Fraenkel-Conrat, Heinz, 1910-
  Reproduction, bacterial DNA viruses.

(Their Comprehensive virology; 7)
Includes bibliographies and index.
1. Viruses–Reproduction. 2. Bacteriophage. I. Wagner, Robert R., 1923-   Joint author. II. Title. III. Series: Fraenkel-Conrat, Heinz, 1910-   Comprehensive virology; 7. [DNLM: 1. DNA replication. 2. Virus replication. QW160 C737 v. 7]
QR357.F72 vol. 7 [QR470]   576'.64'08s   [576'.6482]
ISBN 0-306-35147-1   76-40342

© 1977 Plenum Press, New York
A Division of Plenum Publishing Corporation
227 West 17th Street, New York, N.Y. 10011

Printed in the United States of American

Foreword

The time seems ripe for a critical compendium of that segment of the biological universe we call viruses. Virology, as a science, having passed only recently through its descriptive phase of naming and numbering, has probably reached that stage at which relatively few new— truly new—viruses will be discovered. Triggered by the intellectual probes and techniques of molecular biology, genetics, biochemical cytology, and high-resolution microscopy and spectroscopy, the field has experienced a genuine information explosion.

Few serious attempts have been made to chronicle these events. This comprehensive series, which will comprise some 6000 pages in a total of about 22 volumes, represents a commitment by a large group of active investigators to analyze, digest, and expostulate on the great mass of data relating to viruses, much of which is now amorphous and disjointed, and scattered throughout a wide literature. In this way, we hope to place the entire field in perspective, and to develop an invaluable reference and sourcebook for researchers and students at all levels.

This series is designed as a continuum that can be entered anywhere, but which also provides a logical progression of developing facts and integrated concepts.

Volume 1 contains an alphabetical catalogue of almost all viruses of vertebrates, insects, plants, and protists, describing them in general terms. Volumes 2–4 deal primarily, but not exclusively, with the process of infection and reproduction of the major groups of viruses in their hosts. Volume 2 deals with the simple RNA viruses of bacteria, plants, and animals; the togaviruses (formerly called arboviruses), which share with these only the feature that the virion's RNA is able to act as messenger RNA in the host cell; and the reoviruses of animals and plants, which all share several structurally singular features, the most important being the double-strandedness of their multiple RNA molecules. This grouping, of course, has only slightly more in its favor than others that could have been, or indeed were, considered.

Volume 3 addresses itself to the reproduction of all DNA-containing viruses of vertebrates, a seemingly simple act of classification, even though the field encompasses the smallest and the largest viruses known. The reproduction of the larger and more complex RNA viruses is the subject matter of Volume 4. These viruses share the property of lipid-rich envelopes with the togaviruses included in Volume 2. They share as a group, and with the reoviruses, the presence of enzymes in their virions and the need for their RNA to become transcribed before it can serve messenger functions.

Volumes 5 and 6 represent the first in a series that focuses primarily on the structure and assembly of virus particles. Volume 5 is devoted to general structural principles involving the relationship and specificity of interaction of viral capsid proteins and their nucleic acids, or host nucleic acids. It deals primarily with helical and the simpler isometric viruses, as well as with the relationship of nucleic acid to protein shell in the T-even phages. Volume 6 is concerned with the structure of the picornaviruses, and with the reconstitution of plant and bacterial RNA viruses.

Volumes 7 and 8 deal with the DNA bacteriophages. Volume 7 concludes the series of volumes on the reproduction of viruses (Volumes 2–4 and Volume 7) and deals particularly with the single- and double-stranded virulent bacteriophages.

Volume 8 will be the first of the series on regulation and genetics of viruses, in which the biological properties of the lysogenic and defective phages will be covered, the phage–satellite system P2–P4 described, and the regulatory principles governing the development of selected typical lytic phages discussed in depth.

Volume 8 will be followed by three others dealing with the regulation of gene expression and integration of animal viruses; the genetics of animal viruses; and regulation of plant virus development, covirus systems, satellitism, and viroids. In addition, it is anticipated that there will be two or three other volumes devoted largely to structural aspects and the assembly of bacteriophages and animal viruses, and to special virus groups.

The complete series will endeavor to encompass all aspects of the molecular biology and the behavior of viruses. We hope to keep this series up to date at all times by prompt and rapid publication of all contributions, and by encouraging the authors to update their chapters by additions or corrections whenever a volume is reprinted.

Contents

Chapter 2

Replication of Filamentous Bacteriophages

Dan S. Ray

Chapter 3

Reproduction of Large Virulent Bacteriophages

Christopher K. Mathews

The Isometric Single-Stranded DNA Phages

David T. Denhardt

Department of Biochemistry
McGill University
Montreal, Quebec, Canada

"When you are a Bear of Very Little Brain, and you Think of Things, you find sometimes that a Thing which seemed very Thingish inside you is quite different when it gets out into the open and has other people looking at it."

—A. A. Milne, *The House at Pooh Corner*

1. INTRODUCTION

1.1. A Circular, Single-Stranded DNA Molecule within a Tailless Capsid

The subjects of this chapter have an isometric capsid with icosahedral symmetry enclosing a single-stranded DNA genome. The RNA bacteriophages appear to have a similar structure. Some eukaryotic viruses, but no phages that I know of, contain double-stranded DNA enclosed in an isometric capsid, *sans* tail. Isometric structures can be constructed of subunits arranged with cubic symmetry—either tetrahedral, octahedral, or icosahedral. Each of these symmetries requires a set of identical subunits—12, 24, and 60, respectively—arranged on the surface of a sphere. An attribute of icosahedral symmetry is that a subunit of a fixed size can enclose a larger volume than can be enclosed by using either of the other two point group symmetries

(Caspar and Klug, 1962), and it is this kind of symmetry, or derivatives thereof, that seems to be used generally in virus construction, for example in the heads of the tailed phages.

Viruses with single-stranded DNA are among the smallest forms of "life" known. Those replicating in prokaryotic cells contain fewer than ten genes, while the eukaryotic parvoviruses (Rose, 1974) may contain only a single gene. All of the single-stranded DNA viruses have genomes with molecular weights in the range of 1 to 3 $\times$ 10^6. Larger single-stranded DNAs may have been selected against because of the sensitivity of the single-stranded DNA to environmental hazards; if so, those viruses extant now may be the remnants of a once more diverse primitive life form. One reason for interest in these viruses is that because of the small size of their DNA and their limited genetic content they are very dependent on the host cell. Consequently, they provide a probe for various cell functions—particularly those concerned with replicating the genome.

There is no evidence for an evolutionary relationship between the eukaryotic parvoviruses, of which there may be more than one fundamentally different type, and the prokaryotic phages. I have argued elsewhere that the superficially quite distinct filamentous phages, which also contain single-stranded DNA and are reviewed by Ray in Chapter 2 of this volume, are derived from the same primitive ancestor as the isometric phages and that the isometric phages are variations on a common theme (Denhardt, 1975). For the latter, the single-stranded DNA (always of the same polarity) is enclosed in a protein coat about 32 nm in diameter, composed of multiple copies of four different polypeptides. An electron micrograph of ϕX174 is shown in Fig. 1. The isometric phages all seem to have a common organization of the genome and a set of proteins with equivalent functions. The fact that different isolates are serologically unrelated is not necessarily symptomatic of a lack of relationship since this property may be easily affected by mutations (Bone and Dowell, 1973a). The base sequence of the genome is capable of changing to a surprising degree without losing its ability to produce a functionally equivalent set of proteins (Godson, 1973). Many of the single-stranded DNA phages, including the filamentous phages, have a high (30–35%) molar ratio of thymine in the viral DNA (Marvin and Hohn, 1969; Sinsheimer, 1968), perhaps because codons containing uracil are favored (Denhardt and Marvin, 1969; Sanger, 1975).

The best known isometric phages are S13 (Burnet, 1927) and ϕX174 (Sertic and Boulgakov, 1935); evidence that they are related was first provided by Zahler (1958). Because of the extensive work done

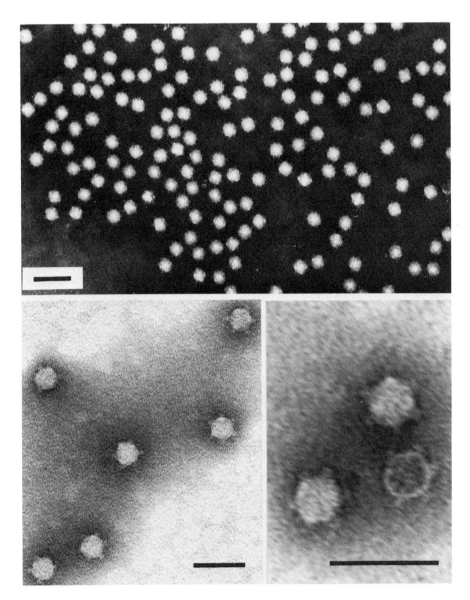

Fig. 1.   Electron micrograph of φX174 negatively stained with phosphotungstic acid. The bar represents 0.05 μm. I thank L. Guluzian and C. Hours for the electron microscopy.

with φX174 (Sinsheimer, 1968), it can be used as the archetype with which the others can be contrasted. These others include φR (Kay and Bradley, 1962; Burton and Yagi, 1968), α3 and St-1 (Bradley, 1970; Bowes and Dowell, 1974), φA and φK (Taketo, 1974, and personal communication), 6SR and BR2 (Lindberg, 1973), U3 (Watson and Paigen, 1971), and the G phages (Godson, 1974b). Host bacteria for these various isolates are appropriate strains of Enterobacteriaceae— *Escherichia, Shigella,* and *Salmonella.* Although some isolates will grow on *E. coli* K (St-1, U3, φK) and others on B (α3), *E. coli* C seems to be the most common host. Insofar as these phages have been studied, there is no reason to think that they differ in any fundamental from φX174. Mutants of φX174 capable of growing on K12 (Bone and Dowell, 1973a,b) and B (Denhardt unpublished, see Razin, 1973) have been isolated. The fact that different isolates made at different times in widely separate parts of the world are all so similar indicates that comparative research should now be concentrated on those we have. I have limited this review to a selected set of references and have concentrated on φX174 except in those cases where the others provide an interesting contrast. For a complete overview of earlier research, see Hoffmann-Berling *et al.* (1966) and Sinsheimer (1968). I offer my apologies to anyone whose work in any specific instance has not been cited. Many facts have been established independently by different individuals and it was not practical to include all possible references.

1.2. Genes and Proteins of the Isometric Phages

φX174 has as its chromosome one molecule of a circular, single-stranded DNA with a molecular weight of about 1.7×10^6, or 5370 nucleotides (Section 1.4.5 and Table 3). The viral DNA has the same polarity as the mRNA and is thus the "plus" strand. A genome of this size can code for about 200,000 daltons of protein assuming that the "average" amino acid has a molecular weight of 120 and all 1670 potential codons are used once, and only once. Eight genes (A–H) have been identified and mapped and the protein products of most of them identified unambiguously. The genetic map (see Fig. 2) is circular (Baker and Tessman, 1967). A list of the genes, their earlier designations, and the molecular weights and functions of the proteins insofar as they are known is presented in Table 1. The direction of transcription and translation is clockwise (Vanderbilt *et al.,* 1971).

Structural proteins found in the virion include the products of genes F, G, and H and have molecular weights of about 50,000, 20,000,

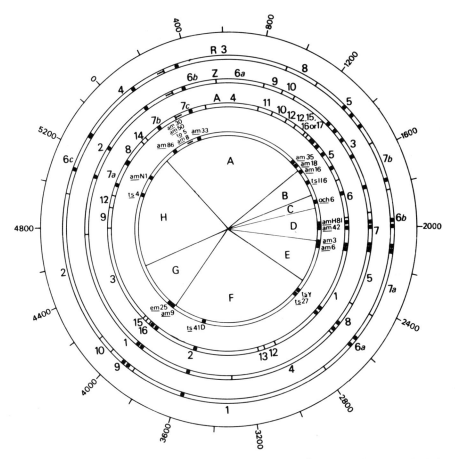

Fig. 2.   Genetic and restriction enzyme maps of the ϕX174 genome. The outer circle is arbitrarily divided into 5500 base pairs; 5370 is probably more accurate. The inner circle is divided into pie-shaped portions each of which is allocated to a gene on the basis of either the known size of the protein or the size estimated from the physical mapping data. The three concentric circles labeled R, Z, and A give the location of the various cleavage products produced by the restriction enzymes *Hind*II, *Hae*III, and *Alu*I, respectively. The sites of various nonsense and temperature-sensitive mutants used to correlate the genetic and physical maps are indicated; *to*5 and *em*25 are tourmaline and emerald mutations, respectively, classified according to their ability to grow on *Shigella sonnei* V64 (Borrias *et al.*, 1969). Reproduced from Weisbeek *et al.* (1976), with permission.

and 37,000, respectively (Burgess, 1969*a*; Mayol and Sinsheimer, 1970; Godson, 1971*a*). Three proteins involved in DNA replication, A, C, and D, have molecular weights of about 60,000, 10,000, and 14,000, respectively (Burgess and Denhardt, 1969; Godson, 1971*a*; Borras *et al.*, 1971; van der Mei *et al.*, 1972*b*). A* results from a translational restart within

TABLE 1

Genes and Gene Functions of the Isometric Phages

Gene designation	Molecular weight of the protein product	Mutant phenotype or function(s) of the protein
A (VI, C, IV)[a]	60,000[b]	RF replication and SS DNA synthesis
B (IV, B, II)	20,000	SS DNA synthesis and virion morphogenesis
C (VIII, H, VI)	12,000	SS DNA synthesis
D (V, D, VII)	14,000	SS DNA synthesis, probably virion morphogenesis
E (I, G, V)	(10,000?)	Lysis of the cell
F (VII, E, I)	50,000	Capsid protein, SS DNA synthesis
G (III, F, IIIa)	20,000	Spike protein, SS DNA synthesis
H (II, A, IIIb)	37,000	Spike protein, pilot protein (?)
A*	37,000	? (the C-terminal portion of A)[c]

[a] The designations in parentheses are those originally given to these genes by Sinsheimer (Benbow *et al.,* 1971), Hayashi (Hayashi and Hayashi, 1971), and Tessman (Tessman *et al.,* 1971), respectively.

[b] The molecular weights given are approximate. Different laboratories have reported slightly different values, and the molecular weights of the corresponding proteins coded for by different isolates of the isometric phages vary somewhat. The relative mobilities of proteins A*/H and B/G can vary with the gel system. (Data compiled from the results of Burgess and Denhardt, 1969; Godson, 1971*a,* 1973; Borras *et al.,* 1971; van der Mei *et al.,* 1972*b*; Linney *et al.,* 1972; Benbow *et al.,* 1972*b*; Siden and Hayashi, 1974.)

[c] A* is part of gene A, and the A* protein is produced as the result of a translational start signal within gene A (Linney *et al.,* 1972; Linney and Hayashi, 1973).

gene A and corresponds to the *C*-terminal portion of the gene A protein (Linney and Hayashi, 1974). The gene B protein is required for virion formation and appears to have a molecular weight of about 20,000 (Benbow *et al.,* 1972*b*; Siden and Hayashi, 1974). The gene E protein has not been clearly identified, but if we assume that the *del*E deletion (see Fig. 10 and Section 7.1) is congruent with that gene then it would have a molecular weight of about 14,000. A protein of about this size was uncovered in SDS gels of virus-coded proteins when the similarly sized gene D protein was eliminated by an amber mutation. The molecular weights of these proteins were determined by electrophoresis in polyacrylamide gels in the presence of sodium dodecylsulfate and mercaptoethanol (see Fig. 11) and there is thus uncertainty in their precise molecular weights. Various substituents on the protein can alter its mobility, and the relative mobilities of certain proteins (H vs. A*, B vs. G) vary with the cross-linker (Linney and Hayashi, 1974; Siden and Hayashi, 1974). These proteins total about 200,000 daltons, and it appears that all of the coding capacity of the genome is accounted for. Two additional genes (gene I, Hayashi and Hayashi, 1971, and gene J, Benbow *et al.,* 1972*b*) have been reported, but current evidence does not confirm their existence (M. Hayashi, personal communication; Weisbeek *et al.*, 1976).

1.3. Enzymatic and Chemical Studies

1.3.1. Restriction Enzyme Maps

A number of researchers have developed restriction enzyme maps of the viral replicative form DNA, and in some cases have assigned particular genetic loci to particular cleavage products. The fairly detailed correlation reported by Weisbeek *et al.* (1976) is illustrated in Fig. 2. Mutations can be assigned to DNA fragments by formation of partial heteroduplexes between intact mutant viral strands and a complementary strand fragment derived from the restriction enzyme cleavage product derived from wild-type RF (Hutchison and Edgell, 1971; Edgell *et al.*, 1972). Wild-type progeny will be produced in spheroplasts infected with these heteroduplexes only when the restriction enzyme fragment carries the relevant portion of the wild-type allele.

Restriction endonucleases that have been used to characterize isometric phage DNA are listed in Table 2 together with a summary of the number of fragments produced from the different genomes. In the literature, the sizes of the individual fragments have usually been calculated assuming that the size of the ϕX174 genome was close to 5500 nucleotides. Since the correct nucleotide content is probably closer to 5370 (Section 1.4.5), the sizes of the individual fragments that have been reported may be some 2% too high. Enzymes which put only one cleavage into viral RF molecules include *Eco*R1, *Mbo*I, *Pst*I, *Ava*I, *Kpn*I, and *Bgl*I. Restriction of ϕX174 replication *in vivo* by F factors (Groman, 1969) and by *Eco*B (Schnegg and Hofschneider, 1969) has been reported.

There is disagreement between Weisbeek *et al.* (1976) (see Fig. 2) and Lee and Sinsheimer (1974*a*) on the relative positions of the *Hae*III 6a and 6b fragments. Grosveld *et al.* (1976) also mapped these fragments, and the *Hin*dII 6a, 6b, 6c, 7a, and 7b fragments, but named them according to their location in the genome. The fragments in each group have similar mobilities in gels and are difficult to separate cleanly. A terminology based on the purported size deduced from relative migration rates in acrylamide and/or agarose may be awkward because differences in base composition or sequence may reverse the relative migration rates of certain fragments under different condi-

TABLE 2
Number of Cleavages of Isometric Phage RF by Restriction Enzymes[a]

Enzyme (cell)	Sequence	ϕX174	S13	G4	St-1
*Hind*II (*Haemophilus influenzae* serotype d)	GTPy/PuAC	13 (a,d,j)	13 (j)	6 (i)	6
*Hae*III (*Haemophilus aegyptius*)	GG/CC	11 (b,d,h)	10 (j)	12	12
*Hae*II (*Haemophilus aegyptius*)	PuGCGC/Py	7	5	3	—
*Hpa*II (*Haemophilus parainfluenzae*)	C/CGG	5 (f,i) 8 (c,d)	7	7 (i)	14
*Hpa*I (*Haemophilus parainfluenzae*)	GTT/AAC	3	3	—	—
*Hap*II (*Haemophilus aphirophilus*)	C/CGG	5 (e)	7 (e)	—	—
*Hin*H (*Haemophilus influenzae* H-I)	PuGCGCPy	8 (e)	3 (e)	—	—
*Hin*f (*Haemophilus influenzae* serotype f)	G/ANTC	16	17	13	15
*Hha*I (*Haemophilus haemolyticus*)	GCG/C	14 (h)	19	12	16
*Hph*I (*Haemophilus parahaemolyticus*)	GGTGA[b]	6	7	10	11
*Hga*I (*Haemophilus gallinarum*)	—	14	15	14	11
*Alu*I (*Arthrobacter luteus*)	AG/CT	23 (g), 24	25	10	20
*Mbo*I (*Moraxella bovis*)	/GATC	0	1	2	4
*Mbo*II (*Moraxella bovis*)	GAAGA[b]	11	17	18	18
*Eco*RI (*Escherichia coli* resistance transfer factor I)	G/AATTC	0 (i)	0 (i)	1 (i)	4
*Pst*I (*Providencia stuartii* 164)	CTGCA/G	1	1	1	0
*Ava*I (*Anabaena varibilis*)	CGPu/PyCG	1	1	0	0
*Bgl*I (*Bacillus globiggi*)	—	0	0	2	1
*Kpn*I (*Klebsiella pneumoniae* OK 8)	—	0	0	1	1

[a] References: (a) Edgell *et al.* (1972), (b) Middleton *et al.* (1972), (c) Johnson *et al.* (1973), (d) Lee and Sinsheimer (1974a), (e) Hayashi and Hayashi (1974), (f) Godson and Boyer (1974), (g) Vereijken *et al.* (1975), (h) Blakesley and Wells (1975), (i) Godson (1975a), (j) Grosveld *et al.* (1976). If no reference is given, the number of cleavages is taken from Godson and Roberts (1976). These workers screened 26 restriction enzymes. (In a few cases, the number of cleavages may be underestimated.) In some of the *Hind*II preparations, *Hind*III was also present but there appear to be no sites in ϕX174 sensitive to this enzyme. Johnson *et al.* (1973) and Lee and Sinsheimer (1974a) used an enzyme preparation from *H. parainfluenzae* that probably contained both *Hpa*I and *Hpa*II activities.

[b] Cleavage is some 8 nucleotides away. See Roberts (1976) for other references and additional details.

tions. Mobilities of fragments in gels are known to be influenced by the nucleotide composition or sequence (Thomas and Davis, 1975).

A few of the enzymes (*Hae*III, *Hha*I, *Sfa*I, *Mbo*II, *Hin*f, *Hpa*II, *Hae*II) will also cleave single-stranded DNA into a set of fragments which at least in some cases correspond to the fragments generated from duplex DNA (Blakesley and Wells, 1975; Godson and Roberts, 1976). Complete digestion may require larger amounts of enzyme and longer incubation times than are needed for duplex DNA.

1.3.2. Pyrimidine Oligonucleotide Analyses

One of the earliest techniques developed for DNA sequence analysis was to generate the tracts of pyrimidines present in the DNA by complete depurination and hydrolysis of the apurinic DNA that resulted (Hall and Sinsheimer, 1963; Cerny *et al.*, 1969; Darby *et al.*, 1970; Delaney and Spencer, 1976). Ling (1972) determined the sequences of some of the longer pyrimidine tracts present in ϕX174 DNA and compared them with previously determined sequences present in f1 DNA. There was some homology between the large pyrimidine tracts—e.g., both phages contained the sequence CTTTTTTT— and the possibility that the two types of phages were related was raised. Harbers *et al.* (1976) extensively characterized the pyrimidine oligonucleotides in S13 DNA and compared the sequences of the larger ones with those present in ϕX174 DNA. Extensive homology was observed in that 10 out of the 14 sequences elucidated were identical in the two phages; however, the largest pyrimidine tract observed, CTTCCTCT-TCT, was unique to S13. Several sequences, e.g., CTCTTTCTC, were found that read the same in both directions—excluding polarity—and were called "true palindromes."

1.4. Properties of ϕX174 Virus and ϕX174 Viral DNA Forms

1.4.1. The Virion

ϕX174 has a particle weight of 6.2×10^6 (Sinsheimer, 1959). The molecular weight of the sodium salt of the DNA is 1.59×10^6. If we add to this the major protein components F ($60 \times 50,000$), G ($60 \times 20,000$), and H ($12 \times 37,000$), we obtain 6.23×10^6. There are also 30–50 copies of a low molecular weight protein (5000–15,000) of unknown origin in the virion (Burgess, 1969*a*; Mayol and Sinsheimer, 1970) and one copy of what is probably A* (Godson, 1971a; Linney and Hayashi, 1974). The number 6.2×10^6 would be on the low side if, as is likely, some of the particles in the virus preparation had lost some of their protein or DNA. In a typical ϕX174 preparation, 60–90% of the particles can be inactive. There is sufficient putrescine and spermidine in ϕX174 virions to neutralize about 0.5% of the DNA phosphates (Bachrach et al., 1975); presumably the rest are neutralized by other cations and positive charges on the capsid proteins. This calculation reveals that the major components of the virion have been identified.

In electron micrographs, the particles appear capable of packing with a minimum separation of about 27 nm in semicrystalline arrays (Daems et al., 1962). The apparent diameter of negatively stained particles is 24–25 nm if the spikes are not included. Under conditions where the spikes can be visualized, the distance between the tips of opposite spikes is 32–36 nm, a value in agreement with the diameter (31.4 ± 0.6 nm) calculated from the translational diffusion coefficient determined by laser self-beat spectroscopy (Bayer and Starkey, 1972; Bayer and DeBlois, 1974). A diameter of 29 nm was estimated from light scattering (Sinsheimer, 1959). These results suggest the presence of a dense core composed of the DNA encased in a shell from which extend by some 5 nm the less dense protein spikes. In high-resolution electron micrographs, spikes can be seen protruding from the virus at the 12 vertices of an icosahedron. Treatment with 4 M urea removes the gene G and gene H proteins and leaves a spherical, "spikeless" particle composed primarily of protein F and the DNA (Edgell et al., 1969).

The proposal (Burgess, 1969a) that 60 copies of the gene F protein formed an icosahedral shell about the DNA and that the 12 spikes occupied the 12 faces with fivefold symmetry is consistent with what we know about the structure of the virion. Each spike would be composed of five copies of the gene G protein, which is known to interact with five copies of the gene F protein (see Section 6.1), and one copy of the gene H protein. In none of the electron microscopic studies has an attempt been made to distinguish the heat-resistant poorly adsorbing particles from the heat-sensitive "activated" particles (see Section 2.1).

None of the other isometric phages has been studied in as much detail as ϕX174. S13 is clearly very similar (Jeng et al., 1970; Spencer et al., 1972; Godson, 1973). Both the St-1 virion and its DNA have slightly higher sedimentation coefficients than ϕX174 and its DNA (Bowes and Dowell, 1974). ϕA (Taketo, 1974) is very similar, whereas U3 (Watson and Paigen, 1971) may be slightly smaller. The various G phages (Godson, 1974b) have physical properties almost identical to those of ϕX174.

1.4.2. "70 S" Particles

"70 S" particles sometimes constitute a significant portion of a virus preparation (Sinsheimer, 1968). They are believed to be degradation products of mature virions formed by an interaction between the virus particles and cell debris after cell lysis (Bleichrodt and Knijnenburg, 1969). However, it is not excluded that some of them are also precursor particles or abnormal intracellular structures (Weisbeek and Sinsheimer, 1974; Section 6.1). In addition to their reduced sedimentation coefficient, these particles are less dense and contain less DNA. The DNA isolated from a population of particles has a molecular weight of about 4×10^5 and is composed of fragments representing most, if not all, of the genome (Weisbeek *et al.,* 1972). The protein composition of the "70 S" particles, in contrast to the defective particles made in gene H mutants, is identical to that of whole phage (Mayol and Sinsheimer, 1970).

1.4.3. Hairpin Loops

The viral DNA is a covalently continuous circular polydeoxynucleotide containing no non-DNA components. It can be completely degraded by nucleases (Schaller, 1969; Radloff and Vinograd, 1971) and has been entirely synthesized *in vitro* (Section 2.3.1). In earlier work, it had been suggested that there was a nonnucleotide component in ϕX174 DNA because of the inability of exonuclease I to degrade linear single-stranded DNA completely under certain conditions; however, this was later shown to result from secondary structure in the DNA (Sinsheimer, 1968). Bartok *et al.* (1975) have partially characterized the regions of single-stranded ϕX174 DNA that are resistant to the *Neurospora crassa* single-strand specific nucleases. By this criterion, there are two or three especially stable hairpin structures in ϕX174 DNA, one composed of approximately 48 nucleotides and one (perhaps two) of about 32 nucleotides. The sequences are specific and yield a very limited number of pyrimidine oligonucleotide tracts after digestion (see Fig. 15). In particular, T_4 and T_5 sequences are highly enriched. The location of these sequences in the genome is not known, nor is their function, if any. It may be a coincidence, but there are also three promoters in ϕX174 (Section 3.1.1). The sequences of several promoter and ribosome-binding sites have been elucidated in the single-stranded DNA phages but there is not enough information available to make any striking correlations (Denhardt, 1975).

1.4.4. Superhelical RF I

A portion of the double-stranded replicative form DNA (RF) that accumulates in the cell after infection is found as a covalently closed duplex circle and is called RF I. Another portion, in which at least one of the strands is not covalently continuous, usually because of a nick or gap, is called RF II. These two forms of DNA differ in their sedimentation coefficients after isolation. RF I sediments more rapidly than RF II because the superhelical twists in the molecule make it more compact. RF I, and other covalently closed circular duplexes, whether superhelical or not, can also be distinguished from RF II in CsCl equilibrium density gradients containing an intercalating dye such as ethidium bromide. Because the number of dye molecules that can be intercalated into the covalently closed circular molecule is restricted relative to nicked or linear molecules, the closed circular duplex bands at a greater density. These properties of RF I are the result of a topological constraint on the closed circular duplex—the number of times one strand winds around the other (α) must remain constant. The winding number (α) can be expressed as the sum of two other numbers, the duplex winding number (β) and the superhelix winding number (τ) (Bauer and Vinograd, 1968). I have attempted to illustrate these and other properties in a simple fashion in Fig. 3 using a linear molecule with constrained ends; this is equivalent to a closed circular duplex and facilitates the depiction of various properties.

The first property is the relation between β and τ. Any change in β must be compensated for by a change in τ. For example, if the pitch of the helix *in vivo* were slightly different from the pitch *in vitro* then a superhelical molecule would be generated (I → II or III). Recent measurements indicate that ethidium intercalation unwinds the duplex by 26° (Wang, 1974). If this measurement is combined with measurements of the amount of ethidium required to remove all superhelical turns [0.055 mol per mol nucleotide in 3 M CsCl (Wang, 1969); 0.04 mol per mol nucleotide in 50 mM tris-HCl (Waring, 1970)] from ϕX174 RF I (10^4 nucleotides), one can calculate that there are 30 (low salt) to 40 (high salt) negative superhelical turns in the duplex (superhelix density of -0.06 to -0.08). It is noteworthy that in this range there is an inverse correlation between the sedimentation coefficient and the superhelix density (Denhardt and Kato, 1973). Campbell and Jolly (1973) have analyzed by light scattering the various structures (Y-shaped, toroidal) that ϕX174 RF assumes as a function of the superhelix density.

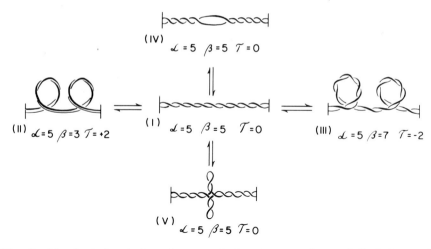

Fig. 3. Topological relations between duplex turns and superhelical turns. A restrained linear duplex is shown rather than a covalently closed circular duplex for ease of representation; the same relations hold. In all cases, the topological winding number (α) is fixed at 5, i.e., the number of times one strand winds about the other. Form I exists in an environment where the duplex winding number (β) is precisely compatible with α. In order to accommodate a more tightly wound duplex, either a region must be partially denatured (IV) or compensating negative superhelical twists (τ) must be formed (III). Note that if the denatured region in IV can be created in a region containing a palindrome then a structure can be established that is stabilized by the formation of base-stacked, hydrogen-bonded hairpin loops (V). The transition from III to V illustrates the interconvertibility of negative superhelical turns and cruciform structures. During replication or transcription when regions of a restrained duplex are forced to wind in order to compensate for the unwinding induced by the polymerase elsewhere in the molecule, the duplex winding number can be kept constant if positive superhelical turns are introduced; the transition from I to II illustrates how the introduction of positive superhelical turns reduces the number of duplex turns. The presence of positive superhelical turns will not favor cruciform formation.

If the *in vitro* superhelix structure is a uniform B form duplex with ten base pairs per turn, then *in vivo* there would be close to 11 base pairs per turn for a completely base-paired nonsuperhelical duplex. Eleven pairs per turn is a property of A form DNA. The "take-home" lesson of this exercise is that we do not know the detailed structure of the DNA *in vivo* and that the conformation of the duplex (pitch, number of base pairs per turn) is sensitive to the environment, to base composition, and to nucleotide sequence.

The second property is that hairpin formation restores much of the base stacking and H-bonding energy lost when a segment of a duplex is denatured; hence in a molecule with a high superhelix density the formation of a cruciform structure (V) would be favored. If such regions were present in RF I *in vivo,* but not *in vitro,* then negative superhelical turns would be generated upon isolation if the pitch of the Watson–Crick helix remained unchanged. Note that the pitch, or number of base pairs per turn, can be the same for the duplex sections in structures III, IV, and V, and can be greater than for structures I and II. There is no evidence for the presence of cruciform structures in ϕX174 RF I (Bartok and Denhardt, 1976).

Whether superhelical molecules exist *in vivo* or not, and if they do not exist as such then why they become negatively superhelical after isolation, is not known. Unwinding of a region of a constrained duplex during replication or transcription will generate positive superhelical molecules (structure II). The act of ligation, the last step in the formation of a closed circular duplex, does not generate superhelical structures. Thus to argue that superhelical DNA exists in the cell, one must postulate a mechanism for supplying the necessary energy. The stress in superhelical molecules is evidenced by the disappearance of superhelical turns when the duplex is nicked. Since both RF I and RF II must have the same compact structure *in vivo,* the intracellular structure is condensed for other reasons—probably related to those responsible for the formation of compact DNA (Lerman, 1974).

1.4.5. Relevant Physical Parameters

Table 3 contains a collection of physical–chemical data on ϕX174 and its DNA. I have tried to be fairly comprehensive and to include as many different determinations of the same property as seemed warranted. The variations in general reflect minor differences in experimental technique or are simply the result of experimental error. It appears that ϕX174 DNA contains about 5400 nucleotides and has a molecular weight of about 1.7×10^6, rather than the previously accepted figure of 5500 nucleotides (Sinsheimer, 1968).

Two discrepancies merit comment. One is the disagreement between Rust and Sinsheimer [see (p) in footnote to Table 3] and Siegel and Hayashi [see (k) in footnote to Table 3] on the density of the complementary strand in neutral CsCl equilibrium density gradients; it appears likely that the lower value is the result of partial renaturation of the complementary strand with the viral strand. The reason for the discrepancy in the figures for the sedimentation coefficient of the linear strand in high salt [16.1 according to Studier (h), 14.3 according to Pouwels *et al.* (l)] is not obvious to me. The variations in the density assigned to RF in neutral CsCl are the result of differences in the choice of reference markers. There is general agreement that the RF is lighter than *E. coli* DNA by 1–7 mg/ml. The disagreement on the density of denatured RF I is probably the result of differences in the completeness of the denaturation. Differences in the density of RF substituted with bromouracil are probably due to differences in the degree of substitution.

2. FORMATION OF THE PARENTAL RF

2.1. Adsorption to the Cell

The mature ϕX174 particle is a fairly stable structure—resistant, for example, to pronase and sodium dodecylsulfate under a variety of conditions—and thus, like other bacteriophages, has had to evolve a strategy for getting its DNA into the cell. It is reasonable that the spikes, each composed of one gene H protein and five gene G proteins, are the adsorption organelles (Brown *et al.*, 1971). This is in agreement with phenotype mixing experiments, which suggest that the adsorption site contains four to six subunits (Hutchison *et al.*, 1967), and with the mapping of certain host range mutants in gene G (Weisbeek *et al.*, 1973). However, the fact that other host range mutants map in gene F (S13 gene I, Tessman, 1965) indicates that the gene F protein also plays an active role in the phage–host interaction. Spikeless capsids, derived by urea treatment of virions, can attach to cells, but in a nonphysiological and unproductive manner (Newbold and Sinsheimer, 1970c).

Although it has not been ruled out that one spike is specifically designated as the adsorption organ, it seems more likely that any one of the 12 spikes can promote attachment. Single-hit antiserum inactivation kinetics and the inability of the phage to cause cell agglutination (Brown *et al.*, 1971) can be explained by assuming that one inactivating antibody molecule irreversibly disrupts the structure of the virion and that when the virus adsorbs to one cell it is hindered from adsorbing to another cell. Mutations in genes F, G, and H can alter physical properties of the virus (Hutchison *et al.*, 1967; Baker and Tessman, 1968) and can affect adsorption rates (Tessman and Tessman, 1968; Newbold and Sinsheimer, 1970c). Mutations in F and G result in the absence of serum blocking power from the infected cell; mutations in B, and to a lesser extent H, reduce the amount of serum blocking power made (Tessman and Tessman, 1968; Sinsheimer, 1968; Iwaya and Denhardt, 1971). Gene A mutants also make little serum blocking

TABLE 3

Physical Data for ϕX174

Data	References[a]
Virion	
Specific absorption at 260 nm: 8.14/mg/ml; 260/280 = 1.53, 25.5% DNA	(a)
Density in CsCl: 1.40 g·cm^{-3}; particle weight: 6.2 × 10^6 daltons	(a)
Translation diffusion constant: 1.96 (± 0.08) × 10^{-7}cm^2·s^{-1} (37°C)	(b)
Sedimentation coefficient: 114 S (a), 120 S (c)	(a,c)
Single-stranded ϕX174 DNA	
$E(P)$ = 8700 in 0.2 M NaCl, 37°C	(d)
Molecular weight: 1.59 (±0.05) × 10^6 daltons[b]	(e)
Sedimentation coefficients (circular/linear strands):	
23.6 ($s_{20,w}$) (corrected from neutral CsCl, only one boundary)	(f)
15.8/13.9 (HCHO-treated, in 0.2 M NaCl +HCHO, neutral)	(d)
23.8 (in 0.2 M NaCl, pH 7, only one boundary)	(d)
18.4/14.3 (s) (centrifuged in 1 M NaCl, 0.3 M phosphate, pH 12.6)	(g)
18.4/16.1 ($s_{20,w}$) (centrifuged in 0.1 M NaOH, 0.9 M NaCl)	(h)
13.1/12.0 (in 40 mM sodium carbonate, pH 11)	(i)
Replicative form	
Number of base pairs: 4800 ± 160 (by comparison with fd RF II DNA)[b]	(e)
5200 ± 100 (by comparison with λc$_{26}$)	(j)
5370 (F. Sanger sequence data)	
Sedimentation coefficients (I = naturally occurring superhelical molecule)	
RF I $s_{20,w}$ = 21.2 (corrected from measurements in neutral CsCl	(f)
RF II $s_{20,w}$ = 16.2 density gradients)	
RF I $s_{20,w}$ = 21.4 (from band sedimentation in neutral 1 M NaCl)	(g)
RF II $s_{20,w}$ = 17.4	
Denatured RF I: $s_{20,w}$ = 53 (measured in 1 M NaCl, pH 12.8)	(g)
= 54.1 (measured in alkaline CsCl gradients)	(f)
= 40 (measured in 1 M NaCl, pH 7)	(g)
= 33 (measured in 20 mM Na$_3$PO$_4$, pH 11)	(f)

Base compositions (mol %)	C	T	A	G	
Viral strand	18.5	32.8	24.6	24.2	(d)
Viral strand	20.9	31.3	24.5	23.3	(k)
Complementary strand	26.1	24.0	30.8	19.1	(k)

power, probably because of a gene dosage effect. Isolation and mapping of a variety of host range mutants using restriction enzyme fragments would reveal what parts of which proteins determine host specificity (Weisbeek *et al.,* 1973).

The ϕX174 virion has at least two stable conformations, a heat-resistant form (Φ*) unable to adsorb to the cell at 4°C and a more heat-sensitive form (Φ) capable of adsorbing efficiently to the cell. The equilibrium between the two is such that moderate temperatures, phosphate concentrations, and a slightly basic pH favor the thermolabile, adsorption-proficient form (Bleichrodt and van Abkoude, 1967, 1968). The nature of the conformational changes between these two structures

TABLE 3 (*continued*)

Data	References[a]
Buoyant densities	
[*E. coli* DNA: 1.708 g·cm^{-3} in neutral CsCl (m), 1.766 g·cm^{-3} in alkaline CsCl]	
Viral strand: 1.722 (g), 1.724 (l), 1.725 (m) g·cm^{-3} in neutral CsCl	(g,l,m)
1.765 g·cm^{-3} in alkaline CsCl	(f,k)
1.431 g·cm^{-3} in neutral Cs$_2$SO$_4$	(n)
1.740 g·cm^{-3}, ^{15}N-substituted, in neutral CsCl	(m)
1.769 g·cm^{-3}, D^{15}N-substituted, in neutral CsCl	(m)
1.83 (o), 1.807 (p) g·cm^{-3}, BrU-substituted, in neutral CsCl	(o,p)
1.511 g·cm^{-3}, BrU-substituted, in neutral Cs$_2$SO$_4$	(n)
Complementary strand: 1.717 (p), 1.724 (k) g·cm^{-3} in neutral CsCl	(p,k)
1.756 g·cm^{-3} in alkaline CsCl	(k)
1.809 g·cm^{-3} BrU-substituted, in neutral CsCl	(q)
1.488 g·cm^{-3} BrU-substituted, in neutral Cs$_2$SO$_4$	(n)
RF (I + II) (viral strand/complementary strand if differently labeled)	
1.703 (f), 1.704 (o), 1.706 (l), 1.708 (k) g·cm^{-3} in neutral CsCl	(f,o,l,k)
1.708 g·cm^{-3} ^{15}N/^{14}N in neutral CsCl	(m)
1.722 g·cm^{-3} D^{15}N/H^{14}N in neutral CsCl	(m)
1.732 (o), 1.747 (q) g·cm^{-3} Thy/BrU in neutral CsCl	(o,q)
1.747 (p), 1.755 (o), 1.761 (r) g·cm^{-3} BrU/Thy in neutral CsCl	(o,p,r)
1.787 g·cm^{-3} BrU/BrU in neutral CsCl	(o)
Denatured RF I (isolated from cells)	
1.744 (s), 1.779 (k), 1.78 (f) g·cm^{-3} in alkaline CsCl	(s,k,f)
1.758 g·cm^{-3} BrU/Thy RF in neutral CsCl	(p)

[a] References: (a) R. L. Sinsheimer, *J. Mol. Biol. 1:*37–42 (1959), (b) M. E. Bayer and R. W. De-Blois, *J. Virol. 14:*975–980 (1974), (c) N. L. Incardona, R. Blonski, and W. Feeney, *J. Virol. 9:*96–101 (1972), (d) R. L. Sinsheimer, *J. Mol. Biol. 1:*43–53 (1959), (e) S. A. Berkowitz and L. A. Day, *Biochemistry 13:*4825–4831 (1974), (f) A. J. Burton and R. L. Sinsheimer, *J. Mol. Biol. 14:*327–347 (1965), (g) P. H. Pouwels, H. S. Jansz, J. van Rotterdam, and J. A. Cohen, *Biochim. Biophys. Acta 119:*289–300 (1966), (h) F. W. Studier, *J. Mol. Biol. 11:*373–390 (1965), (i) W. Fiers and R. L. Sinsheimer, *J. Mol. Biol. 5:*424–434 (1962), (j) J.-S. Kim, P. A. Sharp, and N. Davidson, *Proc. Natl. Acad. Sci. USA 69:*1948–1952 (1972), (k) J. E. D. Siegel and M. Hayashi, *J. Mol. Biol. 27:*443–451 (1967), (l) P. H. Pouwels, C. M. Knijnenburg, J. van Rotterdam, J. A. Cohen, and H. S. Jansz, *J. Mol. Biol. 32:*169–182 (1968), (m) R. L. Sinsheimer, B. Starman, C. Nagler, and S. Guthrie, *J. Mol. Biol. 4:*142–160 (1962), (n) K. Geider, H. Lechner, and H. Hoffmann-Berling, *J. Mol. Biol. 69:*333–347 (1972), (o) D. T. Denhardt and R. L. Sinsheimer, *J. Mol. Biol. 12:*647–662 (1965), (p) P. Rust and R. L. Sinsheimer, *J. Mol. Biol. 23:*545–552 (1967), (q) M. Goulian, A. Kornberg, and R. L. Sinsheimer, *Proc. Natl. Acad. Sci. USA 58:*2321–2328 (1967), (r) H. Muller-Wecker, K. Geider, and H. Hoffmann-Berling, *J. Mol. Biol. 69:*319–331 (1972), (s) C. H. Schröder, E. Erben, and H.-C. Kaerner, *J. Mol. Biol. 79:*599–613 (1973).
[b] This figure has been revised upward (Day, personal communication).

is not known, but it is likely to be primarily a rearrangement of the capsid proteins since the sedimentation coefficients and densities of the two forms are similar. Bleichrodt *et al.* (1968) argued that the Φ/Φ* transition involved one weak noncovalent bond not located in the immediate vicinity of the adsorption site.

In the presence of a suitable receptor, the phage attaches in a reversible manner. Divalent cations are required, either Ca^{2+} or Mg^{2+}, the optimal concentration usually being between 1 and 10 mM depending on the medium. Healthy, exponentially growing cells and a pH of 7–7.5 also favor good infection. If the temperature is above 15°C, irreversible attachment follows; below 15°C, it does not (Newbold and Sinsheimer, 1970a). Treatment of cells with chloroform will block attachment (Brown *et al.*, 1971). Attachment to cell walls, or to a lipopolysaccharide extracted from cell walls with phenol plus chloroform plus ether or by lysozyme treatment, can also be demonstrated (Incardona and Selvidge, 1973). Attachment is first order, with a rate constant of about 8×10^{-9} ml/min/bacterium under the conditions used (Newbold and Sinsheimer, 1970c; Bayer and Starkey, 1972). Defective 110 S particles isolated from a temperature-sensitive gene H mutant infection were incapable of stable attachment (Newbold and Sinsheimer, 1970c).

Bayer and Starkey (1972) have suggested that ϕX174 adsorbs to sites where there are adhesions between the cell wall and the protoplasmic membrane. The possibility that phage adsorption creates an adhesion has not been eliminated. There are about 200–400 adhesions per cell and they make up about 6% of the total surface area of the cell. From the diffusion constant of the virus particle, it was calculated that adsorption occurred at almost the maximal rate predicted. Two different models compatible with the data were presented.

A locus in *E. coli* C that controls the ϕX174 receptor site maps near *xyl* at 79′ and has been designated *phx* (Bachmann *et al.*, 1976). ϕX174 sensitivity can be transduced into many ϕX174-resistant strains by P1 transduction of a *xyl* marker from a ϕX174-sensitive strain.

2.2. Eclipse of the Virion

Eclipse is defined as the irreversible loss of particle infectivity accompanying the injection of the viral DNA into the cell. It normally occurs as the result of an interaction between the virion and an appropriate molecular configuration on the cell surface that accomplishes a derangement of the virus coat. This or an analogous change can be triggered *in vitro* by incubation in 0.1 M $CaCl_2$ (Incardona *et al.*, 1972) or by exposure to an osmotic shock fluid derived from sensitive cells (Neuwald, 1975), to cell walls (Brown *et al.*, 1971; Beswick and Lunt, 1972), or to isolated lipopolysaccharide (Incardona and Selvidge, 1973; Jazwinski *et al.*, 1975a). The resulting particle has a lower S value because the DNA is partially extruded, but it retains its normal density if nuclease action is avoided (Newbold and Sinsheimer, 1970b). This rearrangement of the virion coat has a high energy of activation, some 36 kcal/mol, and does not occur below 15–20°C (Newbold and Sinsheimer, 1970c; Incardona, 1974). The mechanism of the process, what it is that causes the viral proteins to alter their relations with each other, is obviously of interest and is now amenable to study by a combined genetic and physicochemical approach.

Incardona (1974) has begun such studies with mutant and wild-type ϕX174 using Arrhenius plots [$k = A \exp(-Ea/RT)$] to analyze the activation energy and preexponential factor for the eclipse reaction *in vivo* and *in vitro*. Above 30°C, the kinetics are biphasic and suggest the presence of two competing first-order processes. The preexponential term for the faster process was reduced threefold by the *cs*70 mutation. The *cs*70 mutant is a cold-sensitive mutant of ϕX174 that has an altered virion protein and will not undergo eclipse at or below 26°C (Dowell, 1967).

Jazwinski *et al.* (1975a) have characterized the lipopolysaccharide of the outer cell membrane of *Salmonella typhimurium* that is responsible for adsorption and eclipse of ϕX174 and S13. There is a lipid component containing ester-linked fatty acids and a complex carbohydrate polymer. The phage-binding site appears to have the structure

$$(GlcNAc) \quad\quad Gal \quad Hep \quad P\text{-}P \text{ ---} EtN$$
$$\downarrow \quad\quad\quad\quad \downarrow \quad\quad \downarrow \quad\quad |$$
$$Glc \rightarrow Gal \rightarrow Glc \rightarrow Hep \rightarrow Hep \rightarrow KDO$$
$$|$$
$$P$$

(GlcNAc, *N*-acetylglucosamine; Glc, glucose; Gal, galactose; Hep, heptose; KDO, 2-keto-3-deoxyoctulosonic acid; P, phosphate; EtN, ethanolamine). ϕX174, but not S13, requires the *N*-acetylglucosamine at the nonreducing terminus for optimal binding and eclipse. For phage eclipse to follow binding of the virion to this structure, it is essential that the ester-linked fatty acids of the lipid A moiety be present. How this structure differs from the analogous, but not identical, structure in *E. coli* is not known.

Following eclipse of the phage particle in a metabolically active cell, the DNA exits from the virus and is incorporated into a double-stranded structure containing a newly synthesized complementary strand. As discussed in Section 2.3.5, synthesis is initiated at multiple, perhaps randomly located, sites on the single-stranded DNA. This is true for ϕX174, but probably not for G4. If synthesis of the complementary strand is prevented, then the single-stranded DNA is trapped more or less inside the cell. Since single-stranded DNA has an affinity for various proteins (e.g., DNA-binding proteins) and probably also for the hydrophobic membrane surface, it is unclear what the exact status of the DNA is. Knippers *et al.* (1969*b*) showed that in the absence of thymine the viral strand could be found in a comparatively free state in the cell, at least after exposure to concentrated CsCl. Francke and Ray (1971) argued in contrast that DNA synthesis was necessary to extract the DNA from the phage coat in an undegraded state. Most of the phage coat remains outside the cell and can be eluted in an "active" form (Newbold and Sinsheimer, 1970*b*; see also Dumas and Miller, 1974).

The phage does some damage to the cell when it eclipses; however, actual lysis from without has not been observed. At sufficiently high multiplicities of infection (40 plaque-forming units/cell, and note that phage preparations are typically 25% active), the permeability barrier of the cell is broken; DNA, RNA, and protein synthesis are inhibited and the cells are killed, even in the absence of any synthetic activity (shown by using UV-irradiated phage) on the part of the phage (Stone, 1970*a*). This damaging effect of viral infection may explain the inhibition of 23 S RNA synthesis by ϕX174 infection in the presence of chloramphenicol (Palchoudhury and Poddar, 1968) and also the inability of Ishiwa and Tessman (1968) to detect an effect of chloramphenicol on the virus-induced shutoff of host DNA synthesis. Cells that have been infected for 5–10 min become resistant to the lethal effects of high multiplicity infections, probably because of superinfection exclusion (Section 3.3).

2.3. Synthesis of a Complementary Strand

In 1966 it was reasonable to believe that the conversion of single-stranded ϕX174 DNA to RF bore less of a relation to the replication of double-stranded *E. coli* DNA than did RF replication. In 1976 the opposite seems almost to be true. Synthesis of a complement to single-stranded ϕX174 DNA requires many of the functions (e.g., those coded for by the *dna*B, C/D, and G genes) that are also required for the replication of *E. coli* DNA. In contrast, RF replication requires at least two functions (those coded for by the *E. coli rep* gene and the ϕX174 A gene) that are not necessary for *E. coli* DNA replication. The fact that the process of parental RF formation involves many of the reactions that occur during replication of double-stranded DNA helped open up a field that otherwise might still be largely inaccessible. As we shall see in what follows, research with several of the single-stranded DNA bacteriophages has led to the identification and partial characterization of at least one important reaction in DNA replication.

2.3.1. Test Tube Synthesis of φX174 DNA

By the middle 1960s, work in R. Sinsheimer's laboratory and elsewhere had established that single-stranded φX174 DNA was incorporated into a double-stranded replicative form as the result of the *de novo* synthesis of a complementary strand by preexisting host cell enzymes (reviewed by Sinsheimer, 1968). Goulian *et al.* (1967) then showed that this reaction could be accomplished *in vitro* with DNA polymerase I provided that oligonucleotide primers were made available (Goulian, 1968). The complete synthesis of a biologically active DNA molecule showed that the DNA polymerase made few mistakes and that there were no nonnucleotide components in the DNA. This endeavor was successful because of the availability of the then recently discovered polynucleotide ligase.

The discovery of *pol*A mutants, the subsequent uncovering of DNA polymerases II and III, and the demonstration that DNA polymerase III is coded for by the *dna*E gene, and hence essential for DNA replication, laid the foundation for the now firmly established principle that DNA polymerases replicate DNA (Gefter, 1975). But at least one serious problem remained—how did DNA polymerases initiate chains? The abovementioned *in vitro* synthesis of biologically active DNA required that DNA primers be provided. But was this the mechanism *in vivo*? The observation by Brutlag *et al.* (1971) that conversion of M13 single-stranded DNA to RF *in vivo* was sensitive to rifampicin in a rifampicin-sensitive strain, but resistant to rifampicin in a rifampicin-resistant strain, was consistent with an alternative possibility. This was that a short oligoribonucleotide was synthesized by RNA polymerase and then used as a primer by DNA polymerase. More recent *in vitro* work suggests that RNA polymerase III (RNA polymerase I plus a rifampicin-dissociable factor) is the enzyme actually responsible for synthesis since it, unlike RNA polymerase I, is unable to work on single-stranded φX174 DNA complexed with unwinding protein (Wickner and Kornberg, 1974a).

However, in the case of φX174 there was still a puzzle: parental

RF synthesis was not sensitive to rifampicin *in vivo* under conditions where M13 RF formation was (Silverstein and Billen, 1971). Fortunately, research by Kornberg and his collaborators in an *in vitro* system has fitted several pieces of this puzzle together. This work (reviewed by Schekman *et al.*, 1974) developed from the observation that properly prepared, soluble (membrane-free) extracts of *E. coli* cells from early exponential phase cultures had the capacity to synthesize a complement to single-stranded viral DNA *in vitro*. Similar work in Hurwitz's laboratory (Wickner *et al.*, 1972) has progressed in parallel. Jazwinski and Kornberg (1975) found that intact ϕX174 virions could be used instead of DNA if the reaction mix was supplemented with a membrane fraction or certain nonionic detergents. In the case of ϕX174, the synthetic reaction has been found to require some 10 (Schekman *et al.*, 1975) or 11 (Wickner and Hurwitz, 1975b) protein components. This work involved repeated subdivision of a crude extract into two required fractions, as illustrated in Fig. 4; some properties of the isolated proteins are summarized in Table 4 (Schekman *et al.*, 1975).

For the initiation step, proteins i and n, the unwinding protein, and the *dna*B and *dna*C proteins are necessary. Acting together in an ATP-dependent process, these proteins form an intermediate that serves as a substrate for the *dna*G protein (Weiner *et al.*, 1976). The *dna*G protein probably synthesizes an RNA primer which is used by the DNA polymerase III holoenzyme in the presence of unwinding protein to

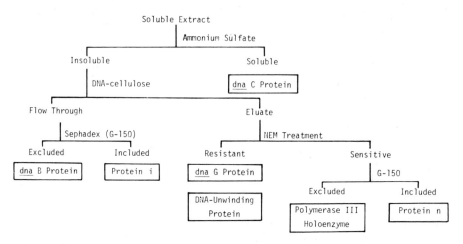

Fig. 4.   Scheme used in Kornberg's laboratory to fractionate various proteins required for the synthesis of a complement to single-stranded ϕX174 DNA *in vitro*. It is designed so that each step yields only two fractions, which are then tested for the relevant activity. Adapted from Schekman *et al.* (1974).

TABLE 4

Summary of Protein Properties[a]

Protein	DNA binding[b]	NEM sensitive	Gene locus	Molecular weight	Function
*dna*C	+	+	*dna*C	20,000	?[c]
*dna*B	−	−	*dna*B	250,000[d]	?
Protein i	±	−	?	40,000	?
Protein n	+	+	?	80,000	DNA binding
DNA polymerase III holoenzyme[e]	+	+	*dna*E	330,000[f]	DNA synthesis
*dna*G	+	−	*dna*G	65,000[g]	RNA synthesis
DNA-unwinding protein	+	−	?	76,000[h]	DNA binding

[a] Adapted from Schekman *et al.* (1975).
[b] Denatured calf thymus DNA-cellulose and 50 mM imidazole-HCl (pH 7.0).
[c] ?, unknown.
[d] M. Wright, S. Wickner, and J. Hurwitz, *Proc. Natl. Acad. Sci. USA* 70:3120–3124 (1973).
[e] DNA polymerase III* (*dna*E locus) + copolymerase III* (77,000 dalton subunit, gene locus unknown).
[f] W. Wickner and A. Kornberg, *J. Biol. Chem.* 249:6244–6249 (1974).
[g] J.-P. Bouché, K. Zechel, and A. Kornberg, *J. Biol. Chem.* 250:5995–6001 (1975).
[h] J. H. Weiner, L. L. Bertsch, and A. Kornberg, *J. Biol. Chem.* 250:1972–1980 (1975).

synthesize a complement to the ϕX174 viral strand template. The DNA polymerase III holoenzyme is composed of the *dna*E gene product and a second protein which Wickner and Kornberg (1974*b*) have called copolIII* and Wickner and Hurwitz (1974) have called elongation factor II. For the maturation step, DNA polymerase I and polynucleotide ligase are required. The $5' \rightarrow 3'$-exonuclease activity of DNA polymerase I is believed to remove whatever RNA primer may be present, while the DNA polymerase activity simultaneously (?) fills in the gap thus created. The final step is ligation of the $5',3'$-termini on the newly synthesized strand by polynucleotide ligase.

Many of these components have been shown also to be required *in vivo*, and it seems likely that the *in vitro* reactions studied in Kornberg's and Hurwitz's laboratories are largely comparable to the *in vivo* reactions. The *in vivo* situation will be discussed below. In the ϕX174 reaction, the absolute necessity for synthesizing an RNA primer remains to be confirmed (Wickner and Hurwitz, 1975*a,b*). An interesting question is why ϕX174 and M13 use different mechanisms for converting single-stranded DNA to RF. Perhaps the answer lies in the fact that M13 replication must coexist with *E. coli* DNA replication in the cell whereas ϕX174 replication is not so restricted. Thus ϕX174 can "afford" to preempt the host cell enzymes whereas M13 cannot.

2.3.2.   G4 and St-1

G4 is an isometric phage isolated using *E. coli* C as its host (Godson, 1974*b*). St-1 was selected for its ability to grow on K12 strains (Bradley, 1970). These phages appear in many respects to be similar to φX174, yet the *in vitro* requirements for the conversion of their DNA to RF are different from those of φX174, and of M13. Although the rest of the discussion concerns only G4, it is possible that St-1 behaves similarly (Wickner and Hurwitz, 1975*a*).

In order to synthesize a complement to G4 DNA, all that is needed is DNA-unwinding protein, the *dna*G protein, and DNA polymerase III holoenzyme (Zechel *et al.,* 1975). In contrast to φX174, there is no requirement for the *dna*B or C protein or for protein i or n. Since this distinction is true for phenol-extracted DNA that has been treated with 10 M urea or centrifuged through alkaline sucrose gradients in the presence of 1 M NaCl, it seems unlikely that virion proteins are responsible for the difference. Somehow the nucleotide sequence or structure of the DNA must select which replication system is used. Clues to what sort of signal is involved should be fairly easily forthcoming, since there is a small "gap" left at a unique position in the parental RF. This "gap" is located as shown in Fig. 5 about 250

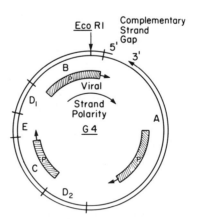

Fig. 5.   Properties of the G4 genome. The DNA is oriented with the same clockwise 5′→3′ viral strand polarity as the other isometric phages. Although no genetic work has been reported on G4 yet, the disposition and functions of the genes will surely be the same as for φX174 since a similar set of proteins is produced (Godson, 1974*b*). The approximate positions of RNA polymerase binding sites are shown in relation to the unique *Eco*R1 cleavage site and the *Hin*d cleavage products (Godson, 1974*b*). The location of the gap is derived from the data discussed in Fig. 6; note that the opposite orientation for the polarity of the viral strand was selected in that work.

nucleotides away from the single *Eco*R1 cleavage site in the RF molecule. (The viral strand is oriented in a clockwise 5′ to 3′ direction like φX174.) This was shown by filling in the gap with radioactive nucleotides, cleaving the molecule with *Eco*R1, and sedimenting the DNA in an alkaline sucrose gradient. Figure 6A shows the result.

Bouché *et al.* (1975) and Zechel *et al.* (1975) have substantially purified the *dna*G protein using as an assay its ability to prime G4 RF synthesis. This enzyme has a molecular weight of 64,000 and consists of a single polypeptide chain. When incubated with G4 DNA, unwinding protein, and ribonucleoside triphosphates, radioactivity from α-^{32}P-labeled ATP and GTP could be incorporated into a BioGel-15m-excludable form. Optimal incorporation of label, and optimal priming activity for DNA synthesis in a subsequent reaction with DNA polymerase III holoenzyme, required all four rNTPs. The *dna*G protein was capable of RNA synthesis in the absence of one or both of the pyrimidine nucleoside triphosphates, and the RNA synthesized could be used as a primer, albeit less efficiently. In the absence of either ATP or GTP, the ability to synthesize an efficient primer was severely curtailed. Not all of the RNA chains synthesized by the *dna*G protein were used as primers; those that were used appeared to be a special subset.

The RNA primer was shown to be covalently attached to the 5′-end of the newly synthesized strand by cleaving the RF II with *Eco*R1 and centrifuging the labeled DNA in a formamide–sucrose gradient after denaturation. The ^{32}P label was observed to sediment with the short 5% piece produced by *Eco*R1, as illustrated in Fig. 6B. The RNA primer was digested with RNase T1 and fingerprinted. Seven oligonucleotides were observed. The data suggested that the primer was 20–25 nucleotides long and contained all four ribonucleotides, nearly one-half of which were GMP. This work provides strong evidence that the *dna*G protein is a rifampicin-resistant RNA polymerase capable of synthesizing a short piece of RNA that can prime DNA synthesis by DNA polymerase III.

2.3.3. Function(s) of the Capsid Proteins

In a natural infection, the virus particle disgorges its nucleic acid into the cell as the result of a complex interaction between a cell receptor and the virus particle. The question here is what are the functions of the viral proteins in this process. Is their function only to convey the viral genome safely to the cell or do they perform additional functions? Kornberg (1974) has argued that the gene H protein does have an addi-

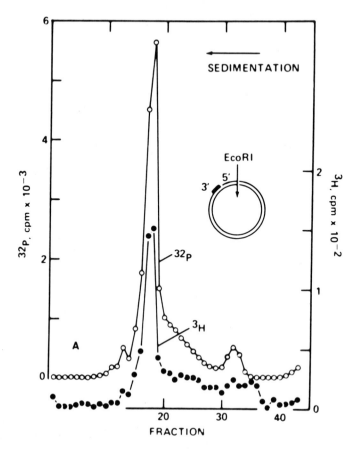

Fig. 6. Relative locations of the unique *Eco*R1 cleavage site in G4 RF and the gap/ RNA primer left at a unique location in the G4 parental RF after synthesis of a complementary strand *in vitro*. (A) The gap of ^{32}P-labeled G4 RF II was filled with DNA polymerase I and [^{3}H]deoxynucleoside triphosphates, cleaved with *Eco*R1, and centrifuged on an alkaline sucrose gradient. The ^{3}H is clearly attached to the larger of the two fragments of the complementary strand generated by cleavage with *Eco*R1. From Zechel *et al.* (1974), with permission.

tional function—that of acting as a "pilot protein" to direct the single-stranded DNA to the appropriate replication apparatus. There is circumstantial evidence in support of this possibility, but strong evidence is lacking. The "pilot protein" cannot be essential since protein-free DNA synthesized *de novo* is infectious (Goulian *et al.*, 1967).

The most interesting support for the "pilot protein" hypothesis is the observation that the gene H protein can be found bound to the RF after infection. Jazwinski *et al.* (1975c) detected several gene H protein molecules bound to RF, and at any of an apparently large number of different locations. The nature of the gene H protein binding and the nature of the RF to which it was bound are not known. That gene H proteins are associated with the RF after infection suggests to me that they may be acting as π proteins (Denhardt, 1972). According to this model, they would function *in vivo* to allow DNA synthesis to be initiated at the sites to which they were bound and they would remain associated with the RF until displaced, causing the formation of gaps in the nascent complementary strand.

The fact that certain gene H temperature-sensitive mutants (e.g., H1068 in S13, Doniger and Tessman, 1969) are able to eclipse but not form parental RF at the restrictive temperature is consistent with the

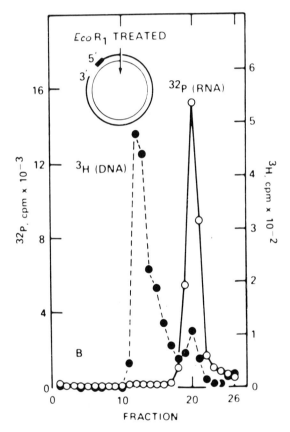

Fig. 6   (B). The strand complementary to the G4 viral strand was synthesized *in vitro* with [α-^{32}P]ribonucleoside triphosphates and [^{3}H]deoxyribonucleoside triphosphates, and the RF II thereby produced was purified, cleaved with *Eco*R1, and centrifuged after denaturation on a sucrose–formamide gradient. The RNA is clearly attached to the smaller of the two fragments of the complementary strand generated by cleavage with *Eco*R1. From Bouché *et al.* (1975), with permission.

"pilot protein" concept. However, the defect could be simply an inability to release the DNA successfully from the virion. There is also a probable gene G mutant (*tss*6 in ϕX174, Dalgarno and Sinsheimer, 1968) that exhibits a similar phenotype, although in this case the temperature-sensitive mutant goes through one cycle of growth at the restrictive temperature and produces phage that are unable to initiate a second cycle of infection at the high temperature even though they can adsorb and eclipse.

2.3.4. Host Functions Required *in Vivo*

Mutants of the host that are incapable of supporting ϕX174 parental RF formation include *dna*B and *dna*G; cells carrying temperature-sensitive alleles in either of these genes are blocked in ϕX174 RF synthesis (Dumas and Miller, 1974; McFadden and Denhardt, 1974). Curiously, mutant hosts defective in the *dna*C or *dna*E gene functions do support RF formation in spite of the fact that *in vitro* these gene functions are required (Kranias and Dumas 1974; Dumas and Miller, 1973; Denhardt *et al.*, 1973). Dumas *et al.* (1975) have shown that in the case of *dna*C mutants an alternative rifampicin-sensitive initiation process using RNA polymerase I comes into play and that this accounts for formation of the parental RF at the nonpermissive temperature by *dna*C mutants. This reaction can occur *in vitro* also unless it is suppressed by the addition of the factor that converts RNA polymerase I to RNA polymerase III (Wickner and Kornberg, 1974a). How *dna*E mutants make RF under restrictive conditions is not understood. Since relatively little synthesis is required (5000 nucleotides), it is possible that there is sufficient activity (even in *pol*A, *pol*B, *dna*E mutants, Denhardt *et al.*, 1973) of one of the three DNA polymerases for the reaction. The observation that *dna*C and *dna*E mutants allow parental RF formation despite the fact that the proteins coded for by these genes are clearly required *in vitro* makes one suspicious of the possibility that even when a particular *dna* mutant allows parental RF formation the function provided by the affected gene may nevertheless still be involved "normally." The inability to form RF would of course implicate the function. But even here there is a puzzle. If RNA polymerase can substitute in a *dna*C mutant, why can it not also substitute in the *dna*G mutant?

One fascinating approach is the study of the requirements of the different isometric phages. G4 and St-1 are clearly distinguishable from ϕX174 in how a complement to their single-stranded DNA genome is formed. As was true *in vitro,* neither *dna*B nor *dna*C is required for the formation of the parental St-1 RF (Bowes, 1974), and none of the *dna* functions (A, B, C, E, and G) appears necessary for G4 RF formation (Dumas, personal communication). Why? Does this represent a profound change in nucleotide sequence and DNA conformation, or is it something that easily can be altered by mutation? It seems unlikely that the differences can be attributed solely to capsid proteins. A careful and systematic investigation of this phenomenon is obviously needed.

Dowell has commenced a relevant study and has isolated what appear to be two different double mutants of ϕX174, called ϕXtB and ϕX$ahb,$ that have acquired the ability to grow in hosts in which ϕX174 is unable to grow (Vito *et al.,* 1975; Haworth *et al.,* 1975). ϕXtB grows in K12 strains and certain *dna* mutants (Bone and Dowell, 1973a,b; Haworth *et al.,* 1975); it resembles St-1. These mutants have suffered changes in their capsid structure since the kinetics of inactivation of the virion by heat or by ϕX174 antiserum is altered. The map positions of the mutations are not known. Vito *et al.* (1975) have argued that these results indicate a function for the capsid proteins in DNA replication.

It has been suggested (Schekman *et al.,* 1974) that the enzyme complex used to synthesize a complement to ϕX174 DNA is related to that used to initiate a round of replication in *E. coli,* whereas the enzyme complex used for synthesis of a complement to G4 DNA is equivalent to that used to initiate synthesis of Okazaki fragments during ongoing *E. coli* DNA replication. M13, it was suggested, used the same replicative system that certain plasmids used. There may be some interesting correlations to be gleaned from these comparisons, but too little is known.

2.3.5.   Synthesis of the ϕX174 Complementary Strand *in Vivo*

The question of whether synthesis of the complementary strand *in vivo* begins at a unique location in the genome and proceeds in an ordered fashion around the genome or whether one or more initiations occur independently of each other has been the subject of several studies. Benbow *et al.* (1974b) argued for the first possibility on the basis of their observation that when UV-irradiated phage were used to infect cells synthesis of a complementary strand proceeded only to a limited extent. This result is consistent with the possibility that synthesis is initiated at a unique site and proceeds unidirectionally around the genome until a UV lesion is encountered. The drawback of this work is that much of the UV-irradiated DNA was not injected into the cell. Zuccarelli (1974) studied the same question by labeling the RF molecule briefly during the formation of the parental RF. Completed molecules were isolated and digested with HindII nuclease, and the amount of pulse label in the various cleavage products was compared with the amount of uniformly distributed label. The expectation was that those portions of the molecule synthesized last would have the greatest ratio of pulse label to uniform label. The data did not fit well with the hypothesis of a single initiation site, but could be explained if there were two or more sites of initiation of synthesis of the complementary strand.

Both Eisenberg et al. (1975) and McFadden and Denhardt (1975) have argued that there are multiple initiation sites for complementary strand synthesis in vivo. They presented evidence that synthesis of the complementary strand was initiated at several sites on any one RF molecule and that in a population of molecules these sites were distributed either randomly or at least among a large number of possible locations in the genome. Gaps separated the nascent 5–12 S pieces from each other, and the activity of a DNA polymerase was necessary to fill them in. Figure 7 shows the distribution among the HindII cleavage products of ^{32}P radioactivity incorporated into the gaps by T4 DNA polymerase. It is evident that in the parental RF molecules gaps can occur in many locations in the genome. In a normal host, DNA polymerase I performs the gap-filling function efficiently; in a polA host (with, however, substantial $5' \rightarrow 3'$-exonuclease activity), the gaps persist for a longer time. At the restrictive temperature in a host carrying a thermosensitive polynucleotide ligase (E. coli ts7), the gaps are filled in but the nascent fragments are not joined together efficiently. These experiments are compatible with the use of an oligoribonucleotide at multiple positions, perhaps randomly located, to prime synthesis of a DNA chain. It would then be removed by the $5' \rightarrow 3'$-nuclease activity of DNA polymerase I. It is not known whether the gene H protein (Jazwinski et al., 1975b,c) is present in these gaps.

3.   EXPRESSION OF THE VIRAL GENOME

3.1.   Transcription

3.1.1.   RNA Polymerase Binding Sites and Polar Mutants

Chen et al. (1973) determined which HindII and HaeIII cleavage products of ϕX174 RF were capable of binding RNA polymerase by making use of the fact that DNA segments bound to RNA polymerase

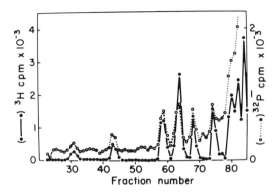

Fig. 7. Distribution of the gaps in the complementary strand of φX174 parental RF synthesized *in vivo*. Cells were infected with a [³H]thymine-labeled gene A mutant (hence unable to replicate its RF) for 3 min and the parental RF was purified. The gaps were filled in with ³²P-labeled triphosphates, the RF was cleaved with *Hind* restriction nuclease, and the fragments were electrophoresed on a polyacrylamide-agarose gel. Electrophoresis is from right to left and the nine peaks of ³H radioactivity contain the *Hind*II fragments 1–9 shown in Fig. 2. ³²P is clearly present in peaks 4–9; the smear at the top is the result of some contamination with fragments of *E. coli* DNA. This experiment, which shows that *in vivo* there is not a single uniquely located gap left in the complementary strand during the formation of the parental RF, was performed by S. Eisenberg.

would be retained by nitrocellulose filters. Additional support for the assignments was obtained by determining to what extent DNA sequences protected by RNA polymerase from digestion with pancreatic DNase would hybridize to different restriction enzyme cleavage fragments. The fragments that would bind *E. coli* RNA polymerase at what appeared to be significant levels were *Hind*II 2, 4, and 6 and *Hae*III 1, 2, and 3. The locations of these fragments are shown in Fig. 2. *Hind*II4 and *Hae*III2 overlap at the gene H/A boundary whereas *Hind*II6c and *Hae*III3 overlap at the gene C/D boundary. These two regions of the genome are where promoters would be expected to map according to the properties of polar nonsense mutants.

Vanderbilt *et al.* (1972) studied a series of *am* nonsense mutants in genes F and G and examined their effect both on the quantities of F, G, and H proteins synthesized and on the amount of phage made in complementation experiments. Different mutants in gene F showed different degrees of polarity, with the most polar mutants mapping, as would be expected, very close to the N-terminal end of the gene. In contrast, a series of mutants in gene G all seemed to map near the center of the gene yet to give widely different degrees of polarity. These experiments suggested that there was no promoter immediately proximal to gene G or H. There appeared to be a promoter before gene A, however, since the polarity of the nonsense mutants in F and G did not extend into gene A. Hayashi and Hayashi (1970) and Benbow *et al.* (1972*a*) made similar observations for ϕX174; the former workers also found a decrease in a large polycistronic mRNA in a polar F mutant. These results and the fact that proteins D and F are made in largest amounts, followed by G, then H, and finally A, B, and C, make it reasonable that the strongest promoter is at the C/D boundary. A promoter just before gene A is likely, but one immediately preceding gene H is not. Thus although the *Hin*dII2 and *Hae*III1 overlap occurs at the gene G/H boundary, a strong promoter at this location seems improbable.

Certain gene D mutants were reported by Benbow *et al.* (1972*a*) to be weakly polar on the basis of a reduced synthesis of F, G, and H proteins. An alternative explanation for the apparent polarity was suggested by Clements and Sinsheimer (1974) when they observed that less ϕX174 mRNA was made in infections with gene D mutants. There was an apparent sixfold decrease in the amount of hybridizable viral mRNA labeled with ^{32}P after a 5-min pulse. Since the profiles of the labeled RNA in gels and gradients appeared similar in both wild-type and mutant infections, they suggested that the gene D protein generally enhanced viral mRNA synthesis. However, if the C/D promoter is the major *in vivo* promoter and leads to the synthesis of most of the *major* size classes of mRNA, then the original interpretation (polarity) could still be valid.

3.1.2.   Stability and Size of the mRNA

The half-life of the ability of S13 mRNA to support the initiation of translation *in vivo* is apparently fairly short. This was demonstrated by Puga *et al.* (1973) in Tessman's laboratory, and a representative experiment is shown in Fig. 8. They showed that after rifampicin was added to a culture of infected cells to block initiation of transcription the capacity for synthesizing S13 specific proteins was rapidly lost. Over 50% of the capacity to synthesize the F protein and the B + G proteins (measured together because they were not well resolved in gels) was lost with a half-life of less than 2 min. In contrast, the physical half-life of the mRNA as measured by hybridization was about 10 min. The kinetics of the decline in the rates of synthesis of both gene F protein and gene B + G proteins fits a two-component curve with 30%

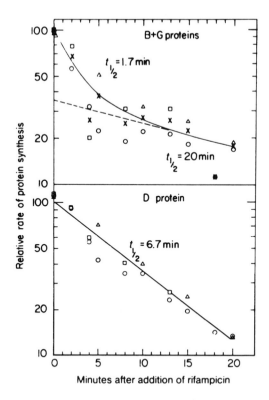

Fig. 8. Functional decay of mRNA for the combined B + G proteins and the D protein of S13. Two-minute pulses of [³H]leucine were given at the indicated times after the addition of rifampicin, which was added 20 min after infection. The proteins were separated on SDS-polyacrylamide gels and the amount of radioactivity incorporated into the various proteins was determined. It was not necessary to use UV-irradiated cells (Section 3.2.1) since by 20 min after infection with S13 host protein synthesis appears to be shut off. From Puga *et al.* (1973), with permission.

of the decay exhibiting a longer half-life of 10–20 min. The decay in the relative rate of synthesis of the gene D protein, in contrast, fit a one-component curve with a half-life of about 6.7 min; however, the data (Fig. 8) are not good enough to absolutely exclude a two-component decay process. It was suggested that the two-component decay curves arose because of heterogeneity in the mRNA population. Those mRNAs with the gene transcript at the proximal end would evince a shorter half-life than those with the gene transcript closer to the distal end. The trivial explanation that the short functional half-life was due to an impairment in the rate with which the aminoacyl tRNA precursor pools became equilibrated with radioactivity after initiating labeling with a radioactive amino acid in the presence of rifampicin was apparently eliminated.

All of the viral mRNA found in infected cells is of viral (plus) strand polarity (Sedat *et al.,* 1969; Hayashi and Hayashi, 1970; Vanderbilt and Tessman, 1970) and is in polysomes (Puga and Tessman, 1973*a*). These polysomes can be found (Puga and Tessman, 1973*c*) in a membrane fraction (the M band), perhaps because of the hydrophobic nature of the viral proteins. The population of mRNA molecules detected *in vivo* is quite heterogeneous in size and contains discrete species ranging from a little less than 10^5 daltons to somewhat over 3×10^6 daltons—roughly twice the size of the genome (Hayashi and Hayashi, 1970, 1972; Warnaar *et al.,* 1970; Puga and Tessman, 1973*a*).

Clements and Sinsheimer (1975) found that both sedimentation velocity centrifugation in denaturing solvents (dimethylsulfoxide) and electrophoresis in polyacrylamide-agarose gels gave similar results except that resolution in the gels was better. A typical electrophoretic pattern is shown in Fig. 9. Arrows show the position of marker RNA

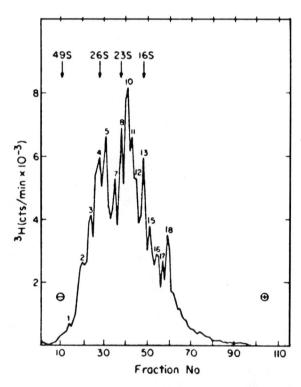

Fig. 9. Polyacrylamide-agarose gel electrophoresis of ϕX174 mRNA labeled with [³H]uracil for 45 s at 20 min after infection. RNA was recovered from gel slices and hybridized to ϕX174 RF in 50% formamide. Arrows show the positions of 16 S and 23 S *E. coli* rRNA and 26 S and 49 S Sindbis RNA. Migration of RNA is toward the right. From Clements and Sinsheimer (1975), with permission.

molecules; peaks 1 and 18 were calculated to have molecular weights at 3.4×10^6 and 2.8×10^5, respectively. The ϕX174 DNA was identified by hybridization to RF. The fact that a short pulse (45 s) of [^{3}H]uracil produced the same distribution of species as a long-term ^{32}P labeling suggested that the major smaller fragments were probably not derived from the larger fragments. However, it is not excluded that some of the discrete size classes are generated by nonrandom (specific sites in the RNA sensitive to an endonuclease) or discontinuous (specific regions in the RNA resistant to an exonuclease) degradation of the mRNA. Warnaar et al. (1970) observed that in the presence of chloramphenicol there was an enrichment for the smaller size classes whereas a pulse-chase experiment led to an enrichment for the larger size classes.

3.1.3. *In Vitro* RNA Synthesis

RF I and RF II, but not denatured RF I or extensively nicked RF II, are asymmetrically transcribed *in vitro* by RNA polymerase (Warnaar et al., 1969). The entire genome can be transcribed by RNA polymerase from uninfected cells in both coupled and uncoupled systems (Bryan et al., 1969). From studies on the size of ϕX174 mRNAs synthesized in the presence and absence of ρ, Hayashi et al. (1970) concluded that there were several sites at which the ρ factor could act. These sites have not been located. The proteins that were synthesized by the RNA made in the presence or absence of ρ were similar, and the predominant product was the gene G protein. In more recent work, Hayashi and Hayashi (1971) used a coupled transcription/translation system to show that both RF I and RF II (randomly nicked RF I or the naturally occurring gapped RF II molecules) could be translated *in vitro* to yield a set of proteins (Section 3.2.1) very similar to that observed *in vivo*. Although RF I was more efficiently transcribed into mRNA than RF II, the size distribution of the mRNA molecules and the efficiency with which they were translated were similar. The major difference was the appearance of a low molecular weight 4 S component among the mRNA molecules transcribed from RF II; the nature of this material and why it was not transcribed from RF I were not understood. Its relation, if any, to the 4 S RNA that can anneal to ϕX174 RF and that is found in uninfected cells is unknown (Warnaar et al., 1970).

Smith et al. (1974) and Grohmann et al. (1975) in Sinsheimer's laboratory identified five different 5′-terminal oligonucleotide sequences at the 5′-ends of the ϕX174 mRNAs synthesized *in vitro* with

RF I. One of the five sequences began with a 5′-C and was not present in the *in vivo* φX174 mRNA whereas the others apparently were. It would be of interest to determine whether nonsuperhelical DNA also yields the C-start mRNA since it is unlikely (Section 1.4.4) that *in vivo* the RF I is as highly negatively superhelical as it is *in vitro*. The high negative superhelical density facilitates the binding of anything that can unwind the duplex and this could lead to artifactual binding/initiation and may account for some ambiguity in the initiation nucleotide (see Table 5).

Smith and Sinsheimer (1976*a,b,c*) determined both the sizes of the various mRNA molecules synthesized in the absence of ρ *in vitro* and the restriction enzyme cleavage fragments to which the 5′-terminal sequences corresponded. Some of their results are summarized in Table 5. The existence of RNA molecules that differed by one genome length yet had the same 5′-terminal oligonucleotide sequence indicated that there was one major ρ-independent terminator in the genome, and it was possible to infer from the data that the terminator was close to the B/C boundary. Readthrough of the terminator must occur to generate molecules greater than one genome in size and to permit gene C protein production. The locations of the *in vitro* promoters and the terminator are shown in Fig. 10. This work reinforces the conclusion (Section 3.1.1) that the RNA polymerase binding site in gene G (Chen *et al.*, 1973) is nonproductive. The parallels between the promoter and terminator locations in the genomes of the isometric phages and the filamentous phages are striking (Fig. 16 in Denhardt, 1975). The approximate locations of RNA polymerase binding sites on G4 RF are shown in Fig. 5.

3.1.4. Synthesis of mRNA *in Vivo*

Puga and Tessman (1973*a*) observed that up to 15–20 RF molecules, but seemingly no more, could be transcribed in the cell. These could be either parental RF molecules (high multiplicity infection with gene A mutants) or progeny RF molecules (resulting from replication of the parental RF). Also, Truffaut and Sinsheimer (1974) showed that progeny RF could be transcribed. The apparent restriction on the number of RF molecules that can be transcribed may be the consequence of a limiting amount of an essential component (RNA polymerase?), of the damaging effects of high multiplicity infections (Stone, 1970*a*), or, in normal infections, of the cessation of RF replica-

TABLE 5

Properties of ϕX174 mRNA Molecules Synthesized *in Vitro* with RF I[a]

Location of the 5'-terminus	Restriction enzyme cleavage fragment overlaps	Length ($\times$ genome)	5'-Terminal sequence
H/A boundary	*Hind*II4/*Hae*III2/*Hpa*1	0.37, 1.37	pppA$_{3-4}$UCUUG(G)
A/B boundary	*Hind*II8/*Hae*III3/*Hpa*1	0.15, 1.15	pppAUCG(C)
C/D boundary	*Hind*II6b/*Hae*III3/*Hpa*3	0.91	pppCG(A) and pppG

[a] Data from Smith and Sinsheimer (1976*a,b,c*). ^{32}P-labeled RNA molecules were synthesized *in vitro* and fractionated according to size. For each size class, the 5'-terminal sequence and the restriction enzyme cleavage fragments to which it would hybridize were determined.

tion after about 15 min (Section 5.1). The data in the Puga and Tessman (1973*a*) paper showed that the ratio of S13 RNA to *E. coli* RNA labeled by a short pulse at multiplicities between 15 and 50 did not change, but no information on the absolute amount synthesized was presented. There is some uncertainty about whether adverse effects of high multiplicity infections are due to phage particles (viable or not) or other extraneous material in a phage preparation. In experiments where high multiplicities of infection are used, attention should be paid to this question.

If replication of the RF is prevented by a mutation in gene A, the RF remains in the closed circular form (Section 4.1) and is transcribed more efficiently (Shleser *et al.,* 1969*a*; Puga and Tessman, 1973*a*). Possibly replication interferes with transcription. Nalidixic acid reduces by 80% (but no further) the amount of S13 mRNA that can be synthesized, although there is no detectable effect on *E. coli* mRNA synthesis (Puga and Tessman, 1973*b*). It was suggested that this was the result of the fact that a large portion of the RF in the cell was in the form of a closed circular duplex and that a metabolite of nalidixic acid acted like an intercalating agent. RF I molecules with a negative super-helix density are more efficiently transcribed than RF II *in vitro* because of their superhelical structure (Hayashi and Hayashi, 1972). However, it is not known if the superhelical structure exists *in vivo* (Section 1.4.4).

The large number of different size classes of viral RNA found *in vivo* is the result of the existence of three different promoters and several ρ-dependent terminators plus one ρ-independent terminator, all of which permit a substantial amount of readthrough. To what extent degradative processes also produce discrete size classes of fragments is unknown.

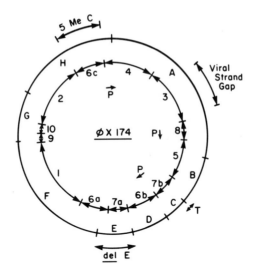

Fig. 10.   Regions of interest in the φX174 genome. The outer circle shows the genetic map of φX174 drawn approximately to scale according to the molecular weights of the proteins as given in Table 1. Transcription and translation proceed clockwise, and this is also the 5′→3′ polarity of the viral (plus) strand. The inner circle indicates the location of the HindII cleavage fragments as determined by Weisbeek et al. (1976). The three promoters (P) and the one ρ-independent terminator (T) are placed according to Smith and Sinsheimer (1976a,b,c). The extent of the delE deletion (Zuccarelli et al., 1972; Kim et al., 1972) is as indicated, but whether it is congruent with gene E has not been established. The 5MeC was shown to be in the HindII6 fragment located between HindII2 and HindII4 by Lee and Sinsheimer (1974b). The gap left in the viral strand during RF replication (and also during single-stranded DNA synthesis, Johnson and Sinsheimer, 1974) is located in the HaeIII6b fragment located within the HindII3 cleavage fragment (Eisenberg et al., 1975).

3.2.   Translation

As is the case for transcription, there appear to be no interesting translational control mechanisms (Sedat and Sinsheimer, 1970). There is no evidence for temporal control, and no "early" or "late" genes have been identified. All the major phage genes are expressed in the absence of RF replication (Shleser et al., 1969b; Denhardt et al., 1972). However, since there are fewer copies of the genome to be transcribed there is a gene dosage effect. What controls there are probably consist of differences in promoter and ribosome-binding-site affinities for RNA polymerase and ribosomes, respectively, and variations in the rates with which the different polypeptides are synthesized. The most abundant φX174-coded proteins *in vivo* are the products of genes D and F; lesser amounts of the other proteins are made.

3.2.1. Synthesis of Viral Proteins *in Vivo* and *in Vitro*

The proteins of the isometric phages have been studied most often by electrophoresis in polyacrylamide gels in the presence of mercaptoethanol and sodium dodecylsulfate since only under these conditions do all of the proteins appear to be completely disaggregated. A typical gel pattern is shown in Fig. 11. It was provided by M. Hayashi, and the correspondence of the peaks of radioactivity with particular gene products was determined in his laboratory. These assignments are deduced from the effect of particular chain-termination codons on the individual proteins. The gene E protein continues to be elusive and may be hidden under the gene D peak (Section 1.2); Benbow *et al.* (1972*b*) tentatively assigned it a molecular weight of 17,500. The peak labeled X may be the gene C protein (Borras *et al.*, 1971, and Table 1) or the small protein in the virion.

In most of the *in vivo* work, UV-sensitive (HCR⁻) cells are irradiated with ultraviolet light prior to infection to reduce endogenous host protein synthesis (Gelfand and Hayashi, 1969; Burgess and Denhardt, 1969). Because these cells are unable to repair UV lesions in their DNA efficiently, low doses of UV radiation effectively destroy their capacity to code for their own proteins within a few minutes. If an undamaged genome is inserted into such cells, it can be transcribed and translated with good, although reduced, efficiency in many cases.

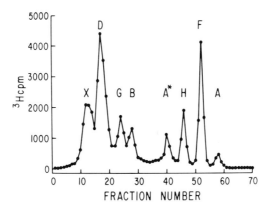

Fig. 11.   Electropherogram of the φX174 proteins. *E. coli* HF4704 was irradiated with ultraviolet light, infected with φX174 at a multiplicity of 10, and labeled with [³H]lysine plus [³H]arginine from 10 to 20 min after infection. The proteins were electrophoresed in the presence of SDS and mercaptoethanol in a 7.5% acrylamide gel using ethylene diacrylate as a cross-linker. Migration is from right to left. I thank Masaki Hayashi for providing this figure.

Godson (1971*a*) and Benbow *et al.* (1972*b*) made a thorough study of the φX174 proteins synthesized in UV-irradiated cells. Seven viral proteins were unambiguously identified and five definitively assigned to cistrons. Most of these assignments confirmed earlier work.

Mayol and Sinsheimer (1970) and van der Mei *et al.* (1972*b*) investigated the φX174-specific proteins synthesized in unirradiated cells using double-label techniques, and their conclusions were mostly in agreement with those of the other studies. There were hints that specific host-coded proteins were induced after infection, but this work has not been followed up. There were slight changes in the relative amounts of the various proteins made in unirradiated as compared with irradiated cells, the greatest change being an increase in the proportion of gene D protein in unirradiated cells.

Bryan and Hayashi (1970) studied the viral proteins synthesized *in vitro* in a coupled system directed by φX174 RF. *N*-Formylmethionine was found in all of the viral proteins synthesized *in vitro*. Several of the proteins comigrated with marker proteins made *in vivo*. The major *in vitro* product was the gene G protein. It was shown to be antigenically similar to the *in vivo* product and to contain the same tryptic peptides (Gelfand and Hayashi, 1970).

In the φX174 literature (and elsewhere), one finds statements to the effect that the gene A protein (or whatever) is "chloramphenicol resistant." This inappropriate term refers to the fact that the process of RF replication, which is dependent on the presence of active gene A protein, is only slightly affected by concentrations of chloramphenicol (30 μg/ml) that severely depress other processes dependent on protein synthesis (e.g., progeny single-stranded DNA synthesis). Godson (1971*b*) used UV-irradiated cells and van der Mei *et al.* (1972*b*) used unirradiated cells to show that the synthesis of gene A protein was inhibited by chloramphenicol to about the same extent as other proteins. From this result, one may infer correctly that more gene A protein is synthesized than is needed for RF replication. In both UV-irradiated and unirradiated cells, the synthesis of the gene F protein seems to be most sensitive to chloramphenicol and the synthesis of gene D protein least sensitive.

Linney *et al.* (1972) made the unexpected discovery that two separate proteins were coded for by gene A. The larger protein (first called A′ but now called A) has a molecular weight of about 60,000 and is the complete product of gene A. The smaller protein (first called A but now called A*) has a molecular weight of about 35,000 and appears to be synthesized because of the presence of a start signal for protein synthesis within gene A. This is diagrammed in Fig. 12. There are two strong arguments supporting this interpretation. One is that nonsense mutants in the distal part of the gene eliminate both proteins. The second is that all but one of the tryptic peptides isolated from A* are contained among the tryptic peptides derived from A (Linney and Hayashi, 1973). Both proteins A and A* bind strongly to single-stranded DNA-cellulose, and this property has been used in their purification. Synthesis of A is more sensitive to rifampicin than is synthesis of A*, presumably because the translational start signal for A is closer to the promoter than is the translational start for A* (Section 3.1.1 and Linney and Hayashi, 1974). It also appears that there is one molecule of the A* protein in the virion (Section 1.4.1) but there is no evidence regarding its function (Section 3.3 and Table VI).

3.2.2. Characteristics of Virus-Coded Proteins; Codon Frequencies

The gene A protein has been partially purified by Linney *et al.* (1972) and Henry and Knippers (1974). It has a molecular weight of about 60,000, binds to DNA-cellulose columns, and may have a specific nicking activity (Section 4.1). It is strongly hydrophobic and tends to aggregate and to associate with membranes (van der Mei *et al.*, 1972*b*). Little is known about the gene B, C, or E proteins. The gene D protein is made in large amounts and has been purified but no enzymatic activity or DNA-binding activity was detected (Burgess, 1969*b*).

The proteins coded for by genes F, G, and H are found in the virion and can be isolated from purified virus. The proteins from

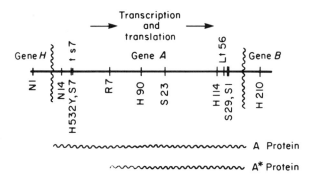

Fig. 12.   Location of different mutations within gene A and their positions relative to the portion of the gene coding for the A* protein. Redrawn from Linney and Hayashi (1974).

ϕX174 and S13 were found to be similar in amino acid and tryptic peptide composition (Poljak and Suruda, 1969). Fractionation in 6 M guanidine permitted the separation of gene F protein (β) and gene G protein (α) and the identification of the N-termini as serine and methionine, respectively (Suruda and Poljak, 1971). Air *et al.* (1975) worked out the sequence of the 67 N-terminal amino acids of the gene G protein and correlated it with the nucleotide sequence contained in the gene G ribosome-binding site and in and around the *Hind*II9 and *Hind*II10 restriction enzyme cleavage fragments. The sequences are shown in Fig. 13a. Figure 13b shows the nucleotide sequence of a portion of gene F and the amino acid sequence of a part of the gene F protein (Sanger, 1975). The number of times each codon is represented in these two sequences is given in Table 6, and it can be seen that there is a preponderance of codons ending in U (Sanger, 1975). Whether this is the cause or the result of the high proportion of T in the viral strand is not known (Denhardt and Marvin, 1969).

3.3. Superinfection Exclusion and Inhibition of Host DNA Synthesis

Two events occur midway through the latent period that may have a common underlying cause. One is superinfection exclusion, the alteration of an infected cell in such a way that a superinfecting phage cannot initiate an infection. The other is inhibition of host cell DNA synthesis and RF replication. Both of these events require that phage

TABLE 6

**Number of Times Specific Codons Are Used
in the Sequences in Fig. 13**[a]

Asp	GAU 5	Glu	GAA 1	Val	GUU 8	Phe	UUU 8
	GAC 5		GAG 3		GUC 1		UUC 3
Asn	AAU 5	Gln	CAG 5		GUA 1	Trp	UGG 1
	AAC 3	Pro	CCU 4	Met	AUG 5	His	CAU 4
Ala	GCU 9		CCA 2	Ile	AUU 8		CAC 2
	GCC 3		CCG 2		AUC 1	Lys	AAA 1
	GCA 2	Gly	GGU 7	Leu	UUA 2		AAG 3
Ser	UCU 7		GGC 5		UUG 1	Arg	CGU 7
	UCC 2	Thr	ACU 9		CUU 7		CGC 1
	UCA 3		ACC 1		CUC 3	Cys	UGC 1
	UCG 2		ACA 3		GUG 1		
	AGU 1		ACG 2	Tyr	UAU 4		Total codons:164

[a] Data from Sanger (1975).

protein synthesis occur (Sinsheimer, 1968; Stone, 1970*b*). Host RNA synthesis and host protein synthesis continue normally after ϕX174 infection, except at high multiplicities. S13 in contrast shuts off host protein synthesis (Puga *et al.*, 1973).

Superinfection exclusion is caused by a block in the synthesis of a complement to the parental single-stranded DNA. The superinfecting phage appears to eclipse normally, but no RF is made (Hutchison and Sinsheimer, 1971). Tessman *et al.* (1971) also studied the exclusion phenomenon and concluded that for physiological reasons of an unknown nature only about 80% of the cells exhibited superinfection exclusion (for both ϕX174 and S13). Representative mutants in different cistrons were tested in two different ways for their ability to cause superinfection exclusion. One made use of the ability of a superinfecting wild-type phage to rescue a preinfecting mutant phage. The other made use of the fact that the superinfecting phage could not make RF. Both of these experiments implicated the gene A function in superinfection exclusion. Hutchison and Sinsheimer (1971) argued that the gene A function could not be responsible because chloramphenicol abolished exclusion under conditions where RF replication still occurred. However, Tessman *et al.* (1971) made the point that these results would be expected if superinfection exclusion required more copious expression of gene A than was necessary for RF replication.

The inhibition of host DNA replication and RF replication coincides with the onset of viral progeny single-stranded DNA synthesis. In contrast to the filamentous phages, where single-stranded and double-stranded DNA syntheses occur simultaneously, the isometric (at least ϕX174) phages appear incapable of supporting both at the same time. However, Dumas and Miller (1976) reported that in a population of ϕX174-infected *dna*C mutant cells RF replication and single-stranded DNA synthesis could continue simultaneously at a slow rate (which was considerably less than normal) at the permissive temperature. Duplex DNA synthesis ceases even if single-stranded DNA synthesis is aborted by mutation in gene B, C, D, F, or G. Stone (1970*b*) found that even though 30 μg/ml chloramphenicol prevented the inhibition of duplex DNA replication, thus suggesting the need for a viral gene product, nevertheless mutants representative of the various known viral genes were still capable of shutting off host DNA synthesis. This dilemma was resolved by the discovery of Martin and Godson (1975) and Funk (personal communication) that only certain amber mutants in gene A would shut off host DNA synthesis. Unfortunately, there was no good correlation with the presence or absence of the A* protein, as

a

Met - Phe - Gln - Thr - 5 Phe - Ile - Ser - Arg - His - 10 Asn -

G-C-G-G-T-A-G-G-T-T-T-C-T-G-C-T-T-A-G-G-A-G-T-T-T-C-A-A-T-C-A-T-G-T-T-T-C-A-G-A-C-T-T-T-C-A-T-T-T-C-T-C-G-C-C-A-C-A-A-T-

⟶ Ribosomal binding site (Donelson et al., unpublished results) ⟶

Ser - Asn - Phe - Phe - 15 Ser - Asp - Lys - Leu - Val - 20 Leu - Thr - Ser - Val - Thr - 25 Pro - Ala - Ser - Ser - Ala - 30 Pro -

T-C-A-A-A-C-T-T-T-T-T-C-T-G-A-T-A-A-G-C-T-G-G-T-T-C-T-C-A-C-T-T-C-T-G-T-T-A-C-T-C-C-A-G-C-T-T-C-T-T-C-T-G-C-G-G-C-A-C-C-T-

⟶ Hind fragment 9 ⟶

⟶ Sequence primed by Hind fragment 10 (Plate III, Fig.1) ⟶

Val - Leu - Gln - Thr - 35 Pro - Lys - Ala - Thr - Ser - 40 Ser - Thr - Leu - Tyr - Phe - 45 Asp - Ser - Leu - Thr - Val - 50 Asn -

G-T-T-T-T-A-C-A-G-A-C-A-C-C-T-A-A-A-G-C-T-A-C-A-T-C-C-A-G-T-A-C-T-T-T-G-A-C-T-C-A-C-T-A-A-C-G-T-T-A-A-T-

⟶ Sequence primed by Hind frag ⟶

Ala - Gly - Asn - Gly - 55 Gly - Phe - Leu - His - Cys - 60 Ile - Gln - Met - Asp - Thr - 65 Ser - Val - Asx -

G-C-T-G-G-T-A-A-T-G-G-T-G-G-T-T-T-T-C-T-T-C-A-T-T-G-C-A-T-T-C-A-G-A-T-G-G-A-T-A-C-C-A-G-T-G-T-C-G T-A / C-G -A-C

⟶ Hind fragment 10 (79 nucleotides) ⟶

⟶ ment 2 (Plate IV) ⟶

⟶ Sequence transcribed (Fig.4) ⟶

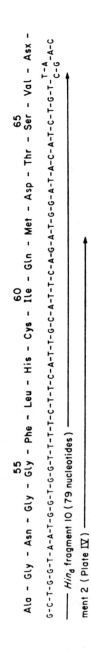

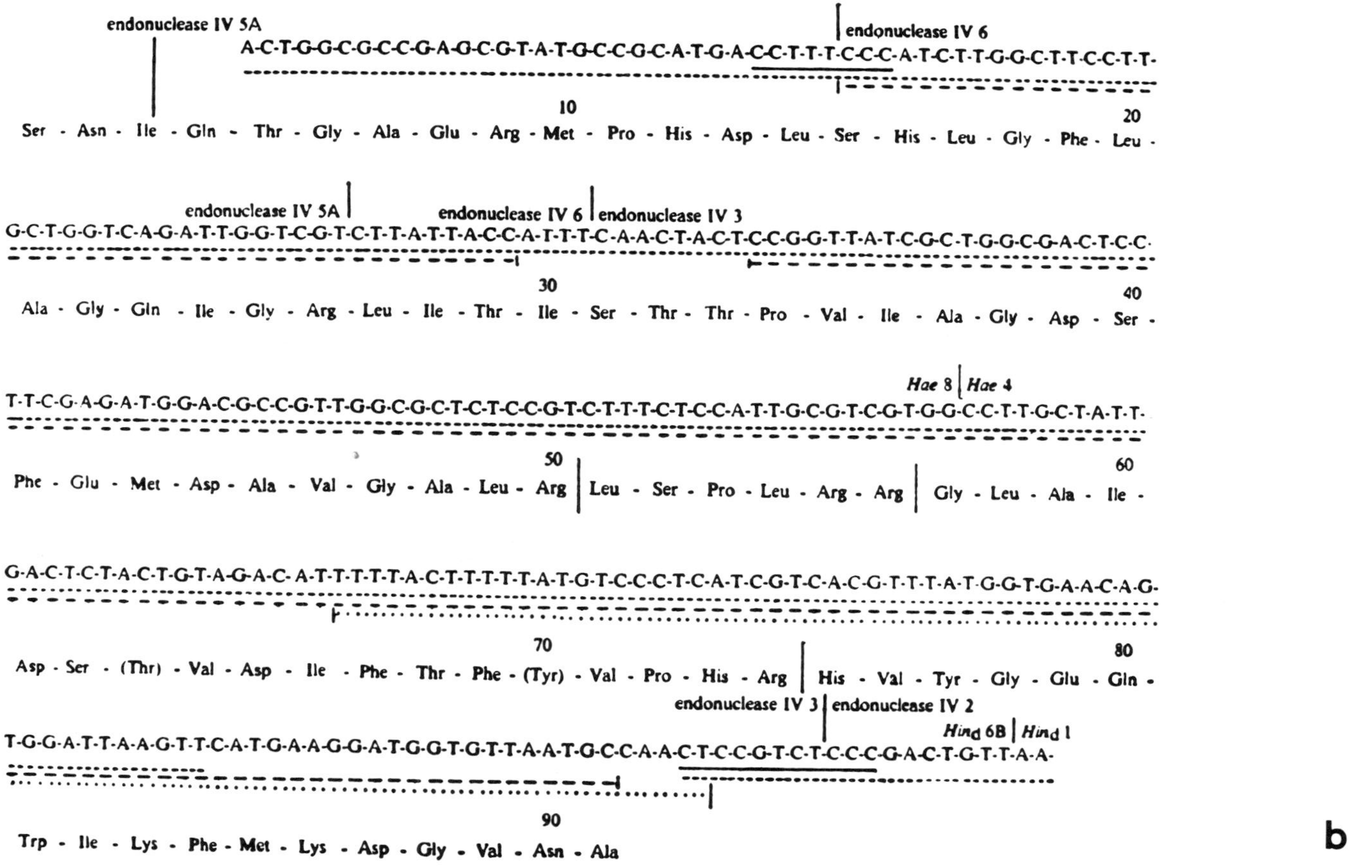

Fig. 13. (a) Amino acid sequence of the *N*-terminal region of the gene G protein and the nucleotide sequence of the portion of the DNA coding for it and for the ribosome-binding site controlling its synthesis. From Air *et al.* (1975), with permission. (b) Amino acid sequence of a portion of the gene F protein (G. M. Air, details to be published) and of the corresponding portion of gene F. The nucleotide sequences were deduced from the work of a number of investigators (A. R. Coulson, E. H. Blackburn, F. Galibert, V. Ling, F. Sanger, J. W. Sedat, and E. B. Ziff) using different methods. From Sanger (1975), with permission.

TABLE 7

Effect of Gene A Mutations on the Shutdown of Host DNA Replication[a]

Amber mutations	A* protein present	Host DNA synthesis blocked
8A, 50, 86	yes	yes
N14, 8tr	yes	no
18, H90	no	no

[a] From Martin and Godson (1975). Mutants 8A and 8tr are heat-insensitive mutants of the original *am*8 mutant that carried a secondary mutation causing temperature-sensitivity.

shown by the data in Table 7 (Martin and Godson, 1975). Amber mutations 8, 50, 86, and N14 map in the proximal part of the gene, H90 near the middle, and 18 near the distal end (see Figs. 2 and 12).

The phenomena of superinfection exclusion and host DNA replication inhibition are of interest because each represents a specific interference with DNA synthesis, perhaps the consequence of the transition from RF replication to progeny single-stranded DNA synthesis. Although it has not been shown, it seems reasonable that suppression of synthesis of complementary strand DNA during both superinfection exclusion and progeny viral strand DNA formation and suppression of synthesis of host DNA are achieved in the same way. The gene A protein, or at least part of it, appears to be responsible. The data are consistent with the hypothesis that the gene A protein combines stoichiometrically with and inhibits a bacterial component that is present in limited amounts and necessary for complementary strand synthesis and host DNA synthesis, but not viral strand synthesis. Some, but not all, gene A mutations would have to yield a product that still inhibits this essential component but is unable to support RF replication. Superinfection exclusion is thought not to be caused by degradation of the viral strand because the superinfecting DNA can be recovered as an infectious molecule (Hutchison and Sinsheimer, 1971).

4. RF REPLICATION

4.1. Function of Gene A

E. Tessman (1966) made a thorough study of suppressible S13 gene A mutants and showed that the gene A protein was required for RF replication. She also showed that its function could not be provided efficiently in *trans* in a complementation experiment between gene A and gene A^+ phage. In this study, the RF was quantitated by an infectivity assay and use was made of the fact that RF was more resistant to inactivation by hydroxylamine than was single-stranded DNA. [Noninfectious RF is not made, either (Shleser *et al.,* 1969a).] In the presence of low concentrations of chloramphenicol (30 μg/ml), RF replication occurred, and continued for a longer time than usual, leading to the formation of larger than normal amounts of RF in the cell; apparently, in the presence of this concentration of chloramphenicol the amounts of the viral proteins required for the synthesis of single-stranded DNA were insufficient to cause the transition from RF replication to progeny single-stranded DNA production. Since synthesis of the gene A protein is reduced by chloramphenicol to about the same extent as that of other proteins (Section 3.2.1), it appears that more gene A protein is synthesized in a normal infection than is needed. High concentrations of chloramphenicol do suppress the expression of gene A function.

Francke and Ray (1971) discovered that under certain conditions the parental RF acquired a nick in the viral strand. These conditions were where the gene A function was active but where RF replication was blocked by using a *rep* host (see next section). When the expression of gene A function was prevented by mutation or by high concentrations of chloramphenicol (100 μg/ml), the viral strand was not nicked. These experiments suggested that the function of the gene A protein was directly or indirectly to cause the nicking of the viral strand in the parental RF. It was argued that the number of RF II molecules formed per cell was fairly constant and independent of the multiplicity of infection. However, this conclusion is probably invalid because only two multiplicities greater than 1 (10 and 100) were used, and at a multiplicity of 100 the cells are likely to be damaged (Section 2.2 and Stone, 1970a). A study of the properties of intermediates in RF formation isolated from cells infected with UV-irradiated phage led Francke and Ray (1971) to propose that the "virus-specified discontinuity" could be made only after the complementary strand was completed and closed. An alternative interpretation, which was mentioned but not ruled out by the data presented, was that the radiation had destroyed the ability of the RF to code for a functional gene A protein by damaging the gene itself.

The gene A protein is considered to be an example of a *cis*-acting protein because of its apparent inability to act in *trans*. This has been shown both in complementation tests and also at the level of *in vivo* nicking of the RF. Thus in simultaneous infections of *rep* cells with [^{3}H]ϕX*am*3 (A^+E^-) and [^{32}P]ϕX*am*8 (A^-E^+) most of the RF II found at 20 min was ^{3}H-labeled; the A$^+$ protein was apparently unable to nick the [^{32}P]RF I produced by the *am*8 phage (Francke and Ray, 1972). Why the gene A protein functions so poorly in *trans* is not known. One possibility is that the substrate is not readily available in the appropriate conformation. This would be the case, for example, if the gene A (or A*) protein derived from the defective mutant phage were capable of binding to the DNA, but not acting, thus preventing access of active gene A protein to the site. A possible test of this proposal would be to construct a double amber mutant of gene A with mutations in the proximal and central parts of the gene so that both gene A *and* gene A* proteins would be more effectively eliminated and an inactive, DNA-binding protein less likely to be made.

Henry and Knippers (1974) substantially purified the gene A protein. In the final purification steps (phosphocellulose chromatography and band sedimentation), there was a good correlation between the presence of an endonucleolytic activity against ϕX174 RF I and the presence of a protein of a molecular weight of about 56,000 in SDS-polyacrylamide gels. The sedimentation rate of the enzyme activity in sucrose gradients was such that if the gene A protein were a typical protein it would have a molecular weight of about 70,000. The nuclease activity present in the preparation put one, and only one, nick into the RF, but it was not determined whether the nick was located randomly or located in a specific region of the genome. The nick was found only in the viral strand. Nuclease activity was also observed with single-stranded ϕX174 and M13 DNAs, but not with the superhelical DNAs of f1, SV40, or PM2. It was suggested that the protein acted at "flipped-out" hairpins in the superhelical DNA. Woodworth-Gutai and Lebowitz (1976) have argued that such cruciform structures (see Fig. 3) exist at palindromic sequences in negatively superhelical DNA because their formation would reduce the superhelix density and lower the free energy of the molecule while retaining much of the energy contained in the stacked, H-bonded duplex (Section 1.4.4). This possibility is attractive because hairpins are known to exist in the single-stranded ϕX174 DNA (Section 1.4.3) and it is conceivable that one is the site in single-stranded DNA that is recognized by the gene A protein. However, if RF I *in vivo* is not negatively superhelical, then "flipped-out" hairpins may not exist intracellularly.

Alternatively, the enzyme could recognize a hairpin, or a specific sequence of nucleotides, in a region of DNA transiently made single-stranded by the act of transcription. This would couple replication to transcription. Since the mRNA is transcribed from the complementary strand, the viral strand would be readily available for gene A action if the necessary sequence were close to the end of that segment of the DNA needed to code for a functional protein. Coupling of transcription to replication is believed to obtain in λ and has been suggested to be the case for M13 (Fidanian and Ray, 1974). Although van der Mei *et al.* (1972*a*) observed that RF replication in the presence of chloramphenicol could proceed for a considerable period after the addition of rifampicin, the above model cannot be eliminated because previously initiated transcription may continue for a period of time, especially in the presence of concentrations of chloramphenicol that slow down the rate of protein synthesis.

Singh and Ray (1975) studied the nuclease activities present in a preparation of gene A protein and observed that single-stranded circular φX174 DNA, but not M13 or G4 DNA, was extensively degraded. Fujisawa and Hayashi (1976*b*) reported that the gene A function was required during single-stranded DNA synthesis to terminate a round of replication and release a monomer-length viral genome (Section 5.1). Tessman *et al.* (1976) found certain S13 gene B mutants that produced an altered gene B protein lacking the *N*-terminal portion. This shortened protein had B protein function but interfered with gene A function, probably by binding to the RF.

4.2.   The *rep* Mutant and Other Required Host Cell Functions

Because it seemed reasonable to me that there should be a host cell function necessary for φX174 replication, but not for *E. coli* replication itself, Hathaway and I undertook the task of discovering it. We selected for mutants that would adsorb but not replicate φX174 and found three. All three, although independently isolated, were apparently blocked at the stage of RF replication. This was a surprise since we had anticipated finding mutants defective in the formation of the parental RF because that seemed at the time to be the step most likely to require a dispensable *E. coli* function. Dressler and I studied one mutant more thoroughly and found that RF I could be formed in the cell but that there was an absolute block to further replication. Although in our first experiments we had found the mutant to be recombination deficient (Denhardt *et al.*, 1967), later work by Calendar *et al.* (1970) and ourselves (Denhardt *et al.*, 1972) indicated that the degree of recombination deficiency was actually quite slight and probably due to the fact that the cell's DNA metabolism was altered. The *rep* mutation maps at 83′, near the origin of replication of the *E. coli* genome, is required for phage P2 replication, and is recessive to the wild-type rep^+ allele (Calendar *et al.,* 1970).

The ϕX174 RF that is formed is transcribed and translated and all the ϕX174 proteins seem to be present in the cell, albeit in reduced amounts, probably because the RF is unable to multiply (Denhardt *et al.,* 1972). The fact that single-stranded DNA synthesis does not occur suggests that the *rep* protein is also necessary for single-stranded DNA synthesis. Alternatively it is possible that there is insufficient production of one or more of the viral proteins necessary to turn on progeny single-stranded DNA synthesis. This latter possibility is supported by the observation that in the presence of low concentrations of chloramphenicol lesser amounts of all the viral proteins are made and single-stranded DNA synthesis, but not RF replication, is suppressed. However, high multiplicity infections still do not engender single-stranded DNA synthesis in the *rep* mutant. One could argue that RF replication must occur before single-stranded DNA can be made, but the molecular basis for such a requirement would be obscure. Mazur and Model (1973) showed that f1 single-stranded DNA synthesis could occur without RF replication if a sufficient amount of gene V protein was permitted to accumulate.

As discussed in the previous section, in the *rep* mutant the gene A protein acts and the viral strand is nicked. The nicked viral strand can be elongated with concomitant displacement of the original viral strand from the template (Francke and Ray, 1971, 1972). Circular RF molecules with one or more single-stranded tails are generated and these molecules sediment at about the same rate as RF I in sucrose gradients. Bowman and Ray (1975) found that in the presence of low concentrations of chloramphenicol formation of viral strands longer than unit length did not occur and they suggested that it was necessary that viral coat proteins be synthesized in the cell before viral strand elongation could occur. Under these conditions, degradation of the viral parental strand still occurred, most likely by nick translation originating at the site of gene A action and performed by DNA polymerase I.

Iwaya (1971) isolated a large number of additional *rep* mutants using, in some cases, a combination of both ϕX174 and P2 to select for them. The advantage of using the two phages is that adsorption mutants are more easily discriminated against since the two phages have different receptor sites. Some of the *rep* mutants supported P2 replication and appeared to permit ϕX174 RF replication, but not progeny single-stranded DNA synthesis or phage maturation. It was not possible to prove that these were not simply leaky *rep* mutants because the mutations all mapped, like *rep,* near the *ilv* locus. At least one can be complemented by a λ prophage carrying the *rep* allele, but little else, from this region (Takahashi, personal communication). Several *rep* mutants were identified as amber mutants on the basis that they could be suppressed by *su*1 or *su*2 suppressors (Denhardt *et al.,* 1972).

The function of the *rep* protein in φX174 replication is not known. *E. coli* can clearly dispense with the *rep* function, but with the result that replication of the chromosome is impaired. Lane and Denhardt (1974, 1975) discovered that there are about twice as many growing forks in a *rep* mutant as in a rep^+ strain and that the velocity with which the growing points move along the *E. coli* chromosome is reduced by about 50%. The chromosome is replicated bidirectionally from the normal origin at about 83′. Exponentially growing cells are larger and have a more massive nucleoid body as the result of having more DNA in the replicating structure. The mutant exhibits a small enhancement in sensitivity to ultraviolet and X-ray radiation, perhaps because of the larger genome. Other phages which are unable to replicate in the *rep* mutant include all the isolates of the isometric phages that have been tested, the filamentous single-stranded DNA phages, and the noninducible phages P2 and 186. It is intriguing that one characteristic these genomes may share is that they are replicated unidirectionally.

Other host cell functions required for φX174 RF replication include *dna*B (Dumas and Miller, 1974), *dna*C (Kranias and Dumas, 1974), *dna*E (Denhardt *et al.,* 1973; Dumas and Miller, 1973), and *dna*G (McFadden and Denhardt, 1974). If a *dna*B, *dna*E, or *dna*G mutant is shifted from the permissive to the restrictive temperature, RF replication is considerably reduced very quickly. It is also reduced in *dna*C mutants, although in this case abnormal forms of RF are synthesized at a low level (Kranias and Dumas, 1975). These abnormal forms appear to be the result of abnormal initiation or termination events; they do not seem to be replicating intermediates.

Taketo (1975*b*) infected spheroplasts of various *dna* mutants with either single-stranded DNA or RF and obtained evidence that the *dna*H (also Sakai and Komano, 1975) and *dna*Z (also Truitt and Walker, 1974) but not *dna*A (also Manheimer and Truffaut, 1974), *dna*I, or *dna*P functions were needed for φX174 replication. Which stage of replication was inhibited was not determined. Derstine and Dumas (1976) observed that the *dna*H phenotype could be reversed by high thymine concentrations and hence probably represented a defect in precursor synthesis. G4 RF replication normally requires the *dna*B, *dna*C, *dna*E, and *dna*G proteins but not the *dna*A protein (Dumas, personal communication). St-1 replication requires *dna*E but not *dna*A, *dna*B, or *dna*C; it was not certain whether *dna*G was required (Bowes, 1974). One point that should be evident is that different varieties of the isometric phages can give different results in a particular *dna* mutant (Vito *et al.*, 1975; Vito and Dowell, 1976) and that different alleles of a particular *dna* gene can give different results with the same phage (Dumas and Miller, 1974; Bowes, 1974). φX174 grows well in *pol*A strains despite the fact that the gaps in φX174 RF persist for a longer time (Schekman *et al.*, 1971). Growth in a *pol*A*ex* strain is, however, inhibited at the restrictive temperature (McFadden, 1975). I suspect that polynucleotide ligase activity is required by all the isometric phages but because of the large amount of enzyme normally present in the cell it may be difficult to demonstrate the requirement (McFadden and Denhardt, 1975; Bowes, 1975).

4.3. Origin of φX174 RF Replication

The first hint as to the location of the origin of φX174 RF replication came from studies of Baas and Jansz (1972*b*) on the frequency of heteroduplex repair after infection of spheroplasts with heteroduplex RF containing mutations at different sites in the genome. The frequency of mixed bursts was higher for mutations ranging from the distal region of gene A through gene E than for mutations situated in gene F through the proximal portion of gene A. It was argued that in order for mixed bursts to be observed replication had to occur before the heteroduplex was converted to a homoduplex by a repair process. If the allele in question were close to the origin of replication, then it would have a high probability of being replicated before being repaired; if it were located far from the origin of replication, then there would be a greater probability of its being reduced to a homozygous state before being replicated. The results suggested that the origin of replication was located in gene A. Weisbeek and van Arkel (1976) refined this study and investigated a series of different gene A mutants which had been physically mapped using restriction enzyme data. As shown in Figure 14a, they observed a sharp jump in the frequency of mixed bursts between *am*35 and *am*18, two mutations which map close together in the distal region of gene A in the *Hin*dII5 cleavage fragment (Fig. 2 and Weisbeek *et al.*, 1976). According to this interpretation, the origin of replication is located between these two alleles and is very close to the A/B junction.

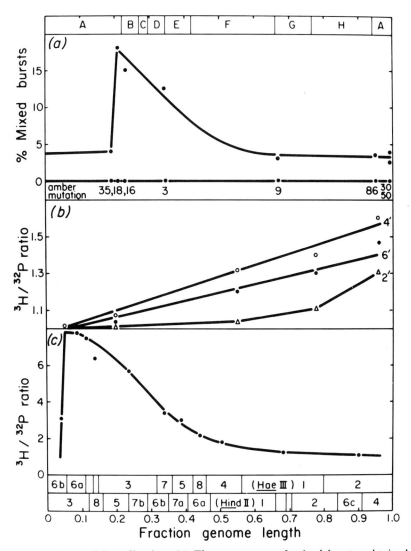

Fig. 14. Origin of RF replication. (a) The percentage of mixed bursts, obtained in single bursts of spheroplasts infected with different heteroduplexes, is plotted against a linear representation of the genetic map. The genetic map is indicated along the top, and the mutants used are placed along the bottom. Redrawn from Weisbeek and van Arkel (1976). (b) Plot of the specific activity of particular HindII fragments (3, 5, 1, 2, and 4) as a function of the position of the fragment in the genome. These fragments were derived from RF I that had been labeled at 16°C for the indicated time during the period of RF replication. Redrawn from Godson (1974a). (c) Plot of the $^3H/^{32}P$ ratio of the HaeIII fragments of ϕX174 RF as a function of the position of the fragment in the genome. The fragments were derived from RF II isolated 30 min after infection of rep cells with ^{32}P-labeled ϕX174 in the presence of [^3H]thymidine. The ratio for HaeIII2 was set equal to 1. Redrawn from Baas et al. (1976). Shown along the bottom are the approximate positions of the HaeIII and HindII cleavage products in the genome; the locations of fragments 9 and 10 are indicated but are not numbered.

Godson (1974a) used a different method to locate the origin of replication. He reasoned that if replicating molecules were labeled with [³H]thymidine for a period of time considerably shorter than that required for a round of replication to be completed then in completed molecules there should be much more ³H in that portion of the genome that was near the terminus of replication. Conversely, that segment of DNA nearest the origin would contain the least amount of radioactivity. Figure 14b shows the data obtained for RF I molecules; clearly there was a gradient of labeling increasing from a low value in HindII3 and HindII5 to a high value in HindII4. Thus by this definition the origin of replication was located in the HindII3 cleavage product. This interpretation ignores the fact that a gap-filling step (next section) intervenes between RF replication and RF I formation.

Baas et al. (1976) made use of the discovery by Francke and Ray (1971) that in rep mutants infected with a gene A⁺ phage nick translation occurs, originating, it is believed, at the nick inserted in the viral strand by the gene A protein. Rep cells were infected with ³²P-labeled φX174 in the presence of [³H]thymidine. The labeled DNA was extracted and digested with the HaeIII restriction nuclease, and the ratio of ³H/³²P in the various cleavage products was examined after separation by gel electrophoresis. Figure 14c shows the result. The largest ratio of ³H/³²P was found in the HaeIII6a fragment. The simplest interpretation of this result is that the origin is immediately counterclockwise to the HaeIII6a fragment and about in the middle of HaeIII6b. Eisenberg et al. (1975) came to a similar conclusion from their study of the location of the gap (see next section) in the viral strand of nascent RF II; HaeIII6b, and to a lesser extent HaeIII6a, was most heavily labeled in the gap-filling reaction. [There is some confusion in the literature about the order of these two fragments (Lee and Sinsheimer, 1974a; Weisbeek et al., 1976).]

There appears to be a dilemma. The heteroduplex repair data suggest that the origin is in HindII5 in the distal region of gene A, whereas the terminus-labeling, nick-translating, and gap-filling data suggest that the origin is in the middle of gene A. Since the conclusion drawn from the genetic data relies heavily on the am35 mutant, it is essential to obtain confirmation with additional independent mutants.

4.4. Nascent RF Molecules Contain Gaps

While performing a control for a series of experiments we were doing, Schekman discovered that intracellular φX174 RF II molecules

could not be converted to alkali-stable RF I molecules by polynucleotide ligase. Further investigation of this phenomenon revealed that
there were gaps in the RF II because when T4 DNA polymerase was
included in the reaction with ligase then RF I was formed. We found
that the gaps were present in newly synthesized RF molecules and that
in a *pol*A mutant the gaps persisted for a longer time than usual
(Schekman *et al.,* 1971). It seems likely that these gaps reflect some
aspect of DNA replication, perhaps the location of an RNA primer or
a π protein, or result from an event occurring during termination of a
round of replication and separation of the sibling molecules. The nature
of the termination process—how the two interlocked parental strands
are finally unwound and how the progeny RF become covalently circular—is not understood (cf. Gefter, 1975).

Eisenberg and Denhardt (1974*a,b*) studied in more detail the
characteristics of the gaps in ϕX174 RF II produced during RF
replication. There was only one gap in the viral strand, and it was
located in the *Hin*dII3 cleavage fragment. When the gap was filled
using radioactive deoxynucleoside triphosphates and then analyzed by
electrophoresis and homochromatography for the pyrimidine oligonucleotides produced after digestion with formic acid and diphenylamine,
a large number were found. There was a fourfold enrichment for the
unique C_6T isoplith (Eisenberg *et al.,* 1975). The pyrimidine oligonucleotides present in the viral strand gap are shown in Fig. 15c and may
be compared with those in the complete viral strand (a) and in the
major hairpin loops (e). The complexity of the pyrimidine tract pattern
was unexpected since a determination of the average size of the gap in
the viral strand had suggested that only some 16 nucleotides were lacking. One interpretation of these data is that there is a gap of variable
size in the viral strand of the nascent RF II that can encompass a siza-
ble region (10%?) of the genome. It is, however, largely restricted to the
region of the *Hin*dII3 fragment and often contains the unique C_6T
oligonucleotide. It does not contain pyrimidine tracts (T_4, T_5) characteristic of the stable hairpin loops in viral DNA (Fig. 15e and Section
1.4.3).

There are also gaps in the newly synthesized complementary
strands of the nascent RF II, about five to ten of them per RF
molecule, separating nascent pieces of DNA of roughly 80,000–800,000
daltons. In contrast to the gap in the newly synthesized viral strand, the
gaps in the complementary strand can be found in many regions of the
genome. This was shown by filling in the gaps with radioactive
nucleotides, digesting the RF with a restriction enzyme, and observing
that all of the restriction enzyme cleavage products contained label

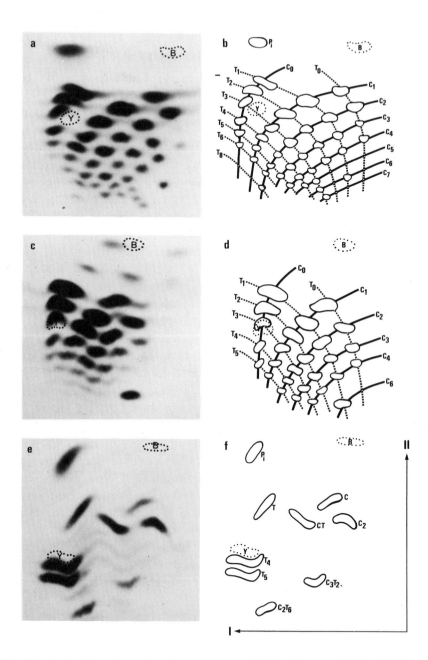

Fig. 15. Pyrimidine oligonucleotides present in ϕX174 viral strand DNA (a,b), in the gap left in the viral strand at the end of a round of replication (c,d), and in the major hairpin loops in ϕX174 DNA (e,f). The ^{32}P-labeled DNA was hydrolyzed with formic acid/diphenylamine and the pyrimidine oligonucleotides were fractionated by two-dimensional ionophoresis/homochromatography. The gap in the viral strands of the RF II population evidently can contain any of a number of pyrimidine oligonucleotides,

roughly in proportion to the size of the fragment. A quantitative study of the base composition of the nucleotides incorporated into the gaps, of the distribution of label among the fragments produced by the combined action of *Hae*III and *Hind*II, and of the oligonucleotide tracts present suggested that the gaps were not randomly located. The gaps appeared to have an average size of about 14 nucleotides (Eisenberg *et al.*, 1975).

These results are for the most part consistent with the results of Geider *et al.* (1972). These workers found that when cells in the process of RF replication were treated with ether and then allowed to continue replication in the presence of density-labeled and isotopically labeled deoxynucleoside triphosphates two types of incorporation could be observed. One type gave rise to labeled viral and complementary strands that had been completely synthesized *in vitro*; these were believed to derive from RF molecules that had been "initiated" *in vivo* but had not accomplished much synthesis at the time of ether treatment. The second type gave rise to labeled strands that were only partially substituted with the density label; these appeared to result from the filling in of gaps in RF II molecules that had just been replicated *in vivo*. From the shift in density of the RF, it was calculated that about 600 nucleotides were incorporated into the RF during the gap-filling/nick-translating process. However, there was considerable heterogeneity. Schröder *et al.* (1973) reported evidence for gaps in the complementary strands of nascent RF II molecules. Their failure to detect a gap in the viral strand and their observation that full-length linear strands labeled during the gap-filling process were almost exclusively of complementary strand polarity stand in contrast to the results of Eisenberg *et al.* (1975) and may be explained by their nonphysiological conditions.

4.5.   Structure of the Replicating Intermediate: The "Reciprocating Strand" Model

The most detailed studies on the structure of the replicating intermediate involved in ϕX174 RF replication have been reported by

---

C_6T in particular (Eisenberg *et al.*, 1975). The hairpins, in contrast, consist of a simpler sequence characterized especially by the presence of C_2, CT, T_4, and T_5 tracts (Bartok *et al.*, 1975). (a,c,e) Actual autoradiograms; (b,d,f) grid pattern from which the identity of the spots can be determined. The RF with the gap in the viral strand was prepared by Shlomo Eisenberg. The hairpin loops were prepared by Katalina Bartok. The pyrimidine tracts were determined by Barbara Harbers in John Spencer's laboratory.

Schröder and co-workers (Schröder and Kaerner, 1972; Schröder *et al.*, 1973). They found that a portion of the pulse-labeled viral strand DNA was present in a linear strand that was longer than one complete genome. The complementary strand in contrast was present in unit-length or shorter strands. The replicating intermediates that sedimented most rapidly (27–28 S) banded in CsCl at a greater density than intact duplex DNA and appeared to contain single-stranded regions. This signified that synthesis of the new viral strand preceded synthesis of the complementary strand. In the culture as a whole, equivalent amounts of viral and complementary strands were labeled by a short pulse. The data were consistent with the rolling circle model (Gilbert and Dressler, 1968).

McFadden and Denhardt (1975) studied the properties of ϕX174 replicating intermediates found under conditions of ligase insufficiency in an *E. coli* mutant possessing a temperature-sensitive polynucleotide ligase. The infected cells were transferred from permissive to nonpermissive conditions during RF replication. A variety of control experiments showed that ligase activity was severely reduced and that no detectable adventitious nicking occurred. When a pulse of [³H]thymidine was administered during RF replication at the restrictive temperature, label was found to flow into viral strands of unit length or longer and into complementary strands of less than unit length. They concluded, as Eisenberg and Denhardt (1974*b*) had earlier, that the complementary strand was synthesized discontinuously. Also, in agreement with the conclusions of Schröder and Kaerner (1972), a portion of the viral strand template in the replicating intermediates was single-stranded, indicating that synthesis of the complementary strand lagged behind synthesis of the viral strand.

Because of the existence of longer-than-unit-length strands, it is widely believed that replication proceeds according to the rolling circle model (Gilbert and Dressler, 1968). However, the linchpin of this model—longer-than-unit-length strands exist because the parental viral strand is used as a primer for many rounds' worth of continuous synthesis—has not been proved. One can argue that initiation occurs by some other device and that the reason a longer-than-unit-length strand is generated is that it is necessary to keep the end of the viral strand near what will be the terminus of replication so that a circular progeny viral strand can be formed. I have outlined in Fig. 16 and elsewhere (Denhardt, 1975) the details of this proposal. In essence, it assumes initiation by an RNA or π protein primer, displacement of the newly synthesized 5'-end by branch migration of the parental viral strand, and covalent joining of the free 5'-end of the displaced, newly

Fig. 16. Reciprocating strand model. The parental viral strand is shown as a thin continuous line, the parental complementary strand is shown as a thick continuous line, and the nascent strands are stippled. (a) Synthesis of a new viral strand is initiated on a closed circular duplex at the origin of replication in the region of gene A. Priming is accomplished either by the synthesis of a short oligoribonucleotide or by the proper placement of a nucleotide by a π protein. After a short sequence of DNA is synthesized, the accumulation of positive superhelical twists in the molecule (not shown) requires that the parental duplex be nicked. The gene A protein together with cellular proteins that are involved in the initiation or priming of a round

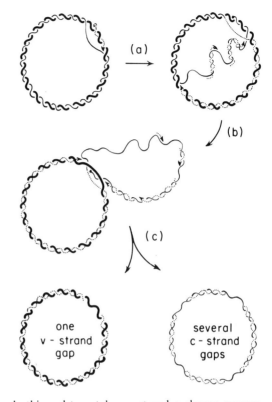

of DNA replication is imagined to do this and to catalyze a strand exchange process. This results in the joining of the 5′-end of the newly synthesized viral strand to the parental viral strand. If the 5′-end is a 5′-OH, then the reaction is not unlike that catalyzed by ribonuclease where the 2′-OH attacks the phosphate and displaces the 5′-linked ribose (see Denhardt, 1975). Excision of 5′-terminal primer ribonucleotides by this process would generate the requisite 5′-OH. Branch migration occurs at the same time so that the 5′-end of the parental viral strand is retained within a duplex structure. (b) Synthesis of the viral strand is unidirectional and continuous and proceeds clockwise around the genome. Synthesis of the complementary strand is discontinuous and lags behind synthesis of the viral strand. The synthesis of complementary strand fragments is presumed to be primed by RNA by a mechanism like that discussed in Section 2.3.1. In order to permit the parental strands to unwind, it is necessary for the exchange reaction between the nascent viral strand and the parental strand to occur repeatedly; in other words, to reciprocate. (c) When synthesis of the viral strand is almost complete, a situation arises where the two parental strands are completely unwound. A strand exchange at this point releases two separate and circular, but incomplete, duplexes. One has a single gap of variable size in the viral strand. The other has several gaps separating nascent pieces of complementary strand DNA. If the final strand exchange reaction should occur before the two parental strands are completely unwound, a catenane would result. If the 3′-end of the nascent viral strand should join the 5′-end of the parental viral strand, and a strand exchange reaction occur between the complementary strands, then a figure-8 molecule (see Section 7.1) or circular dimer would be formed.

synthesized strand (which is envisioned to be still in the process of being synthesized) to the parental viral strand. In order to permit the parental strands to unwind, this strand exchange process may have to occur repeatedly and for this reason I call it a "reciprocating strand" model.

The major points of departure of the reciprocating strand model from the rolling circle model are as follows: (1) Initiation occurs *de novo* with an RNA or π protein primer rather than by elongation of the nicked parental viral strand. (2) The complementary strand template is used not in an "endless" and continuous fashion but rather in a quantized manner requiring a new initiation event for each round of replication. (3) A "free" 5´-end does not exist. There is no covalent attachment to a "membrane site." No linear duplex intermediate is ever formed, however transiently. (4) Strands longer than unit length are formed only subsequent to initiation and are formed by a strand exchange mechanism to allow proper termination and to ensure production of a progeny circular molecule.

The reciprocating strand model is more complex than the rolling circle model and is consistent with a larger body of data, especially the presence of RF II molecules with gaps, the existence of which is not compatible with the rolling circle model. Also, Christian Hours (unpublished work in my laboratory) has looked for a linear molecule of the kind predicted to be excised from the tail of a rolling circle (cf. Schröder *et al.*, 1973) but has been unable to identify any structure with the expected properties. Dressler and Wolfson (1970) found, as predicted by the rolling circle model, that the first RF I molecules to be labeled after a short pulse were labeled in their complementary strands; unfortunately, these workers did not determine whether the entire strand was labeled or whether the label was incorporated as the result of gap filling (cf. Schröder *et al.*, 1973), so that it is not possible to interpret their observations. The "double ring" replicating intermediate and the shorter-than-unit-length nascent viral strands reported by Knippers *et al.* (1969c) are in agreement with the reciprocating strand model. The restriction on the number of dye molecules that can intercalate into the replicating intermediate (Fukuda and Sinsheimer, 1976a) is explained by the fact that the 5´ end is interlocked with the circular duplex.

The reciprocating strand model suggests explanations both for the disparate results on the location of the origin and for the variableness in size and location of the gap in the viral strand of nascent RF II. The key assumption is that the gene A protein nicks the RF in the middle of the A gene but that actual replication only begins some variable distance downstream, closer to the A/B border. Once replication, which requires the *rep* function, initiates, it proceeds around the genome to the site of gene A action. As the replication complex approaches this site, the parental viral strand becomes completely disengaged from the parental complementary strand and both molecules are released as circular structures. As indicated in Fig. 16, the products at this point consist of a parental complementary strand with a continuous, but incomplete, nascent viral strand and a parental viral strand with fragments of nascent complementary strand DNA. Thus the true origin of replication is close to the A/B border (Weisbeek and van Arkel, 1976, and Fig. 14a), but in the absence of the *rep* protein an abnormal nick translation process can begin further upstream at the gene A induced nick (Baas *et al.*, 1976, and Fig. 14c). It is difficult to interpret Godson's (1974*a*) results (Fig. 14b) because of the gap-filling problem.

4.6. Selectivity of Subsequent Replication

As we have seen, there is a profound asymmetry in the semiconservative replication of the RF. The newborn RF molecule with the parental viral strand initially contains a complementary strand consisting of fragments, and as the complementary strand is the template for transcription it is likely that transcription of this RF will be impaired until the fragments are joined. The RF molecule with the newly synthesized viral strand is, in contrast, complete except for a small gap in the gene A region, and this molecule, because of the intactness of the complementary strand, should support normal transcription. However, competition between RNA polymerase and DNA polymerase, one wanting to transcribe the complementary strand and the other wanting to fill in the gap in the viral strand, would have to be resolved. If an intact viral strand in the region of gene A is necessary for gene A function and initiation of a second round of replication, then it is not obvious *a priori* which of the two products of a round of replication will replicate first. According to recent experiments, however, it is the RF with the intact parental complementary strand that is preferentially replicated.

Thus in an elegant experiment Merriam *et al.* (1971*b*) found that when [5-³H]cytosine was incorporated only into the complementary strand of the parental RF it was effective at inducing reversions among the progeny of a particular temperature-sensitive mutant. The mutant used (*ts*163) required a C to T change in the complementary strand. When [5-³H]cytosine was incorporated only in the viral strand of the parental RF of another temperature-sensitive mutant, *ts*41D, which required a C to T change in the viral strand, it was not very effective at inducing reversions among the progeny. Decays in the free virus were effective.

Merriam *et al.* (1971*a*) and Baas and Jansz (1972*a*) characterized the progeny phage produced after infection of spheroplasts with heteroduplex RF. Both groups observed that in single-burst experiments a majority of the spheroplasts yielded only one phage genotype in the progeny. This is presumed to be the result of repair of the heteroduplex and reduction to a homoduplex state prior to replication. The former workers found that among the total progeny there was a preponderance of viral strand genotype, whereas the latter found approximately equal proportions of progeny derived from the two strands. The significant observation in both experiments was that in those bursts which yielded progeny from both strands the predominant genotype was that derived from the complementary strand. Iwaya and Denhardt (1973*a*) provided direct physical evidence for the preferential replication of the RF molecule containing the complementary strand derived from the parental RF by their demonstration that the pool of replicating RF molecules found in the cell after a short period of RF replication only rarely contained the original viral strand.

4.7. Radiobiological Experiments and Parent-to-Progeny Transfer

This state of affairs is incompatible with an earlier concept of ϕX174 replication (Denhardt and Silver, 1966; Sinsheimer, 1970) that ascribed an overriding role to the parental viral strand in the parental RF, even after RF replication had ostensibly occurred. Belief in the importance of the viral strand was founded in part on radiobiological experiments (Denhardt and Sinsheimer, 1965*b*; Datta and Poddar, 1970) that indicated that the decay of a ^{32}P atom contained only in the parental viral strand could efficiently destroy the ability of the infected cell to form a plaque, even after the RF had apparently replicated. Similar, but not identical, results have been obtained with ^{3}H suicide (Denhardt, unpublished) and some illustrative data are shown in Fig. 17.

Despite the lower energy of the β particle emitted by a ^{3}H nucleus (maximum energy 0.018 MeV) as compared with a ^{32}P nucleus (maximum energy 1.7 MeV) and the fact that it is not part of the covalent backbone of DNA, the decay of a tritium atom contained in [^{3}H]thymidine in single-stranded ϕX174 DNA results in the inactivation of infectious phage particles with an efficiency per decay (α) of about 0.2. When the single-stranded DNA enters the bacterium, it becomes less sensitive and is inactivated with an efficiency of 0.1. (The details of this experiment are described in the caption.) The difference

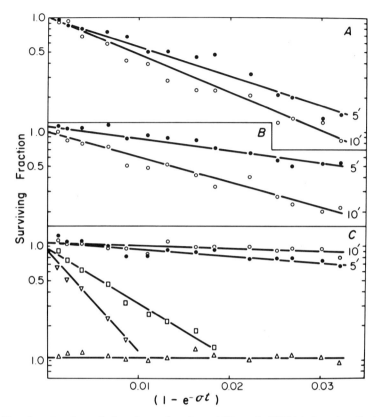

Fig. 17. Inactivation of the plaque-forming ability of φX174-infected cells by the decay of ³H atoms contained in [³H-methyl]thymidine. *E. coli* CR was grown in a defined minimal medium, starved (Denhardt and Sinsheimer, 1965a), and then divided into two portions one of which was infected with unlabeled φX174 and one of which was infected with φX174 labeled with [³H-methyl]thymidine at a specific activity of 15 Ci/mmole. The phage was allowed to eclipse for 10 min and then each culture was split and one portion combined with medium containing nonradioactive thymidine and the other combined with medium containing [³H-methyl]thymidine (15 Ci/mmole, 2 μg/ml final concentration). Aliquots were taken from the cultures at various times (●, 5 min; O, 10 min), divided into small portions, and stored in liquid nitrogen. Replication of the phage in the cultures was monitored by premature lysis, and there was an average of one phage/cell at 14 min after the addition of medium. This is a normal eclipse period under these conditions. At intervals over the following 8 months, a set of samples was thawed and assayed for infectious centers. The data are plotted as the surviving fraction (normalized against the titers observed in the first set of thawed samples) vs. the fraction of ³H atoms that have decayed (cf. Denhardt and Sinsheimer, 1965b). A: Cells were infected with radioactive phage; replication proceeded in the presence of radioactive thymidine. B: Cells were infected with nonradioactive phage; replication proceeded in the presence of radioactive thymidine. C: Cells were infected with radioactive phage; replication proceeded in the presence of nonradioactive thymidine. ∇, Inactivation of [³H]φX174 alone; □, inactivation of the "zero-time" complexes (taken immediately before addition of medium), cells infected with [³H]φX174; Δ, stability of nonradioactive complexes (control).

in sensitivity in these two cases is probably the result of a greater degree of radiation damage inflicted on the DNA molecule in the relatively compact virion.

The three sets of curves (Fig. 17A,B,C) represent the sensitivity of infected cells to inactivation by ^{3}H decays at various stages after infection. Sensitivity was measured by the loss of plaque-forming ability, and complexes were taken at 5 min and 10 min after infection. The eclipse period was 15 min. In A, cells were infected in radioactive medium with radioactive phage. In B, cells were infected in radioactive medium with nonradioactive phage. In C, cells were infected with radioactive phage in nonradioactive medium. The bottom curve in C shows the stability of nonradioactive complexes at 5 min after infection. Collectively, these curves show that if the infection is carried out in radioactive medium the infectious centers are almost as rapidly inactivated when nonradioactive phage is used to infect them as they are when radioactive phage is used. When nonradioactive cells are infected with radioactive phage, the sensitivity of the infectious centers to inactivation at 5 min after infection is much reduced (efficiency of inactivation 0.017) in comparison with the zero-time complex. This probably represents the difference between the efficiency of inactivation of an RF molecule and a single-stranded DNA molecule. By 10 min after infection, essentially all sensitivity has been lost. These inactivation curves do not seem to suggest an important role for the parental viral strand after RF replication has commenced.

The difficulty with this kind of experiment is the interpretation. Although the infection is synchronized and RF replication in the entire culture is in progress from about 5 min on, it is impossible to know what is happening in each individual cell. The apparent paramount importance of the parental viral strand in the ^{32}P suicide experiments probably can be ascribed to a lag in RF replication in some of the cells (especially when starved) and a general damaging effect that radiophosphorus decay has on the cell. In the case of tritium decays, the amount of radiation damage absorbed by the cell is probably greater than in the case of ^{32}P because there is a greater ionization density along the path of the less energetic electron; on the other hand, there is the effect of the recoiling ^{32}P nucleus to consider. In short, it is practically impossible in this type of experiment to sort out a specific effect of radioisotope decay on the molecule involved from a nonspecific effect of the emitted radiation on all the molecules in the vicinity.

The idea that the parental RF was special had been supported also by the low amount of parent-to-progeny transfer of parental DNA that occurred (Knippers et al., 1969b). Schnegg and Hofschneider (1970)

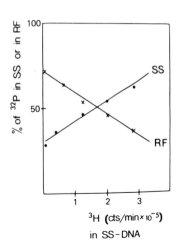

Fig. 18. Transfer of ^{32}P from RF to single-stranded DNA. Nonpermissive cells were infected with ^{32}P-labeled ϕXam3 (lysis-defective) phage in the presence of [^{3}H]thymidine, and the amount of ^{32}P and ^{3}H present in viral DNA forms was determined after separation by velocity centrifugation on neutral sucrose gradients. As single-stranded DNA synthesis proceeded, there was a clear transfer of ^{32}P from RF to single-stranded DNA. From Iwaya and Denhardt (1973b).

and Iwaya and Denhardt (1973b) showed that such transfer could be detected in appropriately designed experiments. Figure 18 illustrates the chase of parental radioactivity out of RF molecules and into progeny single-stranded DNA. These results, and others presented elsewhere in this chapter, suggest that all of the RF molecules in the cell are functionally equivalent once their component strands are complete. Both parental and progeny RF replicate, are transcribed, and can give rise to progeny single-stranded DNA.

4.8. Role of the Membrane

Another concept whose virtue is in jeopardy is that of an "essential membrane site." Yarus and Sinsheimer (1967) first put forward this idea in order to explain the limitation on the number of genomes (usually one, sometimes two) that could father progeny in a previously starved cell. In unstarved cells, no limitation was observed and up to at least four different genomes could multiply. It was suggested that in the cell there were a limited number of "essential membrane sites" at which phage replication could take place. Unfortunately these experiments are complicated by the damaging affects of high multiplicity infections (Stone, 1970a). A parallel was drawn between the number of "sites" for ϕX174 replication and the number of growing forks that could coexist during replication of $E.$ $coli$ DNA in minimal or enriched medium.

Later work by several investigators on the association of pulse-labeled replicating ϕX174 DNA with the membrane (Knippers and Sinsheimer, 1968a; Salivar and Sinsheimer, 1969) has been taken to support the existence of one or more "essential membrane sites."

However, the "essential membrane site" remains elusive, so much so that its existence can be questioned. The fact that more RF molecules could be found associated with the membrane than could supposedly replicate (Salivar and Sinsheimer, 1969) required waffling. Tessman *et al.* (1971) found that up to 40 S13 phage particles could replicate in a cell even though there were only some 15 "sites" for binding RF to the membrane.

Knippers *et al.* (1969a) argued that RF replication occurred on the membrane whereas single-stranded DNA synthesis occurred in the cytoplasm on the basis of the observation that a 20-s pulse given at 5 min after infection yielded a much higher proportion of "membrane-associated" DNA than did a 20-s pulse at 50 min after infection. An alternative explanation of this observation is that DNA synthesis is occurring at a much greater rate at 50 min than at 5 min. It seems to me that more definitive data are needed before anything can be made of the fact that replicating DNA is often found in association with a rapidly sedimenting membrane fraction. Because of the hydrophobic properties of single-stranded DNA, known to be present in replicating intermediates, a nonspecific association can easily occur. In addition, some of the proteins (e.g., the gene A protein, van der Mei *et al.*, 1972b) involved in DNA replication may have hydrophobic properties. The recent experiments (Section 2.3.1) showing that at least some of the proteins known to be required for DNA replication are active in a soluble fraction free of membrane material suggest to me that the "essential membrane site" is a red herring.

5. SINGLE-STRANDED DNA SYNTHESIS

5.1. Asymmetric Displacement Replication

A major advance in our understanding of progeny single-stranded DNA synthesis was made by Lindqvist and Sinsheimer (1968) when they discovered that RF molecules were material precursors to single-stranded DNA. They exploited the discovery that exposure of HCR⁻ (host cell reactivation deficient) cells to mitomycin C reduced host DNA replication more severely than ϕX174 DNA replication (Lindqvist and Sinsheimer, 1967a). Previous work had been complicated by the incorporation of radioactivity into host cell DNA; the labeled *E. coli* DNA masked the labeled ϕX174 DNA. Taketo (1975a) showed that mutations in several different host genes (*uvr* A, B, or C but not *uvr* D or F) that caused the cell to be sensitive to ultraviolet light also caused the capacity of the cell to support ϕX174 replication to be mitomycin-resistant. The biochemical basis of this phenomenon is not understood. (Treated HCR$^+$ cells will not replicate ϕX174.)

Very soon after the discovery that the RF was a material precursor to progeny single-stranded DNA, it was established that the complementary strand was conserved in the RF molecule and that synthesis of a new viral strand in the RF accompanied the displacement of the old viral strand into a progeny virion (Dressler and Denhardt, 1968; Knippers *et al.,* 1968; Komano *et al.,* 1968). It is now established that at a time when net synthesis of RF has largely stopped, and net synthesis of single-stranded DNA is under way, radioactive precursors must flow through the viral strand of an RF molecule. Funk and Sinsheimer (1970*a*) obtained evidence that most, if not all, of the RF molecules in the cell were used repeatedly for single-stranded DNA synthesis and there seemed to be no preferential use of RF made late in infection.

A study of the structure of the replicating intermediates pulse-labeled during the period of single-stranded DNA synthesis revealed that many of the labeled polydeoxynucleotide strands were linear and longer than unit length (Knippers *et al.,* 1969*a*; Dressler, 1970). Espejo and Sinsheimer (1976*a*) found that when RF molecules with such single-stranded tails were isolated from the cell they could exhibit a restricted capability for binding an intercalating dye in a CsCl density gradient. This was believed to result from branch migration and interaction between the two single-stranded tails that resulted so that unwinding of the duplex at the break was hindered. The presence of these long strands suggests covalent attachment of the newly synthesized DNA to a preexisting viral strand, and this in turn provides much of the support for the rolling circle model (Gilbert and Dressler, 1968).

One essential aspect of this model is the insertion of a nick into the viral strand of RF I and the use of the 3′-OH thereby made available as a primer. This may be what happens, but alternative priming mechanisms are known to exist. If another priming mechanism is used, the question then arises: why are there strands longer than unit length? I have suggested elsewhere (Section 4.5 and Denhardt, 1975) that the newly synthesized 5′-end must be joined to the original parental strand in order to provide the proper configuration for termination—i.e., for production of a progeny circular viral strand. In support of the possibility that the replicating intermediate need not obligatorily contain a nascent viral strand longer than unit length is the observation by McFadden and Denhardt (1975) that although much of the DNA pulse-labeled during single-stranded DNA synthesis is longer than unit length some 10% is not. This is illustrated in Fig. 19. Yokoyama *et al.* (1971) also found DNA chains shorter than unit length during single-stranded DNA synthesis.

Fujisawa and Hayashi (1976*a,b*) discovered a 50 S structure that had the properties of an intermediate in progeny single-stranded DNA production. This particle appeared to contain the viral proteins required for single-stranded DNA synthesis (A, D), the proteins in the virion (F, G, H, A*, and X), and an RF molecule comprising a unit-length circular complementary strand and a linear viral strand between one and two times the complete genome. Functional gene A protein was necessary for reduction of twice-unit-length viral DNA to unit-length. The evidence for this was that in cells infected with mutant phage coding for a temperature-sensitive gene A protein single-stranded DNA synthesis stopped after a shift-up and 50 S particles containing linear viral strands of twice unit length could be identified. This result is not the result anticipated from a "rolling circle" process, but is in accord with the reciprocating strand model.

Another fact that is not in agreement with the rolling circle model is that there is a gap in the newly synthesized viral strand in the RF molecules (Schekman *et al.,* 1971). Johnson and Sinsheimer (1974) showed that this gap was in the gene A region of the genome. As

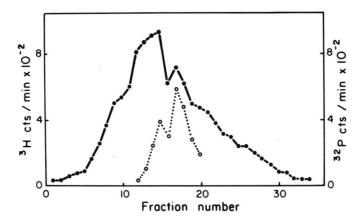

Fig. 19.   Presence of viral strands shorter than unit length during single-stranded DNA synthesis. ϕX174-infected *E. coli* was labeled for 5 s at 60 min after infection during the period of single-stranded DNA synthesis. The viral DNA was purified on a neutral sucrose gradient and then centrifuged on an alkaline sucrose gradient. The distribution of radioactivity is shown in the figure. Sedimentation is toward the left. O, ^{32}P marker circular and linear strands; ●, ^{3}H-pulse-labeled DNA. From McFadden and Denhardt (1975).

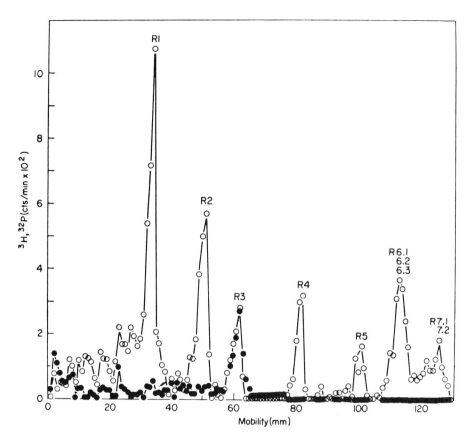

Fig. 20. Location of the gap in RF II found in the cell during single-stranded DNA synthesis. The RF was purified from cells infected for 45 min and pulse-labeled briefly with [³H]thymidine. The RF II fraction was incubated with [α-³²P]dTTP, unlabeled deoxynucleoside triphosphates, DNA polymerase I, polynucleotide ligase, ATP, and other components necessary for conversion to RF I. The RF I was repurified and cleaved with endonuclease R.*Hin*dII, and the resulting fragments were separated by electrophoresis on a 5% polyacrylamide gel. Migration is toward the right. ³H (O) is found in all of the fragments, whereas ³²P (●) is found only in the *Hin*dII3 fragment. Reproduced from Johnson and Sinsheimer (1974), with permission.

illustrated in Fig. 20, radioactivity incorporated into the gap was found only in the *Hin*dII3 fragment. The existence of this gap is incompatible with the hypothesis that a DNA polymerase "rolls" continuously around the complementary strand circle releasing a longer-than-unit-length tail. Instead, each cycle of synthesis of a progeny viral strand must be a separate event involving an initiation, an elongation, and a termination step. Given unidirectional replication, the gap is at the origin/terminus. The pyrimidine tracts present in the gap found in RF

II during single-stranded DNA synthesis appear equivalent to those found in the viral strand of RF II during RF replication (Denhardt *et al.*, 1975).

In many ways, this process resembles the synthesis of a viral strand during RF replication. It differs in that synthesis of a complementary strand is suppressed, a number of additional viral proteins are required, and the viral strand becomes methylated at a unique site.

5.2. Methylation

The methylation phenomenon is intriguing, and one wonders whether it just happens or whether it has significance with regard to DNA replication or maturation and packaging of the DNA into the virion. Razin *et al.* (1970) found 5-methylcytosine together with thymine in the dinucleotide isoplith fraction of ϕX174 DNA at a ratio of about 1 mol/per mol viral DNA. Lee and Sinsheimer (1974*b*) showed that the 5MeC was in the gene H region in the overlap between the *Hae*III2 fragment and the *Hind*II6c fragment (see Fig. 10). ϕX174 DNA apparently is methylated only during single-stranded DNA synthesis. It must be the displaced viral strand in the replicating intermediate during single-stranded DNA synthesis that is methylated because 5MeC is not found in RF I or II (Razin *et al.*, 1973). Evidence that the virus codes for the methylase was obtained by Razin (1973) when he showed that a mutant of ϕX174 (ϕX*h*10) that could grow in *E. coli* B also induced a DNA cytosine methylase. *E. coli* B normally lacks such an activity, in contrast to *E. coli* C. The ability of different mutants to induce this activity has not been tested. If methylation has a function, it probably involves interaction of the viral strand with the viral proteins during morphogenesis since it is that process which most dramatically distinguishes single-stranded DNA synthesis from RF replication. Razin *et al.* (1975) found that nicotinamide interfered with methylation of *E. coli* DNA and reduced the phage yield in ϕX174-infected cells. Although they argued that this meant that DNA methylation was an essential step in progeny viral strand maturation, alternative explanations, such as inhibition of polynucleotide ligase activity, were not ruled out.

5.3. Circularization

How the displaced viral strand is circularized is not known. An attractive hypothesis (Knippers *et al.*, 1969*a*; Iwaya *et al.*, 1973), for which there is no evidence, is that the two ends of a hypothetical linear intermediate fall within the duplex part of one of the hairpins known to exist in ϕX174 DNA (see Section 1.4.3). This would provide a mechanism to bring the two ends together so that ligase, or ligase plus a DNA polymerase, could join them. According to this model, the ends of any linear strand intermediates would be located in a specific region of the genome. In *E. coli ts*7, a mutant with a temperature-sensitive ligase, a portion of the viral DNA found in virions synthesized at the restrictive temperature was found to be linear, and it was suspected that these linear strands might be such intermediates. Iwaya *et al.* (1973) showed that the ends of these linear strands could be covalently joined by ligase plus T4 DNA polymerase, but not ligase alone, a result consistent with the model. However, later work revealed that linear strands with randomly located ends could be circularized equally well (Denhardt *et al.*, 1976). Furthermore, a study of the position of the ends of the DNA molecules generated in the *ts*7 host revealed that they could be located in many different regions of the genome (Miller and Sinsheimer, 1974; Bartok and Denhardt, unpublished results). The origin and significance of the linear strands found under conditions of ligase deficiency are unclear.

Linear viral strands derived from RF II or from single-stranded DNA synthesized under conditions of ligase insufficiency have been reported to be infectious, and this has been taken as evidence for the intrinsic ability of a linear viral strand with appropriately located ends to circularize by forming a hairpin structure (Schekman and Ray, 1971; Schröder and Kaerner, 1974). Miller and Sinsheimer (1974) made similar observations, but concluded that contamination with a low level of complementary strand DNA was responsible for the infectivity since removal of the complementary strands by equilibrium banding in CsCl after annealing the DNA with poly(U,G) resulted in a selective loss of the infectivity associated with the linear viral strand DNA.

The filamentous bacteriophage f1 requires the *dna*A function for growth; progeny DNA is synthesized at the restrictive temperature but it is found to be mostly linear (Bouvier and Zinder, 1974). ϕX174, however, does not require the *dna*A function for growth (Manheimer and Truffaut, 1974; Taketo, 1973), and even if it did it would not bring us any closer to an understanding of how circularization is accomplished. The model presented in the section on RF replication represents an attempt to fill this void. However, speculations of that sort are useful only if they suggest experiments. Perhaps the reader can think of one.

5.4. Viral Proteins Required for Single-Stranded DNA Synthesis

In the presence of moderate amounts of chloramphenicol, or in infections with phage coding for a defective gene A, B, C, D, F, or G protein, progeny single-stranded DNA synthesis does not occur (Lindqvist and Sinsheimer, 1967b; Funk and Sinsheimer, 1970b). The gene B product is required for the assembly of F and G proteins into a subviral particle (see Section 6.1) and it is probable that this complex is necessary for a significant rate of single-stranded DNA synthesis to take place. The gene D protein is also found as a major component of a precursor virus particle and it may be acting together with the gene F and G proteins to activate single-stranded DNA synthesis by packaging the progeny single-stranded DNA. Neither the gene B nor the gene D protein is found in the mature virion. Gene D protein resembles in some ways the DNA-binding gene V protein of the filamentous phages, but no evidence that it is a DNA-binding protein has been obtained (Burgess, 1969b).

As discussed in Section 5.1, one function of one or more of these proteins may be to block synthesis of a complementary strand. That cannot be the only function, however, because in infections with B, D, F, or G mutants one does not see the synthesis of RF at late times that would be expected if displaced single-stranded DNA were being converted to RF (Lindqvist and Sinsheimer, 1967b). Synthesis and simultaneous degradation of the displaced viral strand do not occur because a brief exposure to [^{3}H]thymidine during the time of single-stranded DNA synthesis does not yield asymmetrically labeled RF (Iwaya and Denhardt, 1971). Fukuda and Sinsheimer (1976b) were able to detect a small amount of labeling of the viral strand in RF at late times. This could represent a low level of abortive synthesis of single-stranded DNA or it could result from nick translation.

The gene C product appears to be required in small amounts for single-stranded DNA synthesis. Gene C (then called gene VI) was first identified by Tessman et al. (1967) in S13 as an ochre mutant (suHT205) capable of complementing the other known complementation groups. They showed that this mutant was able to replicate RF normally but was not able to synthesize single-stranded DNA. In later work, a polypeptide of molecular weight about 10,000 was identified as the product of gene C (Borras et al., 1971). Jeng and Hayashi (1970) described a temperature-sensitive mutant in this gene.

Funk and Sinsheimer (1970b) also identified the corresponding gene in ϕX174 as the result of a study of ochre mutants. These ochre mutations were induced by using [5-³H]cytosine decay to cause a C-T transition in the CAA codon, a codon that cannot give rise to amber or opal mutants in one step. It appears that there are no codons in the wild-type gene C that can be mutated to give an amber codon, or if there are the resulting amber mutants are too leaky to be picked up. The ochre mutants in gene C are leaky, and at late times (40 min) after infection a slow synthesis of infectious particles can be detected; to observe this synthesis, it is necessary to use a gene E mutant to prevent lysis of the cell. Both host DNA and RF replication are shut off at the normal time in gene C infections. During the residual synthesis that occurs at late times, much of the labeled RF sediments in neutral sucrose gradients in the RF I position, or even a little faster, and Funk and Sinsheimer (1970b) interpret these results to mean that in gene C mutants there is an accumulation of RF molecules containing single-stranded DNA tails. The leakiness of the gene C mutants, the result of occasional readthrough of the nonsense codon, suggests that very little gene C protein is needed in a normal infection. The gene C function may be involved in a late step of single-stranded DNA synthesis—perhaps involving maturation and packaging of the single-stranded DNA into the virion. Phage particles made under conditions where the gene C ochre mutation was suppressed with different suppressors had normal sensitivities to thermal inactivation, but it has not been proved that the gene C protein is not in the virion. The molecular weight determinations of the gene C protein and the smallest protein component in the virion are not accurate enough to permit the conclusion that they are different.

The gene A protein is also required for single-stranded DNA synthesis (Fujisawa and Hayashi, 1976b). As discussed in Section 5.1, evidence has been adduced that it may be required for proper termination of a round of replication and formation of a circular monomeric viral strand. Although it is plausible to imagine that the gene A protein cleaves a unique sequence in the viral strand at the beginning (to provide a 3´-OH primer) and at the end (to excise the progeny single-stranded DNA) of a round of replication (Henry and Knippers, 1974; Fujisawa and Hayashi, 1976b), it should be noted that this does not yield an RF molecule with a gap (Johnson and Sinsheimer, 1974; Denhardt et al., 1975). It is likely that the origin for single-stranded ϕX174 DNA synthesis is the same as for RF replication, i.e., in the region of gene A. There is disagreement on the location of the origin in G4 (Godson, 1975b; Ray and Dueber, 1975).

6. BIOGENESIS OF THE MATURE VIRION

6.1. Assembly of the Virus Particle

Formation of the ϕX174 particle is closely coupled to the synthesis of progeny single-stranded DNA. Thus no empty phage capsids have been observed in the cell in the absence of single-stranded DNA synthesis. Conversely, the rate of single-stranded DNA synthesis is severely reduced in circumstances where a subviral particle cannot be formed (Lindqvist and Sinsheimer, 1967b; Knippers and Sinsheimer, 1968b; Iwaya and Denhardt, 1971). Proteins that are essential for virus assembly include the products of genes B, D, F, and G.

Weisbeek and Sinsheimer (1974) have shown that the gene D protein is found in a fast-sedimenting 140 S intracellular particulate structure that also contains the F, G, and H proteins in their normal proportions. The gene D protein is made in large amounts in the cell and has been considered possibly to be analogous to the gene V protein of the filamentous phages, although there is no direct evidence in support of this possibility (Denhardt, 1975). The 140 S particle is labile and in the presence of Mg^{2+} ions is efficiently converted into a mature 114 S virion. Conversion in the reverse direction, from a 114 S to a 140 S structure, has not been observed. Approximately 14–20% of the protein content of the 140 S particle is gene D protein (this would be about 80 molecules). Upon conversion to the stable 114 S particle, the gene D protein is lost (or conceivably degraded to yield the small molecular weight proteins in the virion). In a portion of the population, the conversion is defective and "70 S" particles (Section 1.4.2) are formed.

It has been shown in Hayashi's laboratory that the F and G proteins each form a pentameric structure with S values of about 9 and 6, respectively (Tonegawa and Hayashi, 1970; Siden and Hayashi, 1974). In the presence, but not in the absence, of B protein these two pentamers associate to form a 12 S structure. There is no evidence that the B protein itself is part of the 12 S complex or the mature virion. This is interesting because earlier work had been interpreted as indicating that the B protein was part of the mature virion (Sinsheimer, 1968). Siden and Hayashi (1974) have speculated that the gene B protein may modify the F or G protein, e.g., by glycosylation or methylation, so that the FG complex can form.

I am not cognizant of any evidence suggesting that either the A protein or the C protein is involved in ϕX174 morphogenesis. There is evidence that one or two copies of the A* protein are present in the mature particle (Linney and Hayashi, 1974), but the function of this protein is unknown. Possibly it plays a role in circularization of the single-stranded DNA.

The function(s) of the gene H protein is (are) of interest for several reasons. As discussed in Section 5.2, the single methyl group is present in ϕX174 DNA in the gene H region. Also, it has been argued that the gene H protein functions in the initial stages of the infectious cycle by directing the single-stranded DNA to a replication complex (Section 2.3.3). In support of this idea is the association of the gene H protein with the RF after infection and the fact that certain gene H mutants will eclipse but not form parental RF. The importance of the H protein in the virus structure is evidenced by the degradation of the newly synthesized viral single-stranded DNA that occurs in the absence of functional gene H protein. Although single-stranded DNA synthesis occurs at almost a normal rate in gene H amber mutants, the DNA is incorporated into a defective particle and is partially degraded (Siegel and Hayashi, 1969; Iwaya and Denhardt, 1971). From the stoichiometry of the viral proteins (12 gene H proteins with 60 each of F and G proteins), one can surmise that each gene H protein interacts with one of the F + G pentamers.

The coupling between single-stranded DNA synthesis and phage morphogenesis makes for a very complex process, one that is easily perturbed. For example, at 15°C single-stranded DNA synthesis occurs, but is defective (Espejo and Sinsheimer, 1976b). Particles with an S value of 80–90 are produced that appear to contain the normal complement of proteins but only a fragment of DNA representing 20–90% of the genome; all regions of the genome are represented among the fragments derived from a population of particles.

6.2. Lysis of the Cell

In a normal infection, lysis of the cell commences shortly after the appearance of mature phage and well before the full potential of the infection has been realized. Thus any impediment to lysis will increase the yield of phage, provided of course that other steps are not interfered with. Agents that have been successfully used to retard lysis are spermine (Groman and Suzuki, 1966) and 0.2 M MgSO$_4$ (Gschwender and Hofschneider, 1969). Treatment of the cell with high concentrations of mitomycin prior to infection also blocks lysis (Fukuda and Sinsheimer, 1976).

A component with lytic activity against cell walls has not been identified in ϕX174 lysates despite several attempts, and why the cell lyses is not known. What little evidence is available is consistent with the idea that one of the virus-coded proteins—the gene E protein—interferes with cell wall biosynthesis in such a way that the cell wall is progressively weakened and eventually ruptures. Bradley *et al.* (1969) have described the sequence of events during lysis of cells by α3 as follows: First the plasma membrane retracts and indistinct intracellular particles become visible. The cell envelope then swells to form a spheroplast and further membrane retraction occurs. Normal intracellular viral particles become more evident and the cell wall breaks, curling back on the bulge of the spheroplast. Figure 21 shows an electron micrograph of a cell at this stage after infection (27 min). Finally the cell membrane breaks at the bulge and the cell contents are released. The remaining cell ghost gradually disintegrates into cell wall and plasma membrane fragments.

Various antibiotics, e.g., penicillin, seem to act in a similar manner, and with this analogy in mind Iwaya and I sought *E. coli* mutants resistant to ϕX174-induced lysis. In one series of experiments, we isolated *E. coli* mutants resistant to various antibiotics but were unable to demonstrate that any one of these antibiotic-resistant mutants was also refractory to lysis by ϕX174.

If lysis is indeed accomplished by interference with a specific reaction involved in cell wall biosynthesis, then one consequence will be that only exponentially multiplying cells will be lysed. This may explain why UV irradiation or treatment with mitomycin interferes with cell lysis. When cells approach stationary phase they lyse less readily, and concentrated cultures (greater than 5×10^8 cells/ml in usual media) are lysed very poorly. This trait is accentuated in a mutant called ϕXρ^- (Denhardt and Sinsheimer, 1965a). This mutation, whose position in the genetic map is unknown, causes the phage to be even less efficient at lysing cells, and consequently only very "healthy" cells in exponential growth are lysed. Plaques have turbid edges and are smaller than the larger, sharper-edged plaques produced by wild-type phage.

The relation between lysis and phage production actually seems to be more complex than has been manifest so far. Thus Hutchison and Sinsheimer (1966) found that not one of 17 *ts* mutants with altered lysis properties produced progeny phage at the restrictive temperature. A study of reversion rates suggested that one mutation was affecting both lysis and phage production. Tessman (1967) reported that certain temperature-sensitive mutations in genes F, G, and H delayed lysis. One reason for the apparent complexity of the lytic process may be its requirement for actively multiplying cells. In *su*$^-$ cells infected with the

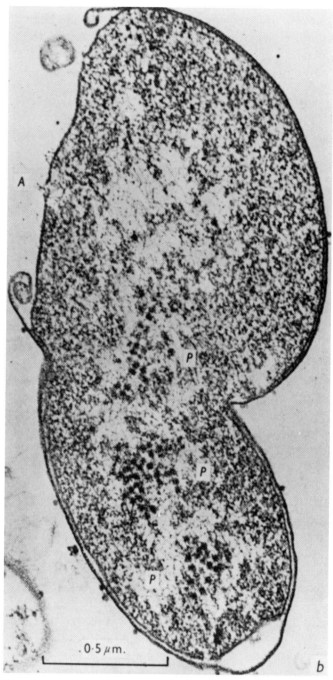

Fig. 21. Electron micrograph of a cell 27 min after infection with α3. The cell wall has broken and the membrane is beginning to disintegrate. There appears to be a small hole at A; P indicates clusters of stained intracellular phage particles. From Bradley *et al.* (1969), with permission.

φX*am*3 gene E mutant, the cells continue to enlarge and to make phage, but cell division is blocked, perhaps because host DNA replication is blocked.

7. RECOMBINATION

7.1. Structural Intermediates

The molecular events occurring during recombination have long been mysterious, and only recently have particular enzymatic functions been directly linked to the recombination process. The small size of the genome of the isometric phages and its dependence on host cell functions have attracted the attention of scientists interested in identifying molecular intermediates and gene functions involved in recombination.

One of the first candidates for an intermediate in recombination between RF molecules was the circular dimer (Rush and Warner, 1968), and evidence was presented that some of the circular dimers might be recombinant molecules. Benbow *et al.* (1972*a*) directly confirmed† that this was the case using the deletion mutant *del*E (Zuccarelli *et al.*, 1972; Kim *et al.*, 1972). The *del*E mutant (see Fig. 10) has suffered a deletion of some 7–9% of its genome in the region of gene E; it is thus unable to lyse cells but otherwise appears to go through a normal life cycle and to make normal, albeit less dense, phage particles. Because of the deletion in this phage DNA, it is possible to distinguish it from normal DNA (contour length of 1.53 μm vs. 1.69 μm). Also, when heteroduplex molecules are formed between wild-type DNA and *del*E DNA a deletion loop is formed. Using these two electron microscopic techniques, Benbow *et al.* (1972*a*) showed that although a few of the circular dimers were recombinant molecules the majority of them were not. Presumably the latter arose either by recombination between sister duplexes or during replication as the result of faulty termination. Most of the recombinant molecules were found instead to be catenated dimers, and as many as 50% of the 1:1 catenated dimers consisted of one normal-length and one *del*E molecule. Catenated dimers, circular dimers, and figure-8 molecules (see below) are illustrated in Fig. 22. Since the preparations of circular dimers analyzed by Rush and Warner (1968) contained catenated dimers, it is possible that many of the recombinant molecules they observed were catenated dimers.

---

† Benbow *et al.* (1972*a*) did not draw this conclusion from their data however (cf. Doniger *et al.*, 1973).

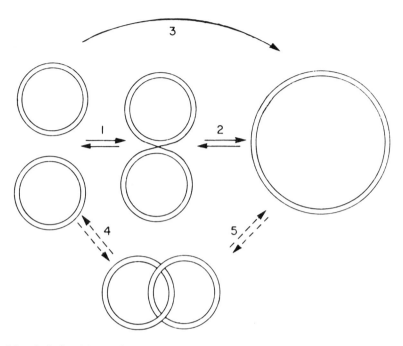

Fig. 22.   Relationship of the dimeric species of S13 RF DNA. The configuration of the figure-8 species is indicated diagrammatically in the center of the figure. Catenanes (two interlocked monomer duplexes, shown at the bottom) could arise either by faulty termination at the end of replication (4) or during the reduction of a circular dimer to two monomers (5). Circular dimers (far right) can also arise during replication (3) or breakdown of the figure-8 (2). The possibility that in some figure-8 molecules the two monomer single-stranded circles are catenated is not excluded. Reproduced from Thompson *et al.* (1975), with permission.

Doniger *et al.* (1973) investigated this question by fractionating the oligomeric molecules into circular dimer and catenated dimer populations and investigating the properties of each class separately. A four-factor cross between two S13 mutants each bearing both an amber and a temperature-sensitive mutation was performed. They found that both circular dimers and catenated dimers yielded about a threefold higher recombination frequency than did the monomer molecules. Further-more, they showed that the frequency of recombinants among dimer DNA molecules was reduced about tenfold in a *rec*A host, the same reduction as was obtained with monomer DNA. Most recombinant cir-cular dimers were heterozygous, because in single-burst experiments almost all of the recombinant circular dimers yielded more than one progeny type. (A homozygous recombinant dimer could, for example, be formed by atypical replication of a recombinant monomer and would not yield more than one recombinant progeny genotype.) The data also indicated that 18 of 21 bursts were composed of two or more nonreciprocal genotypes, a result that implies that more than one event can be involved in reducing the dimer to the monomer. This implies that the dimer usually replicates before reduction to the monomer occurs—a quite reasonable possibility. Although both the circular dimers and the catenated dimers can be intermediates in recombination, it does not follow that they often are. Hofs *et al.* (1972, 1973) presented evidence that both circular and catenated dimers could be formed either by replication or by recombination, and that they were rather stable, showing little tendency to decompose to monomers.

A more attractive intermediate in recombination, and probably also in the formation and breakdown of circular dimers and catenated dimers, is the figure-8. Figure-8 molecules were observed by Gordon *et al.* (1970), and their structures were clearly elucidated by Thompson *et al.* (1975). They consist, as had been expected, of two monomer-length strands and one dimer-length circular strand. All the strands are (or can be) covalently closed. Figure 23 shows electron micrographs of a figure-8 structure and of an α form that is produced when one double-strand scission is inserted into one of the duplex rings. These molecules were spread in the presence of ethidium bromide to stiffen and elongate them so that accidental overlays could be more easily distinguished. An important property of these fused dimers is that branch migration readily occurs at the junction; thus the breakdown of the figure-8 into monomers, perchance catenated, or a circular dimer, can occur at a location far from the initial point of interaction.

7.2. Gene Functions Involved

7.2.1. *recA*

In *recA* mutants, the amount of recombination (ϕX174 and S13) is reduced, but not to the same extent as host cell recombination, and from this result it was deduced that there was a secondary mechanism of recombination, independent of the *recA* function, that permitted about 10% as much recombination as the *recA* pathway (I. Tessman, 1966). The amount of recombination following this second pathway was a function of which genes were involved in the cross. In subsequent work, I. Tessman (1968) discovered that ultraviolet irradiation of the parental phage stimulated recombination 20–40 times in *recA*$^+$ hosts but not in *recA* hosts. Benbow *et al.* (1974*b*) confirmed this work and showed in addition that thymine starvation of the host had the same

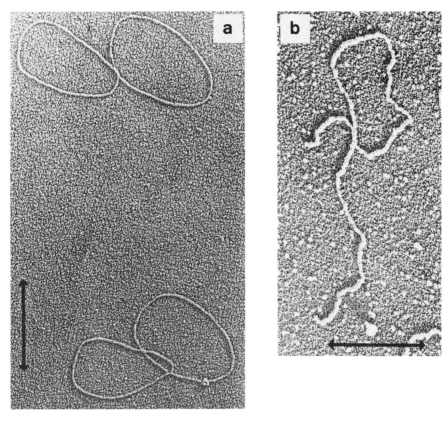

Fig. 23. Electron micrographs of figure-8 molecules (a) and of an α form (b) produced by introducing one double-strand scission into a figure-8 molecule. The molecules were spread in the presence of ethidium bromide. The arrows represent a length of 0.5 μm. Reproduced from Thompson *et al.* (1975), with permission.

effect. They inferred from these results that the single-strand breaks or gaps in RF molecules were substrates for *rec*A-mediated recombination. In *rec*A mutants, the proportions of the recombinant circular dimers (Doniger *et al.,* 1973) and of figure-8 molecules (Benbow *et al.,* 1975) were considerably reduced. Benbow *et al.* (1975) detected figure-8 formation in sonicates of *rec*A⁺ cells and suggested that this could be used as an assay for *rec*A⁺ gene function since in sonicates of *rec*A mutants the frequency of figure-8 formation was much less.

The *rec*A gene product seems to act especially often in the region of gene A. Benbow *et al.* (1974a) compared the genetic map of ϕX174 in a *rec*A⁺ host with that obtained in a *rec*A host and observed a "hot spot" for intragenic recombination in the gene A region under $recA^+$ conditions. A simple interpretation of this is that the $recA$ function both can stimulate recombination between intact duplexes at any point (by nicking?) and can make use of a preexisting nick or gap.

7.2.2. $recB$

$recB$ mutations alone have no effect on ϕX174 recombination; however, in the presence of a $recA$ mutation they reduce the residual recombination five- to tenfold (Benbow *et al.,* 1974a). $recB$ may be involved in the secondary mechanism of recombination, but this has not been shown directly.

7.2.3. Gene A

Baker *et al.* (1971) showed that the gene A function generally stimulated the secondary, but not the primary, mechanism of recombination. They observed that the absolute number of recombinants formed in a $recA$ host between gene A amber mutants was higher when the amber mutants were suppressed than when they were not. In the rec^+ host, roughly the same number of recombinants was observed regardless of whether gene A function, and hence RF replication, occurred. It was necessary to compare the number of recombinants per cell rather than recombination frequency because under nonpermissive conditions phage was made only in cells where recombination reconstituted a functional gene A protein. These results suggest that the primary mechanism of recombination acts as efficiently on the parental RF alone as it does on the parental plus progeny RF present during RF replication.

Benbow *et al.* (1975) have suggested that most $recA$-mediated recombination proceeds via two parental RF molecules bound to an "essential membrane site" (the cap in Fig. 24). This is unlikely because the membrane sites are probably artifacts (Section 4.8), and even if they are not it seems unlikely to me that two parental RF molecules associated with two "essential membrane sites" could form figure-8 molecules and undergo branch migration. The fact that recombination frequently involves the parental RF (the RF containing the parental viral strand) may reflect the large number of gaps present transiently in the complementary strand associated with it.

The primary $recA$-mediated recombination process is stimulated by UV irradiation of the parental viral strand. Since it is only the parental RF that contains the lesions, it is evident that the *rec*A gene product can use the parental RF as an efficient substrate. The presence of an active gene Λ allele also has an effect since in the presence of gene A function in *rec*⁺ cells there is an anomalously high intracistronic recombination frequency in the gene A region that is not reflected in the recombination frequency measured with outside markers (Benbow *et al.*, 1974a). This may be caused by the gap in the viral strand that is left specifically in the gene A region of one of the two products of RF replication. Since the other product has multiple gaps widely distributed about the genome, there would be no noticeable localized effect (Eisenberg *et al.*, 1975).

The secondary mechanism of recombination observed in the absence of the *rec*A function is increased by the presence of an active gene A product. Although it is not excluded that the gene A protein participates directly in this recombinational pathway, it seems more likely to me that the increased recombination detected in *rec*A hosts in the presence of active gene A function is the result of the production of progeny RF containing nicks and gaps. This could be tested by looking at the recombination frequency among the parental RF molecules present in the *rep* host in the presence and absence of gene A function.

Some recombination occurs in *rec*A hosts when gene A function is absent, but the mechanism by which these recombinants arise is not evident (Baker *et al.*, 1971).

7.3. Heteroduplex Repair and Single-Strand Aggression

In the past decade, it has become apparent that many of the puzzling events that occur during recombination (gene conversion, marker effects, nonreciprocal recombination, polarized recombination, and high negative interference) can be explained at least in part by heteroduplex repair. An illustration of the consequences of heteroduplex repair is seen in the model for recombination shown in Fig. 24. The essence of heteroduplex repair is the recognition of a mismatched base pair (or partially base-paired region) by one or more enzymes whose net effect is to excise one of the offending DNA strands and replace it with a strand perfectly complementary to its partner. There is good evidence for heteroduplex repair in a variety of systems, including, as we have discussed earlier, ϕX174.

Formation of heteroduplexes has been demonstrated in a variety of

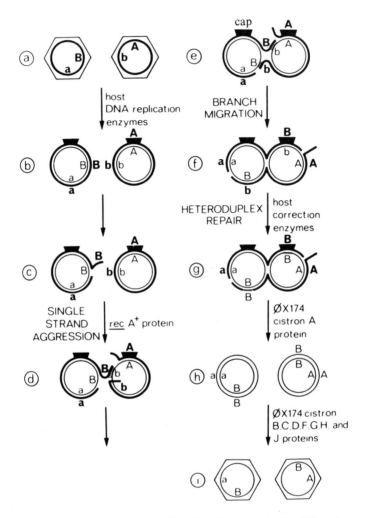

Fig. 24.   Role of the figure-8 in recombination. Two genetically different genomes (a) enter the cell and are converted to RF (b) at a hypothetical membrane site. A nick or gap in one of the molecules (c) initiates an interaction with the other molecule (d) to form a figure-8 structure (e). After branch migration (f) and heteroduplex repair (g), the figure-8 is reduced to two monomers (h), only one of which is recombinant (i). The jagged line indicates the repaired segment. Reproduced from Benbow *et al.* (1974c), with permission.

systems. The presence of a break in one of the strands of an intact duplex, or the presence of a free single-stranded end of a DNA molecule, is generally considered necessary to initiate heteroduplex formation. In the ϕX174/S13 system, nicks or gaps are known to be created both by gene A function alone and by the act of replication. It is likely that the *rec*A function participates in heteroduplex formation.

Benbow *et al.* (1975) have used the term "single-strand aggression" to characterize the phenomenon of heteroduplex formation initiated by a single-stranded end.

Once formation of a heteroduplex structure is initiated, it can rapidly expand over a longer region by strand exchange and branch migration. This migration of the junction occurs with little disruption of the base-stacking and hydrogen-bonding interactions in the duplex, provided that the two duplexes are essentially homologous. Regions of nonhomology, or the presence of a break in one of the DNA chains, will interrupt the process. In the figure-8 molecules formed between wild-type ϕX174 and the ϕX174 *del*E mutant, branch migration would be impaired at the boundary of the deleted region, and this may explain the high frequency of catenated recombinant dimers observed by Benbow *et al.* (1972*a*). In the absence of a break in one of the duplexes, a nuclease will have to act on the figure-8 molecule to permit regeneration of the component monomeric molecules.

The products of this process at this point (Fig. 24f) are symmetrical and complementary, and, if reduction to the monomers and replication followed immediately, equal proportions of parental and reciprocally recombinant duplexes would result. If on the other hand mismatched regions were recognized and eliminated prior to replication, then one or the other of the complementary recombinant or parental genotypes would be lost. The products of this single recombination event would then be asymmetrical and nonreciprocal. The precise outcome would depend on the specific mismatches involved and the capriciousness of the process.

In the specific case of recombination among the isometric phages, the observed products of recombination are (usually) the single-stranded DNA molecules found in progeny virions, and these are separated from the initial recombination event by single-stranded DNA synthesis and perhaps RF replication. If there is any selectivity at either of these two stages as to which RF molecule will be used, then the interpretation will be correspondingly complicated. Thus by judicious invoking of asymmetrical replication and heteroduplex repair it is a simple matter to account for the variety and complexity of recombinant genotypes observed to emanate from recombinational events. But how valid this account is remains to be seen.

NOTE ADDED IN PROOF

Barrell, Air, and Hutchison (1976) have sequenced the gene D region of ϕX174 DNA and have made the startling discovery that it also contains gene E. The nucleotide sequence coding for the last 60% of gene D is also used to code for gene E, but is read in a different phase. There is also a region between genes D/E and F that codes for the small protein found in the virion. The gene that codes for this protein was called (Benbow *et al.*, 1972*b*) gene J on the basis of the properties of the *am*6 mutation, which, however, is not in gene J. Thus Figure 2 should be revised so that gene E is within gene D and so that gene J is inserted between gene D/E and gene F. The molecular weight of the as yet unidentified gene E protein would appear to be around 10,000. The "*del*E" mutants (Zuccarelli *et al.*, 1972; Kim *et al.*, 1972) appear to have been erroneously identified; it is possible that they were simply a mixture of a variety of nonviable deletions maintained as defective phages by passage at high multiplicities of infection.

Fiddes (1976) identified a 111 nucleotide-long intercistronic space between genes F and G and determined its nucleotide sequence. It contained a region of hyphenated two-fold symmetry capable of forming a hairpin loop. The pyrimidine tracts present in this loop were similar to those characterized by Bartok *et al.* (1975) and it was speculated that this loop was one of the major hairpin loops resistant to the *Neurospora crassa* nuclease.

Jeppesen *et al.* (1976) have performed *in vitro* pulse-chase experiments using DNA polymerase I and specific restriction enzyme fragment primers to determine the order of restriction enzyme fragments. The ϕX174 cleavage maps produced by *Hae*II (RGCGCY, 8 fragments), *Hind*II (GTYRAC, 13 fragments), *Hha*I (GCGC, 16 fragments), *Alu*I (AGCT, 23 fragments), *Hap*II (CCGG, 5 fragments), *Hin*fI (GAXTC, 20 fragments), and *Hae*III (GGCC, 11 fragments) were reported. In general there was good agreement with previous maps. They also (cf. Grosveld *et al.*, 1976) noted a positioning of the *Hae*III6 fragments different from Lee and Sinsheimer (1974*a*), and their order of *Hap*II fragments 4 and 5 differed from the order reported by Hayashi and Hayashi (1974). Brown and Smith (1976) have located the unique *Pst* cleavage site in ϕX174 RF near the B/C junction, probably in gene B.

Farber (1976) has extensively purified the ϕX174 gene D protein. It appears to exist normally as a tetramer of molecular weight of about 61,000 and it does not bind to single-stranded DNA. Pollock (1976) was unable to confirm the report of Clements and Sinsheimer (1974) that an amber mutation in gene D reduced the amount of phage-specific mRNA made.

Axelrod (1976*a,b*) has identified three promoters used *in vitro* when ϕX174 RF I is transcribed by *E. coli* RNA polymerase. By employing specific short oligonucleotide primers she was able to initiate transcription selectively at any one of the three promoters. Transcripts starting with A were initiated near the H/A boundary and the A/B boundary. Part of the initiation sequence of the two A start promoters was inferred. The third promoter signaled an RNA transcript starting with G around the C/D boundary. These results accord well with those of Smith and Sinsheimer (1976*a,b,c*). Two rho-independent termination sites were identified, the strongest of which mapped near the H/A boundary. Two rho-dependent termination sites were also identified. Further research is necessary to determine whether the promoters and terminators identified *in vitro* are used *in vivo* and whether the RNA transcripts synthesized using the different promoters and coding for different proteins are equally stable. Kapitza *et al.* (1976) observed that there was a small reduction in the size distribution of ϕX174 RNA molecules synthesized *in vitro* when exposed to RNase III, and they suggested that RNase III participates in the processing of ϕX174 mRNA *in vivo*.

Fukuda and Sinsheimer (1976*a*) studied the structure of pulse-labeled ϕX174 replicating intermediates during RF replication after fractionating the replicating intermediates by CsCl density gradient centrifugation in the presence of propidium diiodide. The viral strand in newly replicated RF II was found as a full-length molecule whereas the complementary strand was present in fragments (see also Eisenberg *et al.*, 1975). They observed pulse-labeled RF molecules that banded at a heavy density in a dye-CsCl density gradient yet were not covalently closed (see also Espejo and Sinsheimer, 1976*a*).

Funk and Snover (1976) found, as did Martin and Godson (1975)—see Table 7—that certain (but not all) gene A mutants failed to terminate host DNA synthesis at later stages of infection. The inability of the host DNA to continue to be replicated did not seem to result from extensive nucleolytic breakdown of the DNA, although one gene A mutant was reported to cause breakdown of the host DNA.

Borrias *et al.* (1976*a*) described a method to produce mutations in selected regions of the genome by mutagenizing specific restriction enzyme fragments, annealing the mutated DNA with a complete viral strand DNA of appropriate genotype and then infecting spheroplasts. Borrias *et al.* (1976*b*) also reported that certain mutants (eg., *to*8, see Figure 2) that map in gene A allowed RF replication but not progeny single-stranded DNA synthesis. These amber mutants mapped in the center of the A gene and were capable of complementing other gene A mutants but not gene B mutants (compare I. Tessman *et al.*, 1976). It appears that gene Bn is contained at least in part within Gene A.

E. Tessman and Peterson (1976) similarly have found a class of *rep* mutations (*gro*L⁻ mutations) that permit RF replication but not progeny single-stranded DNA synthesis. In contrast to the original *rep* mutant, ϕX174 mutants (called *ogr* mutants) can be found that will grow on these *gro*L⁻ strains. The *ogr* mutations were cis-dominant and appeared to map in gene F; it was speculated that a specific complex between the *rep* protein and the genes A and F proteins was involved in progeny single-stranded DNA synthesis and phage maturation.

Studies on *in vitro* ϕX174 DNA synthesis continue unabated. Wickner and Hurwitz (1976) discovered that the *dnaZ* gene product is involved in DNA synthesis on primed single-stranded DNA catalyzed by either DNA polymerase II or III. It was present together with another protein in elongation factor II preparations Eisenberg *et al.* (1976) and Sumida-Yasumoto *et al.* (1976) have reported preliminary studies on the replication of ϕX174 RF *in vitro*. The replication was inhibited by nalidixic acid and novobiocin and required both the ϕX174 gene A protein and the *E. coli rep* protein. Superhelical ϕX174 RF I was one of the products of the *in vitro* replication. Ikeda *et al.* (1976) purified the ϕX174 gene A protein using a complementation assay and obtained evidence that it interacted specifically with superhelical ϕX174 RF I in the region of gene A in the *Hin*dII3 fragment. It appeared to have nucleolytic activity against both superhelical RF and single-stranded viral DNA, but not relaxed RF I (cf. Singh and Ray, 1975, and Henry and Knippers, 1974). Eisenberg (personal communication) has purified the *rep* protein, shown it to be functionally active, and determined its molecular weight to be about 68,000 in SDS polyacrylamide gels. It appears to cause duplex DNA to unwind.

ACKNOWLEDGMENTS

The research performed by myself and my associates over the past dozen years, part of which is summarized in this chapter, has been supported (in the United States) by the National Science Foundation, the United States Public Health Service, and the American Cancer Society and (in Canada) by the Medical Research Council, the National Cancer Institute, and the Conseil de la Recherche Médicale du Québec. We are grateful for this support. I thank Pieter Baas, Larry Dumas, Nigel Godson, Masaki Hayashi, Hank Jansz, Arthur Kornberg, Dan Ray, Fred Sanger, Robert Sinsheimer, John Spencer, Ethel Tessman, Irwin Tessman, Robert Warner, and Peter Weisbeek for the information they provided for this review.

8. REFERENCES

Air, G. M., Blackburn, E. H., Sanger, F., and Coulson, A. R., 1975, The nucleotide and amino acid sequences of the N (5′) terminal region of gene G of bacteriophage φX174, *J. Mol. Biol.* **96**:703.

Axelrod, N., 1976a, *In vitro* transcription of φX174: Selective initiation with oligonucleotides, *J. Mol. Biol.* (in press).

Axelrod, N., 1976b, *In vitro* transcription of φX174: Analysis with restriction enzymes, *J. Mol. Biol.* (in press).

Baas, P. D., and Jansz, H. S., 1972a, Asymmetric information transfer during φX174 DNA replication, *J. Mol. Biol.* **63**:557.

Baas, P. D., and Jansz, H. S., 1972b, φX174 replicative form DNA replication, origin and direction, *J. Mol. Biol.* **63**:569.

Baas, P. D., Jansz, H. S., and Sinsheimer, R. L., 1976, φX174 DNA synthesis in a replication-deficient host: Determination of the origin of φX DNA replication, *J. Mol. Biol.* **102**:633.

Bachmann, B. J., Low, K. B., and Taylor, A. L., 1976, Recalibrated linkage map of *Escherichia coli* K-12, *Bacteriol. Rev.* **40**:116.

Bachrach, U., Fischer, R., and Klein, I., 1975, Occurrence of polyamines in coliphages T5, φX174, and in phage-infected bacteria, *J. Gen. Virol.* **26**:287.

Baker, R., and Tessman, I., 1967, The circular genetic map of phage S13, *Proc. Natl. Acad. Sci. U.S.A.* **58**:1438.

Baker, R., and Tessman, I., 1968, Heat stability of mutants in genes II, IIIa and VI of phage S13, *Virology* **35**:179.

Baker, R., Doniger, J., and Tessman, I., 1971, Roles of parental and progeny DNA in two mechanisms of phage S13 recombination, *Nature (London) New Biol.* **230**:23.

Barrell, D. G., Air, G. M., and Hutchison, C. A., 1976, Overlapping genes in bacteriophage φX174, *Nature* **264**:34.

Bartok, K., and Denhardt, D. T., 1976, Site of cleavage of superhelical φX174 replicative form DNA by the single-strand specific *N. crassa* nuclease, *J. Biol. Chem.* **251**:530.

Bartok, K., Harbers, B., and Denhardt, D. T., 1975, Isolation and characterization of self-complementary sequences from φX174 viral DNA, *J. Mol. Biol.* **99**:93.

Bauer, W., and Vinograd, J., 1968, The interaction of closed circular DNA with intercalative dyes. I. The superhelix density of SV40 DNA in the presence and absence of dye, *J. Mol. Biol.* **33**:141.

Bayer, M. E., and DeBlois, R. W., 1974, Diffusion constant and dimension of bacteriophage φX174 as determined by self-beat laser light spectroscopy and electron microscopy, *J. Virol.* **14**:975.

Bayer, M. E., and Starkey, T. W., 1972, The adsorption of bacteriophage φX174 and its interactions with *E. coli*; a kinetic and morphological study, *Virology* **49**:236.

Benbow, R. M., Hutchison, C. A., III, Fabricant, J. D., and Sinsheimer, R. L., 1971, Genetic map of bacteriophage φX174, *J. Virol.* **7**:549.

Benbow, R. M., Eisenberg, M., and Sinsheimer, R. L., 1972a, Multiple length DNA molecules of bacteriophage φX174, *Nature (London)* **237**:141.

Benbow, R. M., Mayol, R. F., Picchi, J. C., and Sinsheimer, R. L., 1972b, Direction of translation and size of bacteriophage φX174 cistrons, *J. Virol.* **10**:99.

Benbow, R. M., Zuccarelli, A. J., Davis, G. C., and Sinsheimer, R. L., 1974a, Genetic recombination in bacteriophage ϕX174, *J. Virol.* **13**:898.

Benbow, R. M., Zuccarelli, A. J., and Sinsheimer, R. L., 1974b, A role for single strand breaks in bacteriophage ϕX174 genetic recombination, *J. Mol. Biol.* **88**:629.

Benbow, R. M., Zuccarelli, A. J., Shafer, A. J., and Sinsheimer, R. L. 1974c, Exchange of parental DNA during genetic recombination in bacteriophage ϕX174, in:*Mechanisms in Recombination* (R. F. Grell, ed.), pp. 3–18, Plenum, New York.

Benbow, R. M., Zuccarelli, A. J., and Sinsheimer, R. L., 1975, Recombinant DNA molecules of bacteriophage ϕX174, *Proc. Natl. Acad. Sci. USA* **72**:235.

Berkowitz, S. A., and Day, L. A., 1974, Molecular weight of single-stranded bacteriophage fd DNA: High speed equilibrium sedimentation and light scattering measurements, *Biochemistry* **13**:4825.

Beswick, F. M., and Lunt, M. R., 1972, Adsorption of bacteriophage ϕX174 to isolated bacterial cell walls, *J. Gen. Virol.* **16**:381.

Blakesley, R. W., and Wells, R. D., 1975, "Single-stranded" DNA from ϕX174 and M13 is cleaved by certain restriction endonucleases, *Nature (London)* **257**:421.

Bleichrodt, J. F., and Berends-van Abkoude, E. R., 1968, Bacteriophage related to ϕX174 showing a transition between two forms with different heat sensitivity and adsorption characteristics, *Virology* **34**:366.

Bleichrodt, J. F., and Knijnenburg, C. M., 1969, On the origin of the 70 S component of bacteriophage ϕX174, *Virology* **37**:132.

Bleichrodt, J. F., and van Abkoude, E. R., 1967, The transition between the two forms of bacteriophage ϕX174 differing in heat sensitivity and adsorption characteristics, *Virology* **32**:93.

Bleichrodt, J. F., Blok, J., and Berends-van Abkoude, E. R., 1968, Thermal inactivation of bacteriophage ϕX174 and two of its mutants, *Virology* **36**:343.

Bone, D. R., and Dowell, C. E., 1973a, A mutant of bacteriophage ϕX174 which infects *E. coli* K12 strains, *Virology* **52**:319.

Bone, D. R., and Dowell, C. E., 1973b, A mutant of bacteriophage ϕX174 which infects *E. coli* K12 strains, II. Replication of ϕXtB in *ts* DNA strains, *Virology* **52**:330.

Borras, M.-T., Vanderbilt, A. S., and Tessman, E. S., 1971, Identification of the acrylamide gel protein peak for gene C of phages S13 and ϕX, *Virology* **45**:802.

Borrias, W. E., van de Pol, J. H., van de Vate, C., and van Arkel, G. A., 1969, Complementation experiments between conditional lethal mutants of bacteriophage ϕX174, *Mol. Gen. Genet.* **105**:152.

Borrias, W. E., Weisbeek, P. J., and van Arkel, G. A., 1976a, An intracistronic region of gene A of bacteriophage ϕX174 r.ot involved in progeny RF DNA synthesis, *Nature* **261**:245.

Borrias, W. E., Wilschut, I. J. C., Vereijken, J. M., Weisbeek, P. J., and van Arkel, G. A., 1976b, Induction and isolation of mutants in a specific region of gene A of bacteriophage ϕX174, *Virology* **70**:195.

Bouché, J.-P., Zechel, K., and Kornberg, A., 1975, *dnaG* gene product, a rifampicin-resistant RNA polymerase, initiates the conversion of a single-stranded coliphage DNA to its duplex replicative form, *J. Biol. Chem.* **250**:5995.

Bouvier, F., and Zinder, N. D., 1974, Effects of the *dnaA* thermosensitive mutation of *E. coli* on bacteriophage f1 growth and DNA synthesis, *Virology* **60**:139.

Bowes, J. M., 1974, Replication of bacteriophage St-1 in *E. coli* strain temperature-sensitive in DNA synthesis, *J. Virol.* **13**:1400.

Bowes, J. M., and Dowell, C. E., 1974, Purification and some properties of bacteriophage St-1, *J. Virol.* **13**:53.

Bowman, K. L., and Ray, D. S., 1975, Degradation of the viral strand of φX174 parental replicative form DNA in a *Rep⁻* host, *J. Virol.* **16**:838.

Bradley, D. E., 1970, A comparative study of some properties of the φX174 type bacteriophage, *Can. J. Microbiol.* **16**:965.

Bradley, D. E., Dewar, C. A., and Robertson, D., 1969, Structural changes in *E. coli* infected with a φX174 type bacteriophage, *J. Gen. Virol.* **5**:113.

Brown, D. T., Mackenzie, J. M., and Bayer, M. E., 1971, Mode of host cell penetration by bacteriophage φX174, *J. Virol.* **7**:836.

Brown, N. L., and Smith, M., 1976, The mapping and sequence determination of the single site in φX174*am*3 replicative form DNA cleaved by restriction endonuclease *Pst*I, *FEBS Lett.* **65**:284.

Brutlag, D., Schekman, R., and Kornberg, A., 1971, A possible role for RNA polymerases in the initiation of M13 DNA synthesis, *Proc. Natl. Acad. Sci. USA* **68**:2826.

Bryan, R. N., and Hayashi, M., 1970, Initiation of φX174 RF-primed protein with *N*-formylmethionine, *Biochemistry* **9**:1904.

Bryan, R. N., Sugiura, M., and Hayashi, M., 1969, DNA-dependent RNA-directed protein synthesis *in vitro*. I. Extent of genome transcription, *Proc. Natl. Acad. Sci. USA* **62**:483.

Burgess, A. B., 1969*a*, Studies on the proteins of φX174. II. The protein composition of the φX coat, *Proc. Natl. Acad. Sci. USA* **64**:613.

Burgess, A. B., 1969*b*, The proteins of bacteriophage φX174, Ph.D. thesis, Harvard University.

Burgess, A. B., and Denhardt, D. T., 1969, Studies on φX174 proteins. I. Phage-specific proteins synthesized after infection of *E. coli, J. Mol. Biol.* **45**:377.

Burnet, F. M., 1927, The relationship between heat-stable agglutinogens and sensitivity to bacteriophage in the *Salmonella* group, *Br. J. Exp. Pathol.* **8**:121.

Burton, A. J., and Yagi, S., 1968, Intracellular development of bacteriophage φR. I. Host modification of the replicative process, *J. Mol. Biol.* **34**:481.

Calendar, R., Lindqvist, B., Sironi, G., and Clark, A. J., 1970, Characterization of REP⁻ mutants and their interaction with P2 phage, *Virology* **40**:72.

Campbell, A. M., and Jolly, D. J., 1973, Light-scattering studies on supercoil unwinding, *Biochem. J.* **133**:209.

Caspar, D. L. D., and Klug, A., 1962, Physical principles in the construction of regular viruses, *Cold Spring Harbor Symp. Quant. Biol.* **27**:1.

Cerny, R. E., Cerna, E., and Spencer, J. H., 1969, Nucleotide clusters in DNA. IV. Pyrimidine oligonucleotides of bacteriophage S13suN15 DNA and RF, *J. Mol. Biol.* **46**:145.

Chen, C.-Y., Hutchison, C. A., III, and Edgell, M. H., 1973, Isolation and genetic localization of three φX174 promoter regions, *Nature (London) New Biol.* **243**:233.

Clements, J. B., and Sinsheimer, R. L., 1974, Class of φX174 mutants relatively deficient in synthesis of viral RNA, *J. Virol.* **14**:1630.

Clements, J. B., and Sinsheimer, R. L., 1975, Process of infection with bacteriophage φX174. XXXVII. RNA metabolism in φX174-infected cells, *J. Virol.* **15**:151.

Daems, W. T., Eigner, J., van der Sluys, I., and Cohen, J. A., 1962, The fine structure of the 114 S and 70 S components of bacteriophage φX174 as revealed by negative and positive staining methods, *Biochim. Biophys. Acta* **55**:801.

Dalgarno, L., and Sinsheimer, R. L., 1968, Process of infection with bacteriophage φX174. XXIV. New type of temperature-sensitive mutant, *J. Virol.* **2**:822.

Darby, G., Dumas, L. B., and Sinsheimer, R. L., 1970, The structure of the DNA of bacteriophage φX174. VI. Pyrimidine sequences in the complementary strand of the replicative form, *J. Mol. Biol.* **52**:227.

Datta, B., and Poddar, R. K., 1970, Greater vulnerability of the infecting viral strand of replicative form DNA of bacteriophage φX174, *J. Virol.* **6**:583.

Delaney, A. D., and Spencer, J. H., 1976, Nucleotide clusters in deoxyribonucleic acids. XIII. Sequence analysis of the longer unique pyrimidine oligonucleotides of bacteriophage S13 DNA by a method using unlabeled starting oligonucleotides, *Biochim. Biophys. Acta* **435**:269.

Denhardt, D. T., 1972, A theory of DNA replication, *J. Theor. Biol.* **34**:487.

Denhardt, D. T., 1975, The single-stranded DNA phages, *CRC Crit. Rev. Microbiol.* **4**:161.

Denhardt, D. T., and Kato, A. C., 1973, Comparison of the effect of ultraviolet radiation and ethidium bromide intercalation on the conformation of superhelical φX174 replicative form DNA, *J. Mol. Biol.* **77**:479.

Denhardt, D. T., and Marvin, D. A., 1969, Altered coding in single-stranded DNA viruses? *Nature (London)* **221**:769.

Denhardt, D. T., and Silver, R. B., 1966, An analysis of the clone size distribution of φX174 mutants and recombinants, *Virology* **30**:10.

Denhardt, D. T., and Sinsheimer, R. L., 1965a, The process of infection with bacteriophage φX174. III. Phage maturation and lysis after synchronized infection, *J. Mol. Biol.* **12**:641.

Denhardt, D. T., and Sinsheimer, R. L., 1965b, The process of infection with bacteriophage φX174. V. Inactivation of the phage–bacterium complex by decay of ^{32}P incorporated in the infecting particle, *J. Mol. Biol.* **62**:663.

Denhardt, D. T., Dressler, D. H., and Hathaway, A., 1967, The abortive replication of φX174 DNA in a recombination-deficient mutant of *E. coli, Proc. Natl. Acad. Sci. USA* **57**:813.

Denhardt, D. T., Iwaya, M., and Larison, L. L., 1972, The *rep* mutation. II. Its effect on *E. coli* and on the replication of bacteriophage φX174, *Virology* **49**:486.

Denhardt, D. T., Iwaya, M., McFadden, G., and Schochetman, G., 1973, The mechanism of replication of φX174 single-stranded DNA. VI. Requirements for ribonucleoside triphosphates and DNA polymerase III, *Can. J. Biochem.* **51**:1588.

Denhardt, D. T., Eisenberg, S., Harbers, B., Lane, H. E. D., and McFadden, G., 1975, Replication of φX174 in *E. coli*: Structure of the replicating intermediate and the effect of mutations in the host *lig* and *rep* genes, in: *DNA Synthesis and Its Regulation* (M. Goulian and P. Hanawalt, eds.), ICN-UCLA Squaw Valley Symposium, Benjamin, Menlo Park, Calif.

Denhardt, D. T., Eisenberg, S., Bartok, K., and Carter, B. J., 1976, Multiple structures of adeno-associated virus DNA: Analysis of terminally-labeled molecules with endonuclease R.*Hae*III, *J. Virol.* **18**:672.

Derstine, P. L., and Dumas, L. B., 1976, Replication of φX174 in a temperature-sensitive *dna*H mutant of *E. coli* C, *J. Bacteriol.* (in press).

Doniger, J., and Tessman, I., 1969, An S13 capsid mutant that makes no replicative form DNA, *Virology* **39**:389.

Doniger, J., Warner, R. C., and Tessman, I., 1973, Role of circular dimer DNA in the primary recombination mechanism of bacteriophage S13, *Nature (London) New Biol.* **242**:9.

Dowell, C. E., 1967, Cold-sensitive mutants of bacteriophage φX174. I. A mutant blocked in the eclipse function at low temperature, *Proc. Natl. Acad. Sci. USA* **58**:958.

Dressler, D., 1970, The rolling circle for φX DNA replication. II. Synthesis of single-stranded circles, *Proc. Natl. Acad. Sci. USA* **67**:1934.

Dressler, D. H., and Denhardt, D. T., 1968, On the mechanism of φX single-stranded DNA synthesis, *Nature (London)* **219**:346.

Dressler, D., and Wolfson, J., 1970, The rolling circle for φX DNA replication. III. Synthesis of supercoiled duplex rings, *Proc. Natl. Acad. Sci. USA* **67**:456.

Dumas, L. B., and Miller, C. A., 1973, Replication of bacteriophage φX174 DNA in a temperature-sensitive *dna*E mutant of *E. coli* C, *J. Virol.* **11**:848.

Dumas, L. B., and Miller, C. A., 1974, Inhibition of bacteriophage φX174 DNA replication in *dna*B mutants of *E. coli* C, *J. Virol.* **14**:1369.

Dumas, L. B., and Miller, C. A., 1976, Bacteriophage φX174 single-stranded viral DNA synthesis in temperature-sensitive *dna*B and *dna*C mutants of *E. coli*, *J. Virol.* **18**:426.

Dumas, L. B., Miller, C. A., and Bayne, M. L., 1975, Rifampicin inhibition of bacteriophage φX174 parental replicative form DNA synthesis in an *E. coli dna*C mutant, *J. Virol.* **16**:575.

Edgell, M. H., Hutchison, C. A., III, and Sinsheimer, R. L., 1969, The process of infection with bacteriophage φX174. XXVIII. Removal of the spike proteins from the phage capsid, *J. Mol. Biol.* **42**:547.

Edgell, M. H., Hutchison, C. A., III, and Sclair, M., 1972, Specific endonuclease R fragments of bacteriophage φX174 DNA, *J. Virol.* **8**:574.

Eisenberg, S., and Denhardt, D. T., 1974a, Structure of nascent φX174 replicative form: Evidence for discontinuous DNA replication, *Proc. Natl. Acad. Sci. USA* **71**:984.

Eisenberg, S., and Denhardt, D. T., 1974b, The mechanism of replication of φX174 single-stranded DNA. X. Distribution of the gaps in nascent RF DNA, *Biochem. Biophys. Res. Commun.* **61**:532.

Eisenberg, S., Harbers, B., Hours, C., and Denhardt, D. T., 1975, The mechanism of replication of φX174 DNA. XII. Non-random location of gaps in nascent φX174 RF II DNA, *J. Mol. Biol.* **99**:107.

Eisenberg, S., Scott, J. F., and Kornberg, A., 1976, An enzyme system for replication of duplex circular DNA: The replicative form of phage φX174, *Proc. Natl. Acad. Sci. USA* **73**:1594.

Espejo, R. T., and Sinsheimer, R. L., 1976a, The process of infection with bacteriophage φX174. XXXIX. The structure of a DNA form with restricted binding of intercalative dyes observed during synthesis of φX174 single-stranded DNA, *J. Mol. Biol.* **102**:723.

Espejo, R. T., and Sinsheimer, R. L., 1976b, Process of infection with bacteriophage φX174. XLI. Synthesis of defective φX174 particles at 15 C, *J. Virol.* **19**:732.

Farber, M. B., 1976, Purification and properties of bacteriophage φX174, *J. Virol.* **17**:1027.

Fidanian, H. M., and Ray, D. S., 1974, Replication of bacteriophage M13. VIII. Differential effects of rifampicin and nalidixic acid on the synthesis of the two strands of M13 duplex DNA, *J. Mol. Biol.* **83**:63.

Fiddes, J. C., 1976, Nucleotide sequence of the intercistronic region between genes G and F in bacteriophage φX174 DNA, *J. Mol. Biol.* **107**:1.

Francke, B., and Ray, D. S., 1971, Formation of the parental replicative form DNA of bacteriophage φX174 and initial events in its replication, *J. Mol. Biol.* **61**:565.

Francke, B., and Ray, D. S., 1972, *Cis*-limited action of the gene A product of bacteriophage φX174 and the essential bacterial site, *Proc. Natl. Acad. Sci. USA* **69**:475.

Fujisawa, H., and Hayashi, M., 1976*a*, Viral DNA-synthesizing intermediate complex isolated during assembly of bacteriophage φX174, *J. Virol.* **19**:409.

Fujisawa, H., and Hayashi, M., 1976*b*, Gene A product of φX174 is required for site-specific endonucleolytic cleavage during single-stranded DNA synthesis *in vivo*, *J. Virol.* **19**:416.

Fukuda, A., and Sinsheimer, R. L., 1976*a*, Process of infection with bacteriophage φX174. XXXVIII. Replication of φX174, replicative form *in vivo*, *J. Virol.* **17**:776.

Fukuda, A., and Sinsheimer, R. L., 1976*b*, The process of infection with bacteriophage φX174. XL. Viral DNA replication of φX174 mutants blocked in progeny single-stranded DNA synthesis, *J. Virol.* **18**:218.

Funk, F., and Sinsheimer, R. L., 1970*a*, Process of infection with bacteriophage φX174. XXXIII. Templates for the synthesis of single-stranded DNA, *J. Virol.* **5**:282.

Funk, F., and Sinsheimer, R. L., 1970*b*, Process of infection with bacteriophage φX174, XXXV. Cistron VIII, *J. Virol.* **6**:12.

Funk, F. D., and Snover, D., 1976, Pleiotropic effects of mutants in gene A of bacteriophage φX174, *J. Virol.* **18**:141.

Gefter, M. L., 1975, DNA replication, *Annu. Rev. Biochem.* **44**:45.

Geider, K., Lechner, H., and Hoffmann-Berling, H., 1972, Nucleotide-permeable *E. coli* cells. V. Structure of newly synthesized φX174 RF DNA, *J. Mol. Biol.* **69**:333.

Gelfand, D. H., and Hayashi, M., 1969, Electrophoretic characterization of φX174-specific proteins, *J. Mol. Biol.* **44**:501.

Gelfand, D. H., and Hayashi, M., 1970, DNA-dependent RNA-directed protein synthesis *in vitro*. IV. Peptide analysis of an *in vitro* and *in vivo* φX174 structural protein, *Proc. Natl. Acad. Sci. USA* **67**:13.

Gilbert, W., and Dressler, D., 1968, DNA replication: The rolling circle model, *Cold Spring Harbor Symp. Quant. Biol.* **33**:473.

Godson, G. N., 1971*a*, Characterization and synthesis of φX174 proteins in ultraviolet-irradiated and unirradiated cells, *J. Mol. Biol.* **57**:541.

Godson, G. N., 1971*b*, φX174 gene expression in u.v.-irradiated cells treated with chloramphenicol, *Virology* **45**:788.

Godson, G. N., 1973, DNA heteroduplex analysis of the relation between bacteriophage φX174 and S13, *J. Mol. Biol.* **77**:467.

Godson, G. N., 1974*a*, Origin and direction of φX174 double- and single-stranded DNA synthesis, *J. Mol. Biol.* **90**:127.

Godson, G. N., 1974*b*, Evolution of φX174: Isolation of four new φX-like phages and comparison with φX174, *Virology* **58**:272.

Godson, G. N., 1975*a*, Evolution of φX174. II. A cleavage map of the G4 phage genome and comparison with the cleavage map of φX174, *Virology* **63**:320.

Godson, G. N., 1975*b*, A physical map of G4 and the origin of G4 double- and single-stranded DNA replication, in: *DNA Synthesis and Its Regulation* (M. Goulian and P. Hanawalt, ed.), Benjamin, Menlo Park, Calif.

Godson, G. N., and Boyer, H., 1974, Susceptibility of the ϕX-like phages G4 and G14 to *Eco*R1 endonuclease, *Virology* **62**:270.

Godson, G. N., and Roberts, R. J., 1976, A catalogue of cleavages of ϕX174, S13, G4, and St-1 by 26 different restriction enzymes, *Virology* **73**:561.

Gordon, C. N., Rush, M. G., and Warner, R. C., 1970, Complex replicative form molecules of bacteriophage ϕX174 and S13su105, *J. Mol. Biol.* **47**:495.

Goulian, M., 1968, Incorporation of oligonucleotides into DNA, *Proc. Natl. Acad. Sci. USA* **61**:284.

Goulian, M., Kornberg, A., and Sinsheimer, R. L., 1967, Enzymatic synthesis of DNA. XXIV. Synthesis of infectious phage ϕX174 DNA, *Proc. Natl. Acad. Sci. USA* **58**:2321.

Grohmann, K., Smith, L. H., and Sinsheimer, R. L., 1975, New method for isolation and sequence determination of 5′-terminal regions of bacteriophage ϕX174 *in vitro* mRNAs, *Biochemistry* **14**:1951.

Groman, N. B., 1969, Restriction of bacteriophage ϕX174 by F factor, *Biochem. Biophys. Res. Commun.* **37**:691.

Groman, N. B., and Suzuki, G., 1966, Effect of spermine on lysis and reproduction by bacteriophages ϕX174, lambda and f2, *J. Bacteriol.* **92**:1735.

Grosveld, F. G., Ojamaa, K. M., and Spencer, J. H., 1976, Fragmentation of bacteriophage S13 replicative form DNA by restriction endonucleases from *Haemophilus influenzae* and *Haemophilus aegyptius, Virology* **71**:312.

Gschwender, H. H., and Hofschneider, P. H., 1969, Lysis inhibition of ϕX174-, M12-, and Qβ-infected *Escherichia coli* by magnesium ions, *Biochim. Biophys. Acta* **190**:454.

Hall, J. B., and Sinsheimer, R. L., 1963, The structure of the DNA of bacteriophage ϕX174. IV. Pyrimidine sequences, *J. Mol. Biol.* **6**:115.

Harbers, B., Delaney, A. D., Harbers, K., and Spencer, J. H., 1976, Nucleotide clusters in DNA: Comparison of the sequences of the large pyrimidine oligonucleotides of bacteriophages S13 and ϕX174 DNA, *Biochemistry* **15**:407.

Haworth, S. R., Gilgun, C. F., and Dowell, C. E., 1975, Growth studies of three ϕX174 mutants in *ts*DNA mutants of *Escherichia coli, J. Virol.* **15**:720.

Hayashi, M. N., and Hayashi, M., 1972, Isolation of ϕX174 specific messenger ribonucleic acids *in vivo* and identification of their 5′ terminal nucleotides, *J. Virol.* **9**:207.

Hayashi, M. N., and Hayashi, M., 1974, Fragment maps of ϕX174 RF DNA produced by restriction enzymes from *Haemophilus aphirophilus* and *Haemophilus influenzae* H-1, *J. Virol.* **14**:1142.

Hayashi, M., Hayashi, M. N., and Hayashi, Y., 1970, Size distribution of ϕX174 RNA synthesized *in vitro, Cold Spring Harbor Symp. Quant. Biol.* **35**:174.

Hayashi, Y., and Hayashi, M., 1970, Fractionation of ϕX174 specific mRNA, *Cold Spring Harbor Symp. Quant. Biol.* **35**:171.

Hayashi, Y., and Hayashi, M., 1971, Template activities of the ϕX174 replicative allomorphic DNAs, *Biochemistry* **10**:4210.

Henry, T. J., and Knippers, R., 1974, Isolation and function of the gene A initiator of bacteriophage ϕX174: A highly specific DNA endonuclease, *Proc. Natl. Acad. Sci. USA* **71**:1549.

Hoffmann-Berling, H., Kaerner, H. C., and Knippers, R., 1966, Small bacteriophages, *Adv. Virus Res.* **12**:329.

Hofs, E. B. H., van de Pol, J. H., van Arkel, G. A., and Jansz, H. S., 1972, Dimeric circular duplex DNA of bacteriophage φX174 and recombination, *Mol. Gen. Genet.* **118**:161.

Hofs, E. B. H., van Arkel, G. A., Baas, P. D., Ellens, D. J., and Jansz, H. S., 1973, Mechanism of formation of bacteriophage φX174 circular and catenated dimer RF⁺ DNA, *Mol. Gen. Genet.* **126**:37.

Hutchison, C. A., III, and Edgell, M. H., 1971, Genetic assay for small fragments of bacteriophage φX174 DNA, *J. Virol.* **8**:181.

Hutchison, C. A., III, and Sinsheimer, R. L., 1966, The process of infection with bacteriophage φX174. X. Mutations in a φX lysis gene, *J. Mol. Biol.* **18**:429.

Hutchison, C. A., III, and Sinsheimer, R. L., 1971, Requirement of protein synthesis for bacteriophage φX174 superinfection exclusion, *J. Virol.* **8**:121.

Hutchison, C. A., III, Edgell, M. H., and Sinsheimer, R. L., 1967, The process of infection with bacteriophage φX174. XII. Phenotypic mixing between electrophoretic mutants of φX174, *J. Mol. Biol.* **23**:553.

Ikeda, J.-E., Yudelevich, A., and Hurwitz, J., 1976, Isolation and characterization of the protein coded by gene A of bacteriophage φX174 DNA, *Proc. Nat. Acad. Sci. USA* **73**:2669.

Incardona, N. L., 1974, Mechanism of adsorption and eclipse of bacteriophage φX174. III. Comparison of the activation parameter for the *in vitro* and *in vivo* eclipse reactions with mutant and wild type virus, *J. Virol.* **14**:469.

Incardona, N. L., and Selvidge, L., 1973, Mechanism of adsorption and eclipse of bacteriophage φX174. II. Attachment and eclipse with isolated *E. coli* cell wall lipopolysaccharide, *J. Virol.* **11**:775.

Incardona, N. L., Blonski, R., and Feeney, W., 1972, Mechanism of adsorption and eclipse of bacteriophage φX174. I. *In vitro* conformational change under conditions of eclipse, *J. Virol.* **9**:96.

Ishiwa, H., and Tessman, I., 1968, Control of host DNA synthesis after infection with bacteriophage S13 and φX174, *J. Mol. Biol.* **37**:467.

Iwaya, M., 1971, On the mechanism of φX174 DNA replication, Ph.D. thesis, Harvard University.

Iwaya, M., and Denhardt, D. T., 1971, The mechanism of replication of φX174 single-stranded DNA. II. The role of viral proteins, *J. Mol. Biol.* **57**:159.

Iwaya, M., and Denhardt, D. T., 1973a, Mechanism of replication of φX174 single-stranded DNA. IV. The parental viral strand is not conserved in the replicating DNA structure, *J. Mol. Biol.* **73**:279.

Iwaya, M., and Denhardt, D. T., 1973b, Mechanism of replication of φX174. V. Dispersive and conservative transfer of parental DNA into progeny DNA, *J. Mol. Biol.* **73**:291.

Iwaya, M., Eisenberg, S., Bartok, K., and Denhardt, D. T., 1973, Mechanism of replication of single-stranded φX174 DNA. VII. Circularization of the progeny viral strand, *J. Virol.* **12**:808.

Jazwinski, S. M., and Kornberg, A., 1975, DNA replication *in vitro* starting with an intact φX174 phage, *Proc. Natl. Acad. Sci. USA* **72**:3863.

Jazwinski, S. M., Lindberg, A. A., and Kornberg, A., 1975a, The lipopolysaccharide receptor for bacteriophages φX174 and S13, *Virology* **66**:268.

Jazwinski, S. M., Lindberg, A. A., and Kornberg, A., 1975*b*, The gene H spike protein of bacteriophages φX174 and S13. I. Functions in phage-receptor recognition and in transfection, *Virology* **66**:283.

Jazwinski, S. M., Marco, R., and Kornberg, A., 1975*c*, The gene H spike protein of bacteriophage φX174 and S13. II. Relation to synthesis of the parental replicative form, *Virology* **66**:294.

Jeng, Y. C., and Hayashi, M., 1970, A new complementation group of φX174, *Virology* **40**:407.

Jeng, Y., Gelfand, D., Hayashi, M., Shleser, R., and Tessman, E. S., 1970, The eight genes of bacteriophage φX174 and S13 and comparison of the phage-specified proteins, *J. Mol. Biol.* **49**:521.

Jeppesen, P. G. N., Sander, L., and Slocombe, P. M., 1976, A restriction cleavage map of φX174 DNA by pulse-chase labelling using *E. coli* DNA polymerase, *Nucleic Acids Res.* **3**:1323.

Johnson, P. H., and Sinsheimer, R. L., 1974, Structure of an intermediate in the replication of bacteriophage φX174 DNA: The initiation site for DNA replication, *J. Mol. Biol.* **83**:47.

Johnson, P. H., Lee, A. S., and Sinsheimer, R. L., 1973, Production of specific fragments of φX174 replicative form DNA by a restriction enzyme from *Haemophilus parainfluenzae,* endonuclease HP, *J. Virol.* **11**:596.

Kapitza, E. L., Stukacheva, E. A., and Shemayakin, M. F., 1976, The effect of the termination *rho* factor and ribonuclease III on the transcription of bacteriophage φX174 DNA *in vitro, FEBS Lett.* **64**:81.

Kay, D., and Bradley, D. E., 1962, The structure of bacteriophage φR, *J. Gen. Microbiol.* **27**:195.

Kim, J.-S., Sharp, P. A., and Davidson, N., 1972, Electron microscope studies of heteroduplex DNA from a deletion mutant of bacteriophage φX174, *Proc. Natl. Acad. Sci. USA* **69**:1948.

Knippers, R., and Sinsheimer, R. L., 1968*a*, Process of infection with bacteriophage φX174. XX. Attachment of the parental DNA of bacteriophage φX174 to a fast-sedimenting cell component, *J. Mol. Biol.* **34**:17.

Knippers, R., and Sinsheimer, R. L., 1968*b*, Process of infection with bacteriophage φX174. XXIII. DNA synthesis in cells infected by a coat protein mutant, *J. Mol. Biol.* **35**:591.

Knippers, R., Komano, T., and Sinsheimer, R. L., 1968, The process of infection with bacteriophage φX174. XXI. Replication and fate of the replicative form, *Proc. Natl. Acad. Sci. USA* **59**:577.

Knippers, R., Razin, A., Davis, R., and Sinsheimer, R. L., 1969*a*, The process of infection with bacteriophage φX174. XXIX. *In vivo* studies on the synthesis of the single-stranded DNA of progeny φX174 bacteriophage, *J. Mol. Biol.* **45**:237.

Knippers, R., Salivar, W. O., Newbold, J. E., and Sinsheimer, R. L., 1969*b*, Process of infection with bacteriophage φX174. XXVI. Transfer of the parental DNA of bacteriophage φX174 into progeny bacteriophage particles, *J. Mol. Biol.* **39**:641.

Knippers, R., Whalley, J. M., and Sinsheimer, R. L., 1969*c*, The process of infection with bacteriophage φX174. XXX. Replication of double-stranded DNA, *Proc. Natl. Acad. Sci. USA* **64**:275.

Komano, T., Knippers, R., and Sinsheimer, R. L., 1968, The process of infection with bacteriophage φX174. XXII. Synthesis of progeny single-stranded DNA, *Proc. Natl. Acad. Sci. USA* **59**:911.

Kornberg, A., 1974, *DNA Synthesis*, W. H. Freeman and Company, San Francisco.

Kranias, E. G., and Dumas, L. B., 1974, Replication of bacteriophage φX174 DNA in a temperature-sensitive *dnaC* mutant of *E. coli* C, *J. Virol.* **13**:146.

Kranias, E. G., and Dumas, L. B., 1975, Synthesis of complex forms of bacteriophage φX174 double-stranded DNA in a temperature-sensitive *dnaC* mutant of *E. coli* C, *J. Virol.* **16**:412.

Lane, H. E. D., and Denhardt, D. T., 1974, The *rep* mutation. III. Altered structure of the replicating *E. coli* chromosome, *J. Bacteriol.* **120**:805.

Lane, H. E. D., and Denhardt, D. T., 1975, The *rep* mutation. IV. Slower movement of replication forks in *E. coli rep* strains, *J. Mol. Biol.* **97**:99.

Lee, A. S., and Sinsheimer, R. L., 1974a, A cleavage map of bacteriophage φX174 genome, *Proc. Natl. Acad. Sci. USA* **71**:2882.

Lee, A. S., and Sinsheimer, R. L., 1974b, Location of the 5-methylcytosine group on the bacteriophage φX174 genome, *J. Virol.* **14**:872.

Lerman, L. S., 1974, Chromosomal analogues: Long-range order in ψ-condensed DNA, *Cold Spring Harbor Symp. Quant. Biol.* **38**:59.

Lindberg, A. A., 1973, Bacteriophage receptors, *Annu. Rev. Microbiol.* **27**:205.

Lindqvist, B. H., and Sinsheimer, R. L., 1967a, Process of infection with bacteriophage φX174. XIV. Studies on macromolecular synthesis during infection with a lysis-defective mutant, *J. Mol. Biol.* **28**:87.

Lindqvist, B. H., and Sinsheimer, R. L., 1967b, The process of infection with bacteriophage φX174. XV. Bacteriophage DNA synthesis in abortive infections with a set of conditional lethal mutants, *J. Mol. Biol.* **30**:69.

Lindqvist, B. H., and Sinsheimer, R. L., 1968, The process of infection with bacteriophage φX174. XVI. Synthesis of the replicative form and its relationship to viral single-stranded DNA synthesis, *J. Mol. Biol.* **32**:285.

Ling, V., 1972, Pyrimidine sequences from the DNA of bacteriophages fd, f1, and φX174, *Proc. Natl. Acad. Sci. USA* **69**:742.

Linney, E., and Hayashi, M., 1973, Two proteins of gene A of φX174, *Nature (London) New Biol.* **245**:6.

Linney, E., and Hayashi, M., 1974, Intragenic regulation of the synthesis of φX174 gene A proteins, *Nature (London)* **249**:345.

Linney, E. A., Hayashi, M. N., and Hayashi, M., 1972, Gene A of φX174. I. Isolation and identification of the products, *Virology* **50**:381.

Manheimer, I., and Truffaut, N., 1974, Growth of bacteriophage φX174 in *E. coli* strains carrying temperature sensitive mutations for DNA initiation, *Mol. Gen. Genet.* **130**:21.

Martin, D. G., and Godson, G. N., 1975, Identification of a φX174 coded protein involved in the shut off of host DNA replication, *Biochem. Biophys. Res. Commun.* **65**:323.

Marvin, D. A., and Hohn, B., 1969, Filamentous bacterial viruses, *Bacteriol. Rev.* **33**:172.

Mayol, R. F., and Sinsheimer, R. L., 1970, Process of infection with bacteriophage φX174. XXXVI. Measurement of virus-specific proteins during a normal cycle of infection, *J. Virol.* **6**:310.

Mazur, B. J., and Model, P., 1973, Regulation of coliphage f1 single-stranded DNA synthesis by a DNA-binding protein, *J. Mol. Biol.* **78**:285.

McFadden, G., 1975, Studies on the replication of bacteriophage φX174, Ph.D. thesis, McGill University.

McFadden, G. M., and Denhardt, D. T., 1974, Mechanism of replication of φX174 single-stranded DNA. IX. Requirement for the *E. coli dna*G protein, *J. Virol.* **14**:1070.

McFadden, G., and Denhardt, D. T., 1975, The mechanism of replication of φX174 DNA. XII. Discontinuous synthesis of the complementary strand in an *E. coli* host with a temperature-sensitive polynucleotide ligase, *J. Mol. Biol.* **99**:125.

Merriam, V., Dumas, L. B., and Sinsheimer, R. L., 1971*a*, Genetic expression in heterozygous replicative form molecules of φX174, *J. Virol.* **7**:603.

Merriam, V., Funk, F., and Sinsheimer, R. L., 1971*b*, Genetic expression in whole cells of heterozygous replicative form molecules of φX174, *Mutation Res.* **12**:206.

Middleton, J. H., Edgell, M. H., and Hutchison, C. A., III, 1972, Specific fragments of φX174 DNA produced by a restriction enzyme from *H. aegyptius,* endonuclease Z, *J. Virol.* **10**:42.

Miller, L. K., and Sinsheimer, R. L., 1974, Nature of φX174 linear DNA from a DNA ligase-deficient host, *J. Virol.* **14**:1503.

Neuwald, P. D., 1975, *In vitro* system for the study of bacteriophage φX174 adsorption and eclipse, *J. Virol.* **15**:497.

Newbold, J. E., and Sinsheimer, R. L., 1970*a*, The process of infection with bacteriophage φX174. XXXI. Abortive infection at low temperatures, *J. Mol. Biol.* **49**:23.

Newbold, J. E., and Sinsheimer, R. L., 1970*b*, The process of infection with bacteriophage φX174. XXXII. Early stages in the infection process: attachment, eclipse, DNA penetration, *J. Mol. Biol.* **49**:49.

Newbold, J. E., and Sinsheimer, R. L., 1970*c*, Process of infection with bacteriophage φX174. XXXIV. Kinetics of the attachment and eclipse steps of the infection, *J. Virol.* **5**:427.

Palchoudhury, S. R., and Poddar, R. K., 1968, Influence of the viral genome on ribonucleic acid synthesis in *E. coli* infected with φX174, *J. Mol. Biol.* **32**:505.

Poljak, R. J., and Suruda, A. J., 1969, The coat proteins of φX174 and S13, *Virology* **39**:145.

Pollock, T. J., 1976, Gene D of Bacteriophage φX174: Absence of transcriptional and translational regulatory properties, *J. Virol.* (in press).

Puga, A., and Tessman, I., 1973*a*, Mechanism of transcription of bacteriophage S13. I. Dependence of mRNA on amount and configuration of DNA, *J. Mol. Biol.* **75**:83.

Puga, A., and Tessman, I., 1973*b*, Mechanism of transcription of bacteriophage S13. II. Inhibition of phage specific transcription by nalidixic acid, *J. Mol. Biol.* **75**:99.

Puga, A., and Tessman, I., 1973*c*, Membrane binding of phage S13 messenger RNA, *Virology* **56**:375.

Puga, A., Borras, M.-T., Tessman, E. S., and Tessman, I., 1973, Difference between functional and structural integrity of messenger RNA, *Proc. Natl. Acad. Sci. USA* **70**:2171.

Radloff, R., and Vinograd, J., 1971, The absence of a non-nucleotide linker in polyoma and φX174 DNA, *Biochim. Biophys. Acta* **247**:207.

Ray, D. S., and Dueber, J., 1975, Structure and replication of replicative forms of the φX-related bacteriophage G4, in: *DNA Synthesis and Its Regulation* (M. Goulian and P. Hanawalt, eds.), Benjamin, Menlo Park, Calif.

Razin, A., 1973, DNA methylase induced by bacteriophage φX174, *Proc. Natl. Acad. Sci. USA* **70**:3773.

Razin, A., and Sinsheimer, R. L., 1970, Replicative form II DNA of φX174:

Resistance to exonucleolytic cleavage by *E. coli* DNA polymerase, *Proc. Natl. Acad. Sci. USA* **66**:646.

Razin, A., Sedat, J. W., and Sinsheimer, R. L., 1970, Structure of the DNA of bacteriophage φX174. VII. Methylation, *J. Mol. Biol.* **53**:251.

Razin, A., Sedat, J. W., and Sinsheimer, R. L., 1973, *In vivo* methylation of replicating bacteriophage φX174 DNA, *J. Mol. Biol.* **78**:417.

Razin, A., Goren, D., and Friedman, J., 1975, Studies on the biological role of DNA methylation: Inhibition of methylation and maturation of the bacteriophage φX174 by nicotinamide, *Nucleic Acids Res.* **2**:1967.

Roberts, R. J., 1976, Restriction endonucleases, *CRC Crit. Rev. Biochem.* (in press).

Rose, J. A., 1974, Parvovirus reproduction, in: *Comprehensive Virology,* Vol. 3 (H. Fraenkel-Conrat and R. R. Wagner, eds.), Plenum, New York.

Rush, M. G., and Warner, R. C., 1968, Molecular recombination in a circular genome—φX174 and S13, *Cold Spring Harbor Symp. Quant. Biol.* **33**:459.

Sakai, H., and Komano, T., 1975, Bacteriophage φX174 DNA synthesis in *E. coli* HF4704S (*dna*H^{ts}) cells, *Biochim. Biophys. Acta* **395**:433.

Salivar, W. O., and Sinsheimer, R. L., 1969, Intracellular location and number of replicating parental DNA molecules of bacteriophages lambda and φX174, *J. Mol. Biol.* **41**:39.

Sanger, F., 1975, Nucleotide sequences in DNA, *Proc. R. Soc. London* **191**:317.

Schaller, H., 1969, Structure of the DNA of bacteriophage fd. I. Absence of non-phosphodiester linkages, *J. Mol. Biol.* **44**:435.

Schekman, R. W., and Ray, D. S., 1971, Polynucleotide ligase and φX174 single-strand synthesis, *Nature (London) New Biol.* **231**:170.

Schekman, R. W., Iwaya, M., Bromstrup, K., and Denhardt, D. T., 1971, The mechanism of replication of φX174 single-stranded DNA. III. An enzymic study of the structure of the replicative form II DNA, *J. Mol. Biol.* **57**:177.

Schekman, R., Weiner, A., and Kornberg, A., 1974, Multienzyme systems of DNA replication, *Science* **186**:987.

Schekman, R., Weiner, J. H., Weiner, A., and Kornberg, A., 1975, Ten proteins required for conversion of φX174 single-stranded DNA to duplex form *in vitro*: Resolution and reconstitution, *J. Biol. Chem.* **250**:5859.

Schnegg, B., and Hofschneider, P. H., 1969, Mutant of φX174 accessible to host-controlled modification, *J. Virol.* **3**:541.

Schnegg, B., and Hofschneider, P. H., 1970, Transfer of parental φX174 DNA to progeny bacteriophage particles observed at low multiplicities of infection, *J. Mol. Biol.* **51**:315.

Schröder, C. H., and Kaerner, H.-C., 1972, Replication of bacteriophage φX174 replicative form DNA *in vivo*, *J. Mol. Biol.* **71**:351.

Schröder, C., and Kaerner, H.-C., 1971, Infectivity to *E. coli* spheroplasts of linear φX174 DNA strands derived from replicative form (RF II) of φX DNA, *FEBS Lett.* **19**:38.

Schröder, C. H., Erben, E., and Kaerner, H.-C., 1973, A rolling circle model of the *in vivo* replication of bacteriophage φX174 replicative form DNA: Different fate of two types of progeny replicative form, *J. Mol. Biol.* **79**:599.

Sedat, J. W., and Sinsheimer, R. L., 1970, The *in vivo* φXmRNA, *Cold Spring Harb. Symp. Quant. Biol.* **35**:163.

Sedat, J., Lyon, A., and Sinsheimer, R. L., 1969, Purification of *E. coli* pulse-labeled RNA by benzoylated DEAE-cellulose chromatography, *J. Mol. Biol.* **44**:415.

Sertic, V., and Boulgakov, N., 1935, Classification et identification des typhi-phages, *C. R. Soc. Biol.* **119**:1270.

Shleser, R., Puga, A., and Tessman, E. S., 1969a, Synthesis of RF DNA and mRNA by gene IV mutants of bacteriophage S13, *J. Virol.* **4**:394.

Shleser, R., Tessman, E. S., and Casaday, G., 1969b, Protein synthesis by a mutant of phage S13 blocked in DNA synthesis, *Virology* **38**:166.

Siden, E. J., and Hayashi, M., 1974, Role of the gene B product in bacteriophage ϕX174 development, *J. Mol. Biol.* **89**:1.

Siegel, J. E. D., and Hayashi, M., 1969, ϕX174 bacteriophage structural mutants which affect DNA synthesis, *J. Virol.* **4**:400.

Silverstein, S., and Billen, D., 1971, Transcription: Role in the initiation and replication of DNA synthesis in *E. coli* and ϕX174, *Biochim. Biophys. Acta* **247**:383.

Singh, S., and Ray, D. S., 1975, A novel single-strand endonuclease specific for ϕX174 DNA, *Biochem. Biophys. Res. Commun.* **67**:1429.

Sinsheimer, R. L., 1959, Purification and properties of bacteriophage ϕX174, *J. Mol. Biol.* **1**:37.

Sinsheimer, R. L., 1968, Bacteriophage ϕX174 and related viruses, in: *Progress in Nucleic Acid Research and Molecular Biology,* Vol. 8 (J. N. Davidson and W. E. Cohn, eds.), pp. 115–170, Academic Press, New York.

Sinsheimer, R. L., 1970, The life cycle of a single-stranded DNA virus, *Harvey Lect. Ser.* **64**:69.

Smith, L. H., and Sinsheimer, R. L., 1976a, The *in vitro* transcription units of ϕX174. I. Characterization of synthetic parameters and measurement of transcript molecular weights, *J. Mol. Biol.* **103**:681.

Smith, L. H., and Sinsheimer, R. L., 1976b, The *in vitro* transcription units of ϕX174. II. *In vitro* initiation sites of ϕX174 transcription, *J. Mol. Biol.* **103**:699.

Smith, L. H., and Sinsheimer, R. L., 1976c, The *in vitro* transcription units of ϕX174. III. Initiation with specific 5′ end oligonucleotides of in vitro ϕX174 RNA, *J. Mol. Biol.* **103**:711.

Smith, L. H., Grohmann, K., and Sinsheimer, R. L., 1974, Nucleotide sequences of the 5′ termini of ϕX174 mRNAs synthesized *in vitro, Nucleic Acids Res.* **1**:1521.

Spencer, J. H., Cerny, R., Cerna, E., and Delaney, A., 1972, Characterization of bacteriophage S13 suN15 single-strand and replicative form DNA, *J. Virol.* **10**:134.

Stone, A. B., 1970a, General inhibition of *E. coli* macromolecular synthesis by high multiplicities of bacteriophage ϕX174, *J. Mol. Biol.* **47**:215.

Stone, A. B., 1970b, Protein synthesis and the arrest of bacterial DNA synthesis by bacteriophage ϕX174, *Virology* **42**:171.

Sumida-Yasumoto, C., Yudelevich, A., and Hurwitz, J., 1976, DNA synthesis *in vitro* dependent upon ϕX174 replicative form I DNA, *Proc. Natl. Acad. Sci. USA* **73**:1887.

Suruda, A. J., and Poljak, A. J., 1971, Separation and purification of the coat proteins of ϕX174, *Virology* **46**:164.

Taketo, A., 1973, Sensitivity of *E. coli* to viral nucleic acid, VI. Capacity of *dna* mutants and DNA polymerase-less mutants for multiplication of ϕA and ϕX174, *Mol. Gen. Genet.* **122**:15.

Taketo, A., 1974, Properties of bacterial virus ϕA and its DNA, *J. Biochem.* **75**:951.

Taketo, A., 1975a, Effect of mitomycin C on the capacity of *E. coli* to support multiplication of ϕA, *J. Gen. Appl. Microbiol.* **21**:183.

Taketo, A., 1975*b*, Replication of ϕA and ϕX174 in *E. coli* mutants thermosensitive in DNA synthesis, *Mol. Gen. Genet.* **139**:285.

Tessman, E. S., 1965, Complementation groups in phage S13, *Virology* **25**:303.

Tessman, E. S., 1966, Mutants of bacteriophage S13 blocked in infectious DNA synthesis, *J. Mol. Biol.* **17**:218.

Tessman, E. S., 1967, Gene function in phage S13, in: *The Molecular Biology of Viruses* (J. S. Colter and W. Paranchych, eds.), Academic Press, New York.

Tessman, E. S., and Peterson, P. K., 1976, Bacterial *rep*⁻ mutations that block development of small DNA phages late in infection, *J. Virol.* **20**:400.

Tessman, E. S., Borras, M.-T., and Sun, I. L., 1971, Superinfection in bacteriophage S13 and determination of the number of bacteriophage particles which can function in an infected cell, *J. Virol.* **8**:111.

Tessman, I., 1966, Genetic recombination of phage S13 in a recombination-deficient mutant of *Escherichia coli* K12, *Biochem. Biophys. Res. Commun.* **22**:169.

Tessman, I., 1968, Selective stimulation of one of the mechanisms for genetic recombination of bacteriophage S13, *Science* **161**:481.

Tessman, I., and Tessman, E. S., 1968, Gene functions and genetics of phage S13, in: *Molecular Genetics* (H. G. Wittmann and H. Schuster, eds.), Springer-Verlag, Berlin.

Tessman, I., Ishiwa, H., Kumar, S., and Baker, R., 1967, Bacteriophage S13: A seventh gene, *Science* **156**:824.

Tessman, I., Tessman, E. S., Pollock, T. J., Borras, M.-T., Puga, A., and Baker, R., 1976, Reinitiation mutants of gene B of phage S13 that mimic gene A mutants in blocking RF synthesis, *J. Mol. Biol.* **103**:583.

Thomas, M., and Davis, R. W., 1975, Studies on the cleavage of bacteriophage lambda DNA with *Eco*R1 restriction endonuclease, *J. Mol. Biol.* **91**:315.

Thompson, B. J., Escarmis, C., Parker, B., Slater, W. C., Doniger, J., Tessman, I., and Warner, R. C., 1975, Figure-8 configuration of dimers of S13 and ϕX174 replicative form DNA, *J. Mol. Biol.* **91**:408.

Tonegawa, S., and Hayashi, M., 1970, Intermediates in the assembly of ϕX174, *J. Mol. Biol.* **48**:219.

Truffaut, N., and Sinsheimer, R. L., 1974, Use of bacteriophage ϕX174 replicative form progeny DNA as templates for transcription, *J. Virol.* **13**:818.

Truitt, C. L., and Walker, J. R., 1974, Growth of phages lambda, ϕX174 and M13 requires the *dnaZ* (formerly *dna*H) gene product of *E. coli*, *Biochem. Biophys. Res. Commun.* **61**:1036.

Vanderbilt, A. S., and Tessman, I., 1970, Mutagenic methods for determining which DNA strand is transcribed for individual viral genes, *Nature (London)* **228**:54.

Vanderbilt, A. S., Borras, M.-T., and Tessman, E. S., 1971, Direction of translation in phage S13 as determined from the sizes of polypeptide fragments of nonsense mutants, *Virology* **43**:352.

Vanderbilt, A. S., Borras, M.-T., Germeraad, S., Tessman, I., and Tessman, E. S., 1972, A promoter site and polarity gradients in phage S13, *Virology* **50**:171.

van der Mei, D., Brons, J. T., and Jansz, H., 1972*a*, The effect of rifampicin on the replication of the replicative form of bacteriophage ϕX174 DNA, *Biochim. Biophys. Acta* **262**:463.

van der Mei, D., Zandberg, J., and Jansz, H. S., 1972*b*, The effect of chloramphenicol on synthesis of ϕX174-specific proteins and the detection of the cistron A proteins, *Biochim. Biophys. Acta* **287**:312.

Vereijken, J. M., van Mansfeld, A. D. M., Baas, P. D., and Jansz, H. S., 1975, *Arthrobacter luteus* restriction endonuclease cleavage map of φX174 RF DNA, *Virology* **68**:221.

Vito, C. C., and Dowell, C. E., 1976, Novel replicative properties of a capsid mutant of bacteriophage φX174, *J. Virol.* **18**:942.

Vito, C. C., Primrose, S. B., and Dowell, C. E., 1975, Growth of a capsid mutant of bacteriophage φX174 in a temperature-sensitive strain of *E. coli, J. Virol.* **15**:281.

Wang, J. C., 1969, Degree of superhelicity of covalently closed cyclic DNA's from *E. coli, J. Mol. Biol.* **43**:263.

Wang, J. C., 1974, The degree of unwinding of the DNA helix by ethidium. I. Titration of twisted PM2 DNA molecules in alkaline CsCl density gradients, *J. Mol. Biol.* **89**:783.

Waring, M., 1970, Variation of the supercoils in closed circular DNA by binding of antibiotics and drugs: Evidence for molecular models involving intercalation, *J. Mol. Biol.* **54**:247.

Warnaar, S. O., Mulder, G., van der Sluis, I., van Kesteren, L. W., and Cohen, J. A., 1969, The transcription *in vitro* of various forms of φX174 DNA, *Biochim. Biophys. Acta* **174**:239.

Warnaar, S. O., De Mol, A., Mulder, G., Abrahams, P. J., and Cohen, J. A., 1970, The transcription of bacteriophage φX174 DNA, *Biochim. Biophys. Acta* **199**:340.

Watson, G., and Paigen, K., 1971, Isolation and characterization of an *E. coli* bacteriophage requiring cell wall galactose, *J. Virol.* **8**:669.

Weiner, J. H., McMacken, R., and Kornberg, A., 1976, Isolation of an intermediate which precedes *dna*G RNA polymerase participation in enzymatic replication of φX174 DNA, *Proc. Natl. Acad. Sci. USA* **73**:752.

Weisbeek, P. J., and Sinsheimer, R. L., 1974, A DNA–protein complex involved in bacteriophage φX174 particle formation, *Proc. Natl. Acad. Sci. USA* **71**:3054.

Weisbeek, P. J., and van Arkel, G. A., 1976, On the origin of bacteriophage φX174 replicative form DNA replication, *Virology* **72**:72.

Weisbeek, P. J., van de Pol, J. H., and van Arkel, G. A., 1972, Genetic characterization of the DNA of the bacteriophage φX174 70 S particle, *Virology* **48**:456.

Weisbeek, P. J., van de Pol, J. H., and van Arkel, G. A., 1973, Mapping of host range mutants of bacteriophage φX174, *Virology* **52**:408.

Weisbeek, P. J., Vereijken, J. M., Baas, P. D., Jansz, H. S., and van Arkel, G. A., 1976, The genetic map of bacteriophage φX174 constructed with restriction enzyme fragments, *Virology* **72**:61.

Wickner, R. B., Wright, M., Wickner, S., and Hurwitz, J., 1972, Conversion of φX174 and fd single-stranded DNA to replicative forms in extracts of *E. coli, Proc. Natl. Acad. Sci. USA* **69**:3233.

Wickner, S., and Hurwitz, J., 1974, Conversion of φX174 viral DNA to double-stranded form by purified *E. coli* proteins, *Proc. Natl. Acad. Sci. USA* **71**:4120.

Wickner, S., and Hurwitz, J., 1975a, *In vitro* synthesis of DNA, in:*DNA Synthesis and Its Regulation* (M. Goulian and P. Hanawalt, ed.), ICN-UCLA Winter Conference, Benjamin, Menlo Park, Calif.

Wickner, S., and Hurwitz, J., 1975b, Association of φX174 DNA-dependent ATPase activity with an *E. coli* protein, replication factor Y, required for *in vitro* synthesis of φX174 DNA, *Proc. Natl. Acad. Sci. USA* **72**:3342.

Wickner, S., and Hurwitz, J., 1976, Involvement of *Escherichia coli dna*Z gene product in DNA elongation *in vitro, Proc. Natl. Acad. Sci. USA* **73**:1053.

Wickner, W., and Kornberg, A., 1974a, A novel form of RNA polymerase from *E. coli, Proc. Natl. Acad. Sci. USA* **71**:4425.

Wickner, W., and Kornberg, A., 1974b, A holoenzyme form of DNA polymerase III, *J. Biol. Chem.* **249**:6244.

Woodworth-Gutai, M., and Lebowitz, J. 1976, Introduction of interrupted secondary structure in supercoiled DNA as a function of superhelix density: Consideration of hairpin structures in superhelical DNA, *J. Virol.* **18**:195.

Yarus, M. J., and Sinsheimer, R. L., 1967, The process of infection with bacteriophage φX174. XIII. Evidence for an essential bacterial "site," *J. Virol.* **1**:135.

Yokoyama, Y., Komano, T., and Onodera, K., 1971, The presence of short DNA chains in φX174 RF II in the late phase of infection, *Agr. Biol. Chem.* **34**:1353.

Zahler, S. A., 1958, Some biological properties of bacteriophages S13 and φX174, *J. Bacteriol.* **75**:310.

Zechel, K., Bouché, J.-P., and Kornberg, A., 1975, Replication of phage G4: A novel and simple system for the initiation of DNA synthesis, *J. Biol. Chem.* **250**:4684.

Zuccarelli, A. J., 1974, Formation of parental replicative forms of φX174: Synthesis of the first complementary strand, Ph.D. thesis, California Institute of Technology.

Zuccarelli, A. J., Benbow, R. M., and Sinsheimer, R. L., 1972, Deletion mutants of bacteriophage φX174, *Proc. Natl. Acad. Sci. USA* **69**:1905.

CHAPTER 2

Replication of Filamentous Bacteriophages

Dan S. Ray

Molecular Biology Institute and Department of Biology
University of California
Los Angeles, California

1. INTRODUCTION

This chapter will review the current state of knowledge of the reproduction of filamentous bacterial viruses. The area of most intense activity since the filamentous bacterial viruses were reviewed last (Ray, 1968; Marvin and Hohn, 1969; Pratt, 1969; Denhardt, 1975) has been the study of the structure and replication of the viral DNA, and, accordingly, these aspects will be the primary focus of the chapter.

Filamentous bacterial viruses have been isolated for several different bacterial strains. They were first isolated by Loeb (1960) and characterized in more detail by Zinder *et al.* (1963). At the same time, filamentous bacterial viruses were described in many different laboratories. In all cases examined, the virions are relatively heat resistant, contain circular single-stranded DNA, have a diameter of approximately 6 nm, are sensitive to shaking with chloroform, and are extruded into the medium as the host cell continues to grow and divide. Most such viruses are specific for bacteria that harbor sex factors.

Essentially all of the studies on the replication of the DNA of filamentous phage have been performed with the Ff group, one of three classes of *Escherichia coli* specific filamentous phages. The Ff group includes fd, f1, M13, ZJ/2, Ec9, AE2, HR, and δ A (Marvin and

Hohn, 1969). Some of these viruses are serologically related, and a genetic relationship has been demonstrated in some cases. All adsorb to the tip of the F-type sex pilus (Fig. 1) and are about 870 nm long. Ff-infected cells release filamentous virions through the cell wall without lysis (Hoffmann-Berling *et al.,* 1963; Hofschneider and Preuss, 1963; Hoffmann-Berling and Mazé, 1964). In liquid medium, titers of up to $2\text{--}5 \times 10^{12}$ per milliliter are readily obtained. Although the infected

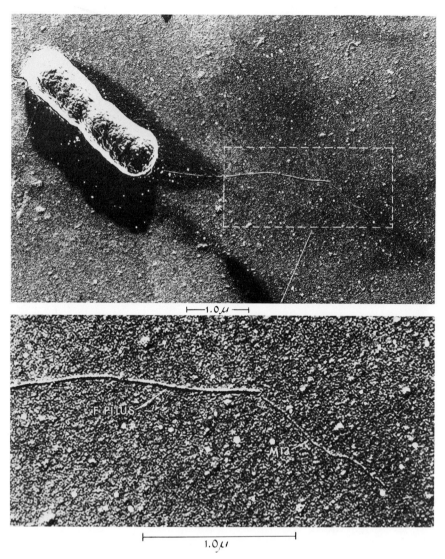

Fig. 1.   Electron micrograph of bacteriophage M13 attached to the tip of an F pilus of *E. coli* Courtesy of J. Griffith.

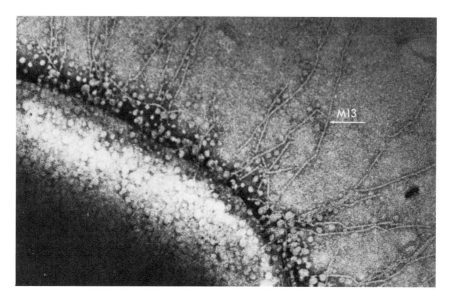

Fig. 2.   Electron micrograph of bacteriophage M13 being extruded from an infected cell. Courtesy of J. Griffith.

cells are not killed, plaque formation based on the reduced growth rate of infected cells permits assay in the standard way under appropriate plating conditions. An electron micrograph of Ff phage being released through the cell wall is shown in Fig. 2.

A second class of filamentous coliphage is defined by its adsorption to I-type sex pili specified by the transmissible drug resistance factor (R factor) of the type that does not inhibit F-promoted fertility (fi⁻). Two such viruses, If1 and If2, have been isolated (Meynell and Lawn, 1968), but they are possibly identical. Physical studies of If1 (Wiseman *et al.,* 1972) show it to have a length 1.5 times that of Ff viruses and to have a distinctly different base composition. However, the capsid proteins are similar to those of Ff phage and some genetic relationship is indicated by DNA-DNA hybridization (Denhardt and Marvin, 1969) and genetic complementation (Kay and Wakefield, 1972).

Bacteriophage IKe may represent a third class of filamentous coliphage (Khatoon *et al.,* 1972). Although it is similar in its physical properties to the Ff phages, it is serologically distinct and has a different host specificity. This phage is specific for strains carrying R fi⁻ sex factors of a type different from those determining the specificity for If phage. Sensitivity to phage IKe appears to define a distinct class of bacterial sex factors.

Two filamentous phages, Pf1 and Pf2, have been isolated for *Pseudomonas aeruginosa* and, like Ff phage, were found to form minute turbid plaques and to be released from growing cells without lysis (Minamishima *et al.,* 1968). Pf appears to be the longest known filamentous phage, with a length of 1915 $\pm$ 77 nm (Bradley, 1973).

A filamentous phage, Xf, from *Xanthomonas oryzae* appears morphologically very similar to the Ff phage but has a significantly different DNA base composition (Kuo *et al.,* 1969). The length of Xf phage is 977 nm, slightly longer than that of Ff phage. In addition, this phage infects at least 16 different strains of *Xanthomonas* and, consequently, is probably not sex specific.

The major coat protein has been sequenced for a number of the filamentous phages (Asbeck *et al.,* 1969; Lin *et al.,* 1971; Snell and Offord, 1972). These results indicate a definite relationship between the major coat proteins of fd, M13, f1, ZJ/2, and If1. Amino acid compositions of the major coat protein of some of the filamentous phages are presented in Table 1. The coat protein of the Xf phage is somewhat smaller and has a distinctly different amino acid composition. A common feature of the composition of the major coat protein of all of these phages is the absence of both histidine and cysteine. Most phages of the Ff group also lack arginine in the major coat protein. These deficits have been used to advantage in detecting minor capsid proteins by labeling with radioactive arginine or histidine (Henry and Pratt, 1969; Jazwinski *et al.,* 1973).

The DNA base compositions of the filamentous bacterial viruses clearly distinguish the Ff phage from the If phage and the Xf phage (Table 2). However, unlike other filamentous phages, the If DNA may contain a fairly large double-stranded portion. On the basis of the physical properties of If1 DNA, Wiseman *et al.* (1972) have speculated that If1 may have arisen by insertion of half a complementary DNA strand into the viral strand of an Ff-like virus.

The small size of Ff viral DNA limits these phages to no more than eight to ten proteins of medium size. Their genome consists of a single-stranded DNA of 5740 $\pm$ 210 nucleotides (Berkowitz and Day, 1974), corresponding to a coding capacity of 1913 $\pm$ 70 amino acids. Plaque-type, conditional lethal, and restriction-modification mutants have been obtained by mutation of the Ff genome with a wide range of physical and chemical agents (Marvin and Hohn, 1969). Several hundred conditional lethal mutants have been assigned to eight complementation groups (Pratt *et al.,* 1966, 1969; Lyons and Zinder, 1972; Mazur and Zinder, 1975*b*) which have been arranged into a circular genetic map by recombination (Lyons and Zinder, 1972). The

TABLE 1

**Amino Acid Compositions of the Major Coat Protein of Some
Filamentous Bacterial Viruses**

Amino acid	Number of residues					
	fd[a]	M13[a]	fl[a]	ZJ/2[b]	Ifl[c]	Xf[d]
Lys	5	5	5	5	4	2
His	0	0	0	0	0	0
Arg	0	0	0	0	1	2
Asp	3	3	3	3	3	2
Thr	3	3	3	2	4	1
Ser	4	4	4	4	4	2
Glu	3	3	3–4	3	3	1
Pro	1	1	1	1	0	1
Gly	4	4	4	4	3	9
Ala	10	10	9–10	11	10	6
Cys	0	0	0	0	0	0
Val	4	4	4	4	6	8
Met	1	1	1	1	1	2
Ile	4	4	4	4	1	3
Leu	2	2	2	2	4	1
Thy	2	2	2	2	1	1
Phe	3	3	3	3	3	0
Trp	1	1	1	1	1	1
Total	50	50	49–50	50	49	42

[a] Modified from Asbeck *et al.* (1969) to include an additional alanine
residue (Snell and Offord, 1972; Nakashima and Konigsberg, 1974).
[b] Snell and Offord (1972).
[c] Wiseman *et al.* (1972).
[d] Lin *et al.* (1971).

availability of these mutants has been an important factor in the
progress of much of the research with Ff phage. Table 3 lists the known
genes along with their physiological roles and the molecular weights of
the corresponding proteins, when these are known.

2. STRUCTURE OF THE Ff VIRION

The molecular structure of the rod-shaped Ff virion must differ
significantly from that of a rod-shaped virus like tobacco mosaic virus.
The nucleic acid of the Ff virion is a single-stranded DNA ring, even
though the virion itself is a linear filament. Also, there are two virion
proteins, the A protein (or gene 3 protein), a minor protein probably
present in only a few copies at one tip of the virion, and the B protein
(or gene 8 protein), the major capsid protein (Pratt *et al.,* 1969). The

TABLE 2

DNA Base Compositions of Some Filamentous Bacterial Viruses

Virus	Host	Base composition (in mol %)			
		Thymine	Adenine	Guanine	Cytosine
fd[a]	E. coli	34.1	24.4	19.9	21.7
M13[a]	E. coli	35.8	23.3	21.1	19.8
Ec9[a]	E. coli	34.3	24.4	20.6	20.7
AE2[a]	E. coli	32	26	21	21
δA[a]	E. coli	33.1	25.7	21.2	20.0
Ifl[b]	S. typhimurium	28.4	27.1	23.1	21.7
Xf[c]	Xanthomonas oryzae	19.3	20.6	32.6	27.5

[a] Marvin and Hohn (1969).
[b] Wiseman et al. (1972).
[c] Kuo et al. (1969).

presence of a full amount of A protein in half-size defective phage strongly supports its location at the end(s) of the phage filament (Marco, 1975).

The B protein is a small protein only 50 residues in length and largely α-helical (Marvin, 1966; Day, 1969). The amino acid sequence of the major capsid protein of Ff phage shows a distinctly nonrandom distribution of acidic, basic, and hydrophobic residues (Fig. 3), suggesting that the acidic amino-terminal portion of the capsid protein might be on the surface of the capsid and the basic carboxyl-terminal portion might interact with the viral DNA.

TABLE 3

Gene	Physiological role	Protein molecular weight
1	Morphogenesis	35,000,[a] 36,000[b]
2	DNA replication	40,000,[a] 46,000[b]
3	Minor capsid protein	56,000,[b] 68,000[c]
4	Morphogenesis	48,000,[b] 50,000[a]
5	SS synthesis	9,688[d]
6	Morphogenesis	3,000[e]
7	Morphogenesis	?
8	Major capsid protein	5,196[f,g]

[a] Model and Zinder (1974).
[b] Konings et al. (1975).
[c] Henry and Pratt (1969).
[d] Nakashima et al. (1974) and Cuypers et al. (1974).
[e] Bertsch et al. (1974).
[f] Asbeck et al. (1969).
[g] Snell and Offord (1972).

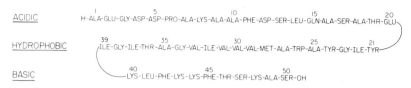

Fig. 3. Amino acid sequence of the major capsid protein (gene 8 protein) of bacteriophage fd. From Asbeck *et al.* (1969) and Nakashima and Konigsberg (1974).

The arrangement of the circular DNA in the filamentous virion has been a subject of considerable controversy. Some electron micrographs have been interpreted in terms of a two-stranded structure in which each strand is separately encapsulated in its own protein coat (Marvin, 1966; Frank and Day, 1970; Griffith and Kornberg, 1972). Alternatively, Bradley (1967) interpreted his electron micrographs in terms of a one-strand model in which both DNA strands are encapsulated in a central core by a single sheath of protein.

More recently, two independent lines of evidence have added further support to the one-strand model. First, it has been found that the two DNA strands can be cross-linked at a small number of points by ultraviolet irradiation of the Ff virion (Francke and Ray, 1972). These results suggest that the two DNA strands are probably in physical contact rather than separated by two layers of coat protein. Second, it now appears that no two-strand model can account for the X-ray diffraction pattern obtained from fibers (Marvin *et al.*, 1974*b*; Wachtel *et al.*, 1974). The only model consistent with the radial electron density distribution and the heavy-atom replacement data is one in which the protein coat forms a hollow tube encasing the DNA with little or no interpenetration of DNA and protein. The protein shell appears to be of 2.5 nm inner diameter and 6 nm outer diameter. In this model, the major capsid proteins are arranged in a left-handed helix of 1.5 nm pitch with 4.5 units per turn. Each protein molecule is elongated in the axial direction, and the molecules slope radially so as to overlap each other similarly to scales on a fish. The structure of the Pfl and Xf bacteriophages appears to be similar to that of the Ff bacteriophages (Marvin *et al.*, 1974*a*).

In addition to its role in phage adsorption (Rossomando and Zinder, 1968; Pratt *et al.*, 1969; Marco *et al.*, 1974), the A protein appears to be involved in viral DNA replication (Jazwinski *et al.*, 1973). Since this minor capsid protein remains associated with the viral DNA even after conversion to the duplex replicative form, it is of interest to know whether the A protein is associated with a specific site on the viral DNA. Such a specific localization of the A protein on the viral DNA would imply that the DNA has a specific orientation in the virion since the A protein appears to be located at only a single tip of the filamentous virion. Experiments to look for a preferred orientation of the circular DNA within the filament have exploited the capacity of sonic fragments of the virus to bind to host cells (Fareed *et al.,* 1966). Only the fragments bearing the adsorbing end of the virus bind to the host receptor site. Using quarter-length fragments derived presumably only from the adsorbing end of the virion, Tate and Petersen (1974*c*) found that the distribution of pyrimidine oligodeoxyribonucleotides from these fragments is identical to that from intact phage DNA. This result implies that there is no preferred orientation of the viral DNA in the filamentous virion and that the A protein is not associated with a specific site on the phage DNA. However, studies on phage attachment in the presence of rifampicin (to be discussed later) appear to be incompatible with a random, fixed orientation of the DNA in the virion.

Studies on the disassembly of Ff virions suggest that the interactions of the gene A and gene B proteins in the virion are qualitatively different. The interaction of the B protein with the viral DNA appears to be highly cooperative since numerous physical and chemical agents cause an all-or-none disassembly of the virion (Rossomando and Zinder, 1968; Rossomando and Bladen, 1969; Rossomando, 1970; Frank and Day, 1970; Ikehara and Utiyama, 1975; Ikehara *et al.,* 1975). The B protein is a highly hydrophobic protein with a high α-helix content. Loss of infectivity of Ff phage in alkali was found to correlate directly with α-helix content (Frank and Day, 1970). The alkali-induced disassembly of the virion appears to be initiated by an ionization of the gene A protein followed by titration of the bulk coat protein (Rossomando and Zinder, 1968). The high cooperativity of the disassembly process has been taken to suggest that the phage structure in aqueous media at neutral pH is stabilized primarily by protein–protein interactions of hydrophobic origin (Ikehara *et al.,* 1975). Exposure of hydrophobic groups upon removal of a single protein molecule is thought to increase the free energy for the surrounding molecules sufficiently to induce dissociation of these molecules. Thus the removal of a single B protein molecule would trigger a rapid and sequential disorganization of the entire virion.

The f1 gene A amber mutant R4 was found to have a decreased alkali stability when grown in either a *su*I (serine) or *su*II (glutamine) host as compared to mutant phage grown in *su*III (tyrosine) host. These results suggest a role for the gene A protein in maintaining the structural integrity of the virion. However, X-ray diffraction data on oriented fibers from R4(Tyr) and R4(Ser) phages show no significant differences between them (Dunker *et al.*, 1974). Furthermore, the gene A protein can be selectively removed from the virion by treatment with 2-chloroethanol without the complete disassembly of the phage particle (Ikehara and Utiyama, 1975). The resulting defective particle lacks infectivity but cannot be distinguished from intact virions by UV absorption, circular dichroism, sedimentation velocity, or CsCl buoyant density. Since the conditions for removal of the A protein from the virion affect the stability of hydrophobic bonding only slightly, it was suggested that the selective loss of the A protein is a reflection of a difference in the electrolytic properties of this protein as compared to the B protein. Segawa *et al.* (unpublished data, cited by Ikehara and Utiyama, 1975) have found that 20% of the amino acid residues of the A protein are acidic while less than 10% are basic. Thus the chloroethanol-induced disassociation could have been induced by the enhancement of the electrostatic repulsion between the DNA and the A protein as a result of the decreased dielectric constant in the presence of the alcohol.

Selective removal of the A protein has also been observed for subtilisin-treated phage (Marco *et al.*, 1974). The particles retain the buoyant density in CsCl of untreated phage but are noninfectious. Heat treatment of phage f1 shows a structural alteration at one end of the virion and suggests that thermal disassembly of the phage begins at one end of the filamentous particle where the A protein is located (Rossomando and Bladen, 1969; Rossomando, 1970; Marco, 1975). These latter experiments have been interpreted to mean that the A protein is located at only one of the two ends of the filamentous virion.

Up to about 5–6% of the phage in a preparation consists of diploid particles of double length and carrying two unit-length DNA molecules (Scott and Zinder, 1967; Salivar *et al.*, 1967). Such diploid particles can be separated from unit-length phage by polyacrylamide gel electrophoresis (Beaudoin *et al.*, 1974; Beaudoin and Pratt, 1974). Infection of nonpermissive cells with gene 3 amber mutants leads to the production of large amounts of noninfectious "polyphage" particles which contain infectious DNA but are much longer than normal phage particles (Pratt *et al.*, 1969). Polyphage have the same UV absorption spectrum and buoyant density in CsCl as normal phage but fail to attach to host cells. Velocity sedimentation of the DNA from polyphage indicates that the DNA is identical in size to that of unit-length phage. The specific infectivity of DNA from polyphage is also equal to that of normal phage, showing that the defectiveness is in the polyphage particle rather than in the DNA contained in such particles.

The yield of diploid phage particles is also increased in infections with phage carrying a mutation in gene 6, a noncapsid protein (Salivar *et al.*, 1967). In mixed infections between amber mutants in nonpermissive hosts, half of the diploid phage are heterozygous, carrying one DNA molecule of each genotype (Scott and Zinder, 1967; Salivar *et al.*, 1967). The highest yield of diploid and heterozygous phage is obtained in crosses between gene 3 and gene 6 mutants. In contrast, mutations in genes 1 and 5 depress the frequency of such particles. The high frequency of heterozygotes in crosses between phage mutants has greatly hindered studies on genetic recombination of the phages of the Ff group.

3. STRUCTURE OF Ff DNA

3.1. Single-Stranded Ring Structure of Ff DNA

The DNA of Ff bacteriophages is judged to be single-stranded on the basis of its noncomplementary base ratio, broad melting profile, unchanged buoyant density after heating to 100°C followed by rapid cooling, and increased sedimentation rate in solutions of high ionic strength (Hoffmann-Berling *et al.*, 1963; Salivar *et al.*, 1964; Marvin and Hohn, 1969). The viral DNA is a covalently closed ring structure (Marvin and Schaller, 1966; Ray and Schekman, 1969*b*) consisting of a single polynucleotide chain linked by phosphodiester bonds (Schaller, 1969). Measurements of the molecular weight of Ff DNA have ranged from 1.7 to 2.5 $\times$ 10^6 (for a review, see Berkowitz and Day, 1974). However, this parameter has been reinvestigated recently by three independent absolute methods (light scattering, equilibrium sedimentation, and sedimentation and diffusion). These measurements are all in close agreement (Table 4) and give a weighted average molecular weight of 1.90 $\pm$ 0.07 $\times$ 10^6 for the sodium salt of Ff DNA (Berkowitz and Day, 1974; Newman *et al.*, 1974). This molecular weight corresponds to 5740 $\pm$ 210 nucleotides. Based on these measurements, the circular duplex replicative form (RF) would have a molecular weight of 3.8 $\pm$ 0.14 $\times$ 10^6.

Thymine accounts for more than one-third of the bases in the viral DNA, leading to a 1.54-fold greater thymine content than that calculated for the complementary strand using the conventional base-pairing rules (Salivar *et al.*, 1964). This large asymmetry in the thymine distribution between the two strands of RF provides the basis for separation of viral and complementary single strands in alkaline CsCl gradients (Ray, 1969).

TABLE 4

Physical Properties of Ff DNA

Diffusion coefficient, $D_{20,w}(10^{-8}cm^2 \cdot s^{-1})$	6.63 ± 0.18^a
Sedimentation coefficient, $s_{20,w}(10^{-13} s)$	24.6 ± 0.4^a
Molecular weight, M ($10^6 g \cdot mol^{-1}$)	
By sedimentation and diffusion	1.87 ± 0.06^a
By equilibrium sedimentation	1.92 ± 0.06^b
By light scattering	1.96 ± 0.12^b
Weighted average	1.90 ± 0.07^b
Number of nucleotides	5740 ± 210^b
Buoyant density in CsCl ($g \cdot cm^{-3}$)	1.722^c
Buoyant density in Cs_2SO_4 ($g \cdot cm^{-3}$)	1.426^c
Radius of gyration, R_G (nm)	41.6 ± 3.5^b
Density increment, $(\partial \rho / \partial c)_\mu$	0.483 ± 0.010^b
Refractive index increment at 436 nm, $(\partial n / \partial c)_\mu (g^{-1} \cdot cm^3)$	0.175 ± 0.019^b
Refractive index increment at 546 nm, $(\partial n / \partial c)_\mu (g^{-1} \cdot cm^3)$	0.170 ± 0.015^b

[a] Newman *et al.* (1974).
[b] Berkowitz and Day (1974).
[c] Szybalski (1968).

3.2. Conformations of Ff DNA

Ff single-stranded viral DNA can exist in at least two different metastable states with characteristic sedimentation rates and conformations (Forsheit and Ray, 1970). Either conformation can be obtained from phage or from infected cells depending on the ionic strength, pH, and temperature during isolation. Interconversion of these two forms occurs at near-physiological conditions, suggesting the possibility of a biological role for the conversion. The faster-sedimenting form observed in high salt appears very compact by electron microscopy while the slower-sedimenting form observed in low salt appears more rigid and elongated with the appearance of single-strand "bushes" separated by short double-stranded regions.

3.3. Self-Complementary Regions in Ff DNA

Further details of the structure of Ff DNA have been obtained from studies of specific regions of the DNA. A DNA core of high GC content remains after digestion of Ff DNA with *Neurospora* endonuclease and *E. coli* exonuclease I (Schaller *et al.,* 1969). This portion of the genome represents only about 150 nucleotides and has a simple distribution of pyrimidine runs. The average chain length of core fragments is around 40 nucleotides, suggesting the existence of three or four such regions per viral DNA molecule. The core also has double-strand-like spectral properties. Its secondary structure recovers rapidly following exposure to denaturing conditions. These data are interpreted in terms of a GC-rich hairpin structure in the viral DNA. Such singularities in the DNA might play important roles in the recognition of the DNA (Gierer, 1966) by one or more enzymes involved in either the replication of the DNA or the morphogenesis of the virion. The probable occurrence of the termini of linear single-strand intermediates in such a hairpin region in the synthesis of ϕX174 circular single strands has been postulated as a mechanism for allowing closure of the termini by the host ligase (Schaller et al., 1969; Schekman and Ray, 1971; Iwaya et al., 1973).

A region of similar size but rich in AT base pairs has been isolated by digestion with an endonuclease which preferentially splits the dG-dG and dG-dA bonds in DNA (Shishido and Ikeda, 1971). Further digestion of this material with the single-strand-specific endonuclease S1 yielded a core fraction with a near-equivalence of dA and dT residues and dG and dC residues. This fraction also exhibited reversible thermal denaturation, suggesting that it too may represent a hairpin structure. The dAT-rich core fragments are in the range of 45–50 nucleotides long and occur at a frequency of about two per viral strand.

3.4. Pyrimidine Tracts in Ff DNA

Degradation of DNA by diphenylamine in acid solution yields a mixture of free purine bases, inorganic phosphate, and pyrimidine oligodeoxyribonucleotides. The pyrimidine tracts released from Ff viral DNAs have been obtained and separated on the basis of chain length in several laboratories (Petersen and Reeves, 1969; Shishido and Ikeda, 1970a,b; Ling, 1972; Tate and Petersen, 1974a,b).

Fractionation of pyrimidine tracts from Ff DNA on a two-dimensional thin-layer system resolves the depurination products on the basis of both size and base composition (Ling, 1972). The polypyrimidine tracts of nine base residues or greater have been sequenced by a technique employing partial digestion with spleen and snake venom phosphodiesterases and fractionation of the partial digests on a two-dimensional thin-layer system. The largest pyrimidine tract contains 20 residues and has the sequence of 5′-C-T-T-T-C-T-T-C-C-C-T-T-C-C-T-T-T-C-T-C-3′. Since the amino acid sequences of the major coat protein (Asbeck et al., 1969; Snell and Offord, 1972; Nakashima and Konigsberg, 1974) and the gene 5 protein (Nakashima et al., 1974; Cuypers et al., 1974) are known, it is possible to decide whether this polypyrimidine sequence could arise from the genes corresponding to either of these proteins. From the amino acid sequences, it can be concluded that neither of the genes for these proteins contains this exceptionally long pyrimidine tract.

The existence of poly(dA) tracts in Ff DNA has been inferred on the basis of a 15 mg per ml density increase of Ff DNA in the presence of a tenfold excess of poly(U) (Sheldrick and Szybalski, 1967). Correspondingly, the complementary strand of Ff RF would be expected to contain some dT-rich clusters.

3.5.   RNA Polymerase Binding Sites

Another method by which a small and unique portion of the Ff DNA has been isolated is by nuclease digestion of complexes of the *E. coli* RNA polymerase and Ff RF (Okamoto *et al.*, 1972; Heyden *et al.*, 1972). There appears to be one strong RNA polymerase binding site per RF, as well as a second weaker binding site. Protection of these specific binding sites by RNA polymerase is not observed in the absence of the σ factor (Shishido and Ando, 1974). The protected DNA in the first binding site contains approximately 40 base pairs. This fragment is double-stranded and upon denaturation yields two distinct single strands with electrophoretic mobilities corresponding to chain lengths of 41 ± 2 and 36 ± 2 nucleotides. The protected DNA from the stronger binding site contains 20 pyrimidines in the viral strand and 21 pyrimidines in the complementary strand. Both binding sites are enriched in AT base pairs just as has been observed for RNA polymerase protected regions in λ DNA (Le Talaer and Jeanteur, 1971). The two binding sites contain none of the previously identified structural peculiarities of Ff DNA, *viz.*, self-complementary hairpin structures or long polypyrimidine tracts. However, nucleic acid sequencing of the stronger binding site (Sugimoto *et al.*, 1975; Schaller *et al.*, 1975) has recently established that this site contains a sequence having twofold rotational symmetry just preceding the point of initiation of a pppGUA-initiated RNA chain (Fig. 4). The point of initiation of the RNA transcript is located in the center of the binding site.

3.6.   DNA Sequence Studies

The C_9T_{11} polypyrimidine tract from Ff phage has been used as a unique primer for the initiation of DNA synthesis by DNA polymerase I on Ff complementary strands (Oertel and Schaller, 1972). By pulse

```
3'- - - - C G A A G A C T G A T A T T A T C T G T C C C A T T T C T G G A C T A A A A A C T A A A - - - - 5'
5'- - - - G C T T C T G A C T A T A A T A G A C A G G G T A A A G A C C T G A T T T T T G A T T T - - - - 3'
            -20              -I0             0           I0            20
```
```
              ppp G U A A A G A C C U G A U U U U U G A U U U A U G G U C A U U C U U C G U U U U - - - - -
```

Fig. 4. Nucleotide sequences of an RNA polymerase binding site and the 5′-pppG-initiated message of bacteriophage fd. The polymerase-binding site contains a sequence having twofold rotational symmetry just preceding the point of initiation of the RNA chain. From Sugimoto *et al.* (1975).

labeling for short time intervals and analyzing the pyrimidine tracts of the reaction products, it was concluded that the reaction products consist of homogeneous single species of DNA growing from a unique point on the DNA template. This approach may prove of value in sequence analysis of limited portions of the Ff genome, particularly with restriction endonuclease fragments which are available now. The sequence of 81 residues of an Ff DNA has been obtained by extension of a chemically synthesized octadeoxyribonucleotide primer (Schott *et al.*, 1973) by DNA polymerase I using labeled nucleoside triphosphates and viral strand template (Sanger *et al.*, 1973, 1974). The octadeoxyribonucleotide A-C-C-A-T-C-C-A functioned as an efficient primer for a specific sequence in the viral DNA. This particular primer sequence was selected as a predicted sequence in the complementary strand from the amino acid sequence Trp-Met-Val in positions 26–28 of the major coat protein. Since the entire sequence of the major coat protein is known (Asbeck *et al.*, 1969), it was expected that the DNA sequence obtained could be checked against the known amino acid sequence and that the intercistronic DNA sequence could be obtained. Unfortunately, the sequence obtained did not correspond to that expected but rather to some other unique sequence in the viral genome. Recent reports of the amino acid sequence of the major coat protein of the Ff phage group (Snell and Offord, 1972; Nakashima and Konigsberg, 1974) suggest that the sequence in the selection region is actually Trp-Ala-Met-Val and thus the hybridization of the primer to a unique site on the viral DNA may have been entirely fortuitous. Nonetheless, the octadeoxynucleotide provided a unique primer which allowed the development of methods for DNA sequencing. The first 12 residues of the synthetic material were determined by use of a two-dimensional "homochromatography" system. Additional sequences were obtained by using the ribo-substitution method, which Salser *et al.* (1972) have adapted for DNA sequencing. This method takes advantage of the ability of DNA polymerase I to incorporate ribonu-cleotides into DNA in the presence of manganese (Berg *et al.*, 1963).

The resulting product can be cleaved specifically with either ribonuclease or alkali and then analyzed by a two-dimensional system.

Extensive additional sequence information has been obtained for several intercistronic regions of Ff DNA by analysis of (1) ribosome-protected initiation sites in mRNA transcribed from duplex Ff DNA (Pieczenik *et al.*, 1974), (2) RNA polymerase protected regions of duplex Ff DNA molecules (Sugimoto *et al.*, 1975; Schaller *et al.*, 1975), and (3) mRNA molecules synthesized on restriction endonuclease fragments of duplex Ff DNA (Sugimoto *et al.*, 1975). These sequences are shown in Fig. 5. Sequences (1) to (3) were derived from RNA synthesized with $\alpha[^{32}P]$ribonucleoside triphosphates using f1 RF DNA as template. The RNA was bound to ribosomes and the initiation complexes were digested with ribonuclease. The protected regions of the labeled mRNA were purified and sequenced by conventional techniques, taking advantage of the ability to determine nearest neighbors.

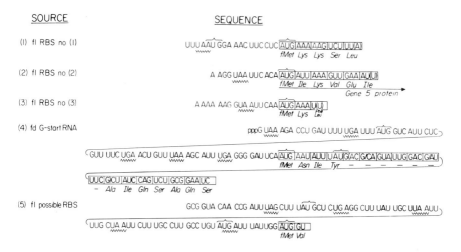

Fig. 5.   Nucleotide sequences of some identified and possible Ff ribosome-binding sites and adjacent sequences. Hypothetical amino acid sequences are given beginning at potential AUG initiator triplets within the sequences. Possible termination triplets are indicated by a sawtooth underline. Sequences (1) to (3) were derived from *in vitro* synthesized RNA protected from pancreatic RNase digestion by ribosomes (Pieczenik *et al.*, 1974). Sequence (4) shows the 5′-terminal sequence of an fd G-start RNA (Sugimoto *et al.*, 1975) and a conjectured point of initiation and sequence of the corresponding protein. Sequence (5) is derived from the DNA sequence obtained by the *in vitro* extension of a chemically synthesized octadeoxyribonucleotide primer (Sanger *et al.*, 1973, 1974). These authors suggest that the AUG triplet at positions 54–56 might be the initiation site for a protein since the sequence GAUUUA shortly before that is similar to sequences characteristically found in this position relative to initiation sites for several known proteins.

Sequence (4) was derived from mRNA synthesized off a restriction endonuclease fragment containing a strong promotor and was also sequenced by conventional RNA sequencing techniques. The RNA polymerase binding site just preceding the start of this chain has also been sequenced and is presented in Fig. 4. Sequence (5) is the expected RNA transcript from the region of f1 DNA sequenced by Sanger *et al.* (1973, 1974) by extension of a chemically synthesized primer.

A common feature of all of these sequences is the presence of an AUG codon preceded by one or more termination codons. In addition to the AUG triplet likely to serve as initiator for translation of the nucleotide sequence, three of the sequences contain one or more other AUG triplets. The selection of the appropriate triplet corresponding to formylmethionine is based on considerations of the presence of in-phase terminators to the right of the AUG and/or the proximity of sequences usually preceding the start of a protein sequence.

Further similarities between these sequences and those of some other ribosome-binding sites are shown in Fig. 6. There appear to be two classes of sequences common to these regions, those containing an AGG triplet and those containing a UUU triplet. For the first class of sequence, there is extensive homology between long sequences containing the AGG triplet. Where data are available for these sequences, a string of purines followed by the triplet CAU precedes the AGG triplet, which is then followed by either AUU or UAA. The sequence homology around the UUU triplet is less extensive. Most often the UUU triplet is surrounded by one or two purines on each side. The biological significance of these sequence homologies and particularly that of the variation on a common sequence remain to be determined.

Another approach to the sequence of Ff ribosome-binding sites has been developed recently (Robertson, 1975). *E. coli* ribosomes were found to bind directly to Ff DNA and to protect a specific region of the DNA from pancreatic DNase digestion. Such fragments can be sequenced by present methods.

So far, only one of the five Ff nucleotide sequences has been identified with a known protein. Seq ence (2) corresponds to the amino terminus of the gene 5 protein. None of the sequences corresponds to the known amino-terminal sequence of the major coat protein. However, Pieczenik *et al.* (1974) have suggested that sequence (1) may correspond to the initiation site for the coat protein since an RNA transcript of less than 1000 nucleotides and containing only ribosome-binding site (1) efficiently directs *in vitro* protein synthesis to yield greater than 90% coat protein. This result suggests the possibility that there may be a precursor form of the coat protein with the amino acid

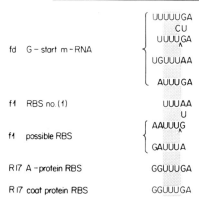

SEQUENCES AROUND AGG PRECEDING AUG

SOURCE	SEQUENCE
	UU GG
fd G−start m−RNA	AAAGCAUGAGGAUUCAAUG
	CC
RI7 Replicase RBS	AAACAUG AGG AUUAC AUG
	CCAA
T7 Early m−RNA RBS	AACAUG AGGUAACA AUG
	UU CA
f1 RBS no. (2)	A AGGUAACA AUG
	UU A
f1 RBS no. (3)	AAAAAAGGUAACA AUG
	AUU
ØX Gene G RBS	AGGUAAUCAUG

SEQUENCES AROUND UUU PRECEDING AUG

fd G − start m − RNA	UUUUUGA
	CU
	UUUUGA
	UGUUUAA
	AUUUGA
f1 RBS no. (1)	UUUAA
	U
f1 possible RBS	AAUUUG
	GAUUUA
RI7 A −protein RBS	GGUUUGA
RI7 coat protein RBS	GGUUUGA

Fig. 6.   Comparison of sequences around possible translation initiation sequences from some DNA and RNA bacteriophages. Data are from the following references: R17, Kozak and Nathans (1972); T7, Arrand and Hindley (1973); fd, Sugimoto *et al.* (1975); f1, Pieczenik *et al.* (1974); φX174, Robertson *et al.* (1973).

sequence predicted by the nucleotide sequence of the f1 ribosome-binding site (1).

Another interesting feature of the known Ff nucleotide sequences is the presence of "true" palindromes (Pieczenik *et al.*, 1974) to the right of the AUG triplet. In f1 ribosome-binding site (2), the "true" palindrome AUUAAAGUUGAAAUUA appears immediately adjacent to the initiator triplet. Similarly, the palindromic sequence UGAAAAAGU overlaps the AUG initiator in the f1 ribosome-binding site (1). The similar presence of a "true" palindrome 11 bases long in the φX174 gene G ribosome-binding site (Robertson *et al.*, 1973) suggests that such sequences may be of some general biological significance. The presence of symmetry elements within coding sequences would greatly restrict the possible amino acid sequences in that region of the gene and could impose a second constraint on allowable nucleic acid sequences in addition to the requirement for the formation of a functional protein.

3.7. *E. coli* B-Specific Modification and Restriction Sites

Ff DNA contains a few methylated bases, as a result of the action of bacterial DNA methylases on intracellular forms of the viral DNA (Benzinger, 1968; Kühnlein *et al.,* 1969; Kühnlein and Arber, 1972; Lautenberger and Linn, 1972; Smith *et al.,* 1972; Hattman, 1973; Van Ormondt *et al.,* 1973; May and Hattman, 1975*a,b*). The bacterial genes controlling the methylation of Ff DNA are the modification genes of the bacterial restriction-modification system of *E. coli* (Arber and Linn, 1969; Boyer, 1971). Ff phages lacking B modification (i.e., unmethylated at B-specific sites) have a lower plating efficiency on *E. coli* B strains. The proportion of infected cells capable of yielding progeny appears to depend on the precise balance between the activities of the restriction endonuclease and the modification methylase.

The *E. coli* B-specific restriction of Ff phages M13 and fd clearly distinguishes between them. Unmodified M13 and fd plate on *E. coli* B with efficiencies of approximately 2×10^{-2} and 4×10^{-4}, respectively (Arber, 1966). This difference appears to result from a different number of *E. coli* B modification (methylation) sites in these viral nucleic acids. M13 contains only a single site while fd and f1 each contain two such sites (Arber and Linn, 1969; Boon and Zinder, 1971; Boyer *et al.,* 1971; Lautenberger and Linn, 1972; Lyons and Zinder, 1972; Kühnlein and Arber, 1972; Smith *et al.,* 1972; Horiuchi *et al.,* 1975). Each site can receive two methyl groups, presumably one on each strand.

Mutants of f1 and fd lacking one or both sites have been isolated. Sites conferring susceptibility to the B-specific restriction endonuclease are indicated by the symbols SB_1 and SB_2. Mutants of fd and f1 which have lost either of the sites (SB_1 or SB_2) are less restricted in their growth on an *E. coli* B strain than wild type. M13 appears to contain only a single such site since it is restricted to the same degree as an fd or f1 phage which has lost one of its sites. Mutants lacking both sites are not restricted in their growth on B strains. The B-specific restriction-modification sites divide the circular genome into two segments with a size ratio of approximately 2:1 (Boon and Zinder, 1971; Lyons and Zinder, 1972). These sites have been located within specific restriction fragments of the f1 genome (Horiuchi *et al.,* 1975). The primary sequence of both strands of the RF appears to be involved in the formation of a functional recognition site for the restriction nuclease since modification or mutation of either strand of a DNA duplex at the SB sites protects the resulting hybrid molecule from restriction (Vovis *et al.,* 1973).

Methylation of fd RF DNA *in vitro* with highly purified B-specific modification methylase and [³H-methyl]-S-adenosylmethionine and partial digestion of the labeled DNA suggest that the sequence surrounding the methylated adenine residue may not contain a twofold rotational symmetry as do the sites for the large number of type II restriction endonucleases (Van Ormondt *et al.,* 1973). However, other lines of evidence support such a symmetrical sequence. First, single-stranded f1 DNA isolated from phage grown on *E. coli* B contains a single *N*-6-methyladenine per SB site (Smith *et al.,* 1972; Hattman, 1973) while f1 RF isolated from *E. coli* K accepts two B-specific methyl groups per SB site as a result of *in vitro* modification (Kühnlein and Arber, 1972; Vovis and Zinder, 1975). Second, f1 hybrid RF molecules in which one strand is modified and the other unmodified accept only one methyl group per SB site regardless of which strand was originally unmodified (Vovis and Zinder, 1975).

Although the SB sites also serve as the recognition sites for the B-specific restriction endonuclease (Linn and Arber, 1968; Boyer *et al.,* 1971; Lautenberger and Linn, 1972; Eskin and Linn, 1972), cleavage of unmodified RF containing only a single restriction site appears to occur at a single random site on the circular molecule since denaturation and renaturation of restricted RF yield circular molecules (Horiuchi and Zinder, 1972). The formation of the circles is not due to the insertion of staggered nicks by the restriction endonuclease since renaturation alone did not circularize the restricted DNA. In addition, the recognition site appears not to be modified by the restriction endonuclease since restricted RF molecules that have been circularized by denaturation and renaturation can be cleaved again by the restriction enzyme.

3.8. Type II Restriction Sites

The use of restriction endonucleases from a variety of bacterial strains has proven to be an exceedingly powerful tool for the analysis of the structure and function of Ff DNA molecules (Takanami, 1973;

Sugisaki and Takanami, 1973; van den Hondel and Schoenmakers, 1973, 1975; Seeburg and Schaller, 1975; Tabak *et al.*, 1974; Horiuchi *et al.*, 1975; Vovis *et al.*, 1975). Many bacterial strains carry one or more restriction endonucleases, each of which recognizes a specific base sequence. These sequence-specific nucleases are designated as type II restriction endonucleases. The high specificity of these enzymes allows the cleavage of DNA molecules into a unique set of fragments. Table 5 lists the number of cleavage sites in Ff RF for some of the known restriction endonucleases.

At least some of the restriction endonucleases are capable of cleaving viral single strands as well as duplex RF molecules (Horiuchi and Zinder, 1975; Blakesley and Wells, 1975). The sites of cleavage in viral single strands appear to be identical to those in the duplex RF.

The order of the specific fragments produced by a single enzyme can be determined from partial digestions followed by redigestion of individual fragments or from the digestion of the product produced using specific fragments as primers for *in vitro* DNA synthesis on a viral template (Seeburg and Schaller, 1975; Takanami *et al.*, 1975; van den Hondel and Schoenmakers, 1975; Horiuchi *et al.*, 1975). A physical map of the Ff genome has been constructed using the single *Hind*II site in Ff RF as a reference point. By hybridization of the com-

TABLE 5

Cleavage of Ff RF by Restriction Endonucleases

Enzyme	Source	Number of cleavage sites			References[a]
		fd RF	M13 RF	f1 RF	
Endo R · *Hind*II	*H. influenzae* Rd	1	1	1	(a–e)
Endo R · *Hin*f	*H. influenzae* Rf	>20	21	>20	(e)
Endo R · *Hin*H-I	*H. influenzae* H-I	3	—	—	(a)
Endo R · *Hae*II	*H. aegyptius*	3	3	3	(c,e)
Endo R · *Hae*III	*H. aegyptius*	11	10	9	(a,b,c,e)
Endo R · *Hap*II	*H. aphirophilus*	13	13	13	(a,b,e)
Endo R · *Hpa*II	*H. parainfluenzae*	13	13	13	(d)
Endo R · *Hha*	*H. haemolyticus*	17	15	16	(e)
Endo R · *Hga*	*H. gallinarum*	6	—	—	(a)
Endo R · *Hsu*	*H. suis*	0	0	0	(e)
Endo R · *Eco*RI	*E. coli*	0	0	0	(e)
Endo R · *Eco*RII	*E. coli*	2	—	2	(f)
Endo R · *Eco*P1	*E. coli*	—	—	5	(c,g)
Endo R · *Alu*	*A. luteus*	15	18	18	(e)
Endo R · *Sma*	*S. marcescens*	0	0	0	(e)

[a] References: (a) Takanami (1973), (b) van den Hondel and Schoenmakers (1973), (c) Horiuchi *et al.* (1975), (d) Seeburg and Schaller (1975), (e) van den Hondel and Schoenmakers (1976), (f) Vovis *et al.* (1975), (g) Model *Et al.* (1975).

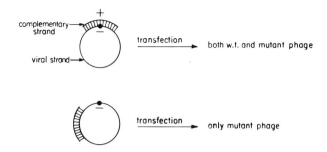

Fig. 7.   Bioassay of complementary strand fragments by hybridization to mutant viral
          strands and transfection of bacterial cells (Middleton *et al.*, 1972).

plementary strands of individual fragments from wild-type RF to different mutant viral strands and infection of bacterial spheroplasts with
these hybrids, known genetic markers have been assigned to specific
fragments (Fig. 7). These results allow a correlation to be made
between the genetic map and the physical map of Ff DNA (Lyons and
Zinder, 1972; Seeburg and Schaller, 1975; van den Hondel *et al.*, 1975;
Horiuchi *et al.*, 1975; van den Hondel and Schoenmakers, 1976).
Physical and genetic maps of Ff DNA are shown in Figs. 8, 9, and 10.
However, since not all of the gene sizes are known, the location of
restriction sites relative to gene boundaries is also only approximate.
The correlation between cleavage maps generated with different restriction enzymes is considerably better since such maps can be constructed
with much greater precision than the genetic map at present. It may be
hoped that the precise localization of more known genetic markers to
specific restriction fragments will eventually refine the correlation
between the physical and genetic maps. Comparison of the restriction
cleavage maps of f1, M13, and fd reveals only slight differences
between these phages, confirming the close relationship of the members
of this group of filamentous phages.

   An interesting feature revealed in the correlation of genetic
markers with specific restriction fragments is the presence of an
apparently noncoding intergenic space between genes 2 and 4 (Fig. 8).
This space is located in the region containing the origin of replication
(Tabak *et al.*, 1974; Suggs and Ray, 1976).

3.9.   Miniature Forms of Ff DNA

   Filaments ranging from 0.2 to 0.5 of the unit length of the Ff
virion have been observed in Ff preparations (Griffith and Kornberg,
1974; Hewitt, 1975; Enea and Zinder, 1975*a*). These particles appear to

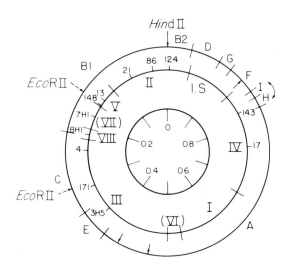

Fig. 8. Physical and genetic map of the f1 genome. The outer circle, representing the physical map, shows the order of the endo R · HaeIII fragments. Arrows on the outside of the circle indicate the cleavage sites for endo R · HindII and endo R · EcoRII; those on the inside of the circle indicate the cleavage sites of endo R · HaeII. The middle circle represents the genetic map with the genes indicated by Roman numerals. Gene sizes were estimated on the basis of the known sizes of the gene products except for genes VI and VII where the gene sizes are unknown. I.S. represents an intergenic space for which no protein is known. The locations of several mutant sites are shown, based on the sizes of the amber fragments synthesized in vitro. From Vovis et al. (1975).

be virions in which a large fraction of the genome has been deleted. The DNA isolated from such particles represents an overlapping series of circular single strands beginning in a common region of the genome near the Hind site and extending in only one direction. The common region shared by all miniphages in the population contains the site for the origin of replication.

Since all of the Ff viral genes are necessary for a productive infection, miniphage are capable of replication only in the presence of a wild-type genome. However, attempts to complement amber mutants in each of the Ff cistrons by mixed infection with amber mutant phage and miniphage have been unsuccessful, suggesting that the genetic content of miniphage cannot be expressed. Yet specific markers can be rescued from miniphage by recombination with two different amber mutant phages, f1 R124 (II_{124}) and f1 R143 (IV_{143}). These two mutants are well mapped: II_{124} is in the proximal portion of gene 2 and IV_{143} is in the distal portion of gene 4 (Horiuchi et al., 1975). This region of the genome is also known to contain the origin of replication (Tabak *et al.*, 1974; Suggs and Ray, 1976). Other gene 2 and gene 4 mutants were not rescued by the miniphage, nor were mutants in other genes. Thus, at least in the case of f1 miniphage, the lack of complementing ability could be explained by the absence of any intact cistrons (Enea and Zinder, 1975*a*).

In cells coinfected with full-length Ff and miniphage, miniature forms of both RF and viral single strands are observed (Griffith and Kornberg, 1974). Figure 11 shows an electron micrograph of M13 unit-length and mini-RF molecules. In coinfections with Ff *am*5 mutants, neither full-length nor mini-forms of single strands are synthesized, although both full-length and mini-forms of RF are made. Similarly, replication of both full-length and mini-RF is inhibited in coinfections with Ff *am*2 mutants. Mini-RF has been observed in nonpermissive cells infected with one particular unit-size gene 5 mutant but not with

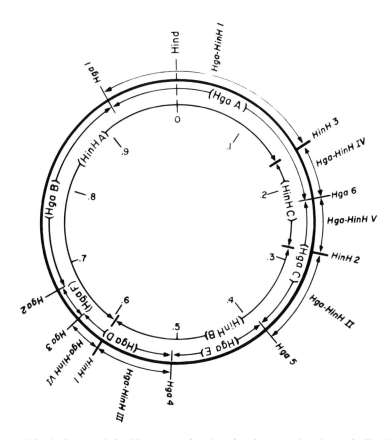

Fig. 9.   Physical map of the fd genome showing the cleavage sites for endo R · *Hind*II, endo R · *Hga*, and endo R · *Hin*H. From Takanami *et al.* (1975).

mutants in other genes (Grandis and Webster, 1973*b*). Although this particular gene 5 lesion might enhance the generation of miniphage DNA, other workers have reported that particles in *am*5 phage preparations are full length (Hewitt, 1975). The subsequent finding of miniphage particles in the *am*5 phage preparation used by Grandis and Webster leaves open the likely possibility that their results could be specific to that particular phage preparation rather than to the specific gene 5 defect (Enea and Zinder, 1975*a*).

Miniphage were first observed in phage preparations obtained after multiple passages beyond the original single plaque isolation (Griffith and Kornberg, 1974). In a study of the phage produced on repeated serial transfer, it was found that the yield of infectious phage particles drops sharply upon serial transfer (Enea and Zinder, 1975*a*). This apparent loss of titer can be accounted for by the concomitant production of miniphage particles. In reconstruction experiments, it was found that miniphage particles can outgrow the intact virion by a factor of about 10 in 2 h. When miniphage particles first appear in an infected culture, they are remarkably uniform in size, but upon additional serial transfers they become very heterogeneous.

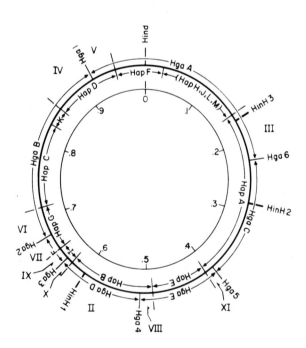

Fig. 10. Localization of the endo R·*Hap* fragments on the fd physical map. Fragments produced by cleavage with both *Hap* and *Hga* endonucleases are indicated by Roman numerals (II to XI). From Takanami *et al.* (1975).

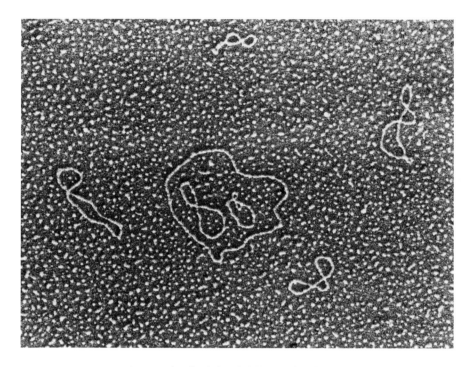

Fig. 11.   Electron micrograph of M13 mini-RF molecules and a single unit-length
RF II molecule. Courtesy of J. Griffith.

Unlike most deletion mutants in other bacteriophages, the Ff mini-phage particles are of the same density as intact virions. This is probably due to the filamentous nature of the virion. The length of Ff virions, like that of rod-shaped RNA viruses, appears to be determined solely by the length of DNA to be encoated. Thus the loss of structural proteins is directly proportional to the loss of DNA in the deletion mutants.

Propagation of miniphage in the presence of a helper phage seems to require only that the mini-form of the DNA be packaged into a fila-mentous particle and that it contain the origin of replication. The minimum size of miniphage particles observed so far is about 20–25% of the genome. It will be of interest to see if still smaller variants can be obtained. In principle, such mutants may need only the origin of replication, a segment of DNA considerably less than that contained in the smallest particles obtained thus far.

The generation of miniphage may be the result of an error in replication or recombination of the unit-size viral genome. Large amounts of mini-forms of viral DNA have been observed in infections of *E. coli* $polA_{ex-1}$, a conditional lethal mutant having a temperature-sensitive $5' \rightarrow 3'$-exonuclease activity associated with polymerase I (Chen and Ray, 1976). This strain was isolated originally on the basis of its hyperrecombinant phenotype (Konrad and Lehman, 1974).

3.10. Multiple-Length Forms of Ff DNA

In addition to the unit-length progeny and replicative forms of Ff DNA, both double-length single-stranded and double-stranded forms of DNA have been detected in small amounts (Jaenisch *et al.,* 1969; Wheeler *et al.,* 1974). By zonal ultracentrifugation of nucleic acid extracts of infected cells, a small amount of double-length and catenated forms of RF can be observed. The origin and significance of these rare forms are unknown. By electron microscopic examination of viral single strands extracted from phage particles, it was found that 0.03% of the single-strand rings were of double length. Such double-length progeny single strands might well arise by an error in processing of the nascent single strands.

4. PHAGE ATTACHMENT AND INITIATION OF INFECTION

Attachment of Ff phage particles to the host cell has long been regarded to occur at the tip of the F pilus of male cells (Marvin and Hohn, 1969). Both the presence of F pili on sensitive cells and the electron microscopic observations of filamentous phage particles attached to the end of the F pilus in male cells have provided the basis for this concept (Caro and Schnös, 1966; Jacobson, 1972). Furthermore, the number of adsorption sites on a sensitive cell is very limited, as are the number of F pili per cell (Tzagoloff and Pratt, 1964). However, the recent work of Marco *et al.* (1974) has raised serious doubts concerning the accepted role of the F pilus. These workers have found that the binding of phage to sensitive cells is inhibited under the conditions of low temperature or cyanide poisoning used in earlier electron microscopic studies and that phage binding and conversion to the parental replicative form occur as efficiently in disrupted cell preparations from F$^-$ cells, lacking F pili, as in preparations from F$^+$ cells. Furthermore, decapsidation and penetration of the DNA into the cell were found to be tightly coupled to formation of the parental RF. These results raise the possibility that the phage particles observed bound to the tips of pili may not lead to productive infections. This view is supported by the electron microscopic observation of phage binding at 37°C in the absence of cyanide to the cell surface rather than to pili (Jacobson, 1972). Marco and colleagues suggest the possibility that the phage receptor may be located in the inner membrane such that it is masked in intact F^- cells but revealed in F^+ cells, perhaps by shedding of the F pilus.

Injection of the viral DNA into the host cell is inhibited by thymine starvation of a thymine-requiring host (Forsheit and Ray, unpublished results); treatment with rifampicin, a specific inhibitor of RNA polymerase (Brutlag et al., 1971; Marco et al., 1974); or infection at nonpermissive temperature with a mutant in the gene 3 protein (Jazwinski et al., 1973). The kinetics and binding of Ff phage to sensitive cells are not altered by rifampicin except for the accumulation of noninfectious (eclipsed) phage particles which retain the size and appearance of infectious phage. However, these eclipsed filamentous particles are sensitive to DNase attack after removal from the cell membrane. It therefore appears that infection can proceed up to the point of RNA polymerase attachment to the DNA origin of replication while still preserving the phage structure. Parental RF formation also does not occur in cells infected at nonpermissive temperature with a temperature-sensitive gene 3 mutant. Thus in the absence of either a functional A protein or an active form of RNA polymerase the viral DNA is neither decapsidated nor converted to the parental RF. The amount of viral DNA in an eclipsed phage particle available for interaction with cellular enzymes must be extremely small, suggesting that the exposed portion of the DNA must carry both the RNA polymerase attachment site required for the unique initiation of the complementary strand (Tabak et al., 1974) and the binding site for the A protein. Since the complementary DNA strand is not initiated in the absence of either a functional A protein or RNA polymerase, both proteins may interact with the viral DNA at overlapping or adjacent sites. These results imply that the viral DNA has a unique orientation in the filamentous virion and is incompatible with models of the virion in which the DNA is fixed in a random orientation (Tate and Petersen, 1974c). It also conflicts with earlier models in which the F pilus served to conduct free phage DNA into the cell (Brinton, 1972).

Infection of cells with phage labeled in the coat proteins as well as in the DNA results in the essentially complete retention of the coat protein label by the cells relative to the DNA label (Trenkner et al., 1967; Smilowitz, 1974; Marco et al., 1974). The major capsid protein (gene 8 protein) enters the cytoplasmic membrane, where it is subsequently reutilized in the assembly of new phage. However, the kinetics and efficiency of utilization of parental coat protein monomers in phage assembly clearly distinguish parental coat proteins from newly synthesized monomers. Eighty percent of the label in newly synthesized coat proteins is released from the cell as phage by 6 min after synthesis, whereas 75% of the label derived from parental phage coat is released from the cell by 2 h after infection and only one-third of the counts are in phage (Smilowitz, 1974). The remainder of the parental label can be recovered from the medium as phage coat protein molecules. Since the parental coat protein is inserted into the cytoplasmic membrane from the outside and the newly synthesized coat protein is inserted from the inside, this difference may determine the rate of utilization of each. However, both the parental and newly synthesized coat proteins are located in the cytoplasmic membrane (Smilowitz *et al.,* 1972; Smilowitz, 1974), and in the same orientation (W. Wickner, 1975). From studies of the binding of ^{125}I-labeled anticoat antibody to spheroplasts or to inverted vesicles, the parental and newly synthesized coat protein were both found to be exposed only on the outer surface of the cytoplasmic membrane. The different rates of utilization of parental and newly synthesized capsid proteins therefore may reside in more subtle differences in these proteins which have not yet been detected.

The A protein (gene 3 protein) is also transferred on infection to the host cell, where it is found in tight association with the viral DNA even after conversion to a double-stranded replicative form (Jazwinski *et al.,* 1973). However, during either the binding or eclipse of the phage the A protein is reduced to a low molecular weight form, at least as judged by a radioactive histidine label (Marco *et al.,* 1974).

5. PARENTAL RF FORMATION (SS→RF)

5.1. Involvement of a Minor Capsid Protein

The first step in the Ff DNA synthetic process is the conversion of the infecting viral DNA to a duplex replicative form. This reaction appears to occur in association with the inner membrane of the bacterial cell (Jazwinski *et al.,* 1973). When gently lysed Ff-infected cells were sedimented to equilibrium in a sucrose gradient, both the viral DNA and the Ff adsorption protein, the gene 3 or A protein, cosedimented with DPNH oxidase, a marker for the inner membrane. RF molecules labeled in their DNA with ^{32}P and in the gene 3 protein with [^{3}H]histidine showed a ^{3}H/^{32}P ratio close to that of the intact virions.

This close association of the gene 3 protein with the viral DNA even after conversion to the duplex replicative form suggests that the gene 3 protein may be involved in intracellular events in the Ff replication cycle.

The gene 3 protein has been hypothesized to play a role in the formation of the parental RF by attaching the infecting viral DNA to the inner cell membrane or, perhaps, to a membrane-associated cellular replicative system (Jazwinski *et al.*, 1973). Ff phage carrying a temperature-sensitive mutation in gene 3 fails to form the parental RF at nonpermissive temperature. However, this failure could have resulted either from a block in parental RF formation at the nonpermissive temperature or from an inability of the mutant phage to attach to or penetrate the host cell at elevated temperature.

It should be noted that viral DNA is synthesized and released from infected cells as noninfectious "polyphage" particles in infections of nonpermissive hosts with gene 3 amber mutant phage (Pratt *et al.*, 1969). The phage particles initiating such infections carry a functional gene 3 protein as a result of propagation of the mutant phage on an amber-suppressing host cell. Replication of this gene 3 defective phage might depend on the presence of a functional A protein on the parental RF molecule. However, the noninfectious "polyphage" particles produced in this case are apparently totally lacking the A protein, yet their DNA is fully infectious to spheroplasts. This result is inconsistent with an essential role for the A protein in M13 DNA replication in spheroplasts. It is unclear, at present, whether this apparent difference in the requirement for the A protein in spheroplasts relative to intact cells represents a different mechanism of replication in the two cases or whether there might be a substantial conflict in the interpretation of these experiments.

5.2. Drug Sensitivity of Parental RF Formation

Conversion of infecting Ff viral DNA to RF is prevented by rifampicin, an inhibitor of the *E. coli* RNA polymerase, but not by chloramphenicol, an inhibitor of protein synthesis (Brutlag *et al.*, 1971). Yet an *E. coli* mutant having a rifampicin-resistant RNA polymerase forms the parental RF even in the presence of the drug. These results suggested a direct involvement of RNA polymerase in the formation of the M13 parental RF and led to the *in vitro* demonstration of the RNA-primed initiation of the complementary strand (W. Wickner *et al.*, 1972).

The formation of M13 parental RF in the presence of high concentrations of chloramphenicol indicates that phage-specific protein synthesis is not required for parental RF formation (Pratt and Erdahl, 1968; Fidanián and Ray, 1972). This result is consistant with the observation that the complementary strand of the RF is the coding strand (Jacob and Hofschneider, 1969).

Synthesis of the Ff complementary strand is resistant to nalidixic acid, an inhibitor of bacterial DNA replication, during formation of the parental RF (Fidanián and Ray, 1972). Cells infected in the presence of nalidixic acid express at least one viral function, that of gene 2, indicating that the complementary strand of the parental RF formed in the presence of the drug is of high fidelity and is capable of being expressed. In contrast, complementary strand synthesis is preferentially inhibited by the drug during RF→RF replication (Fidanián and Ray, 1974). The basis for this clear distinction between the reactions leading to complementary strand synthesis in these two cases is unknown. Perhaps RF replication involves a nalidixic acid sensitive component not required for parental RF formation. Alternatively, parental RF formation may occur at a protected site within the cell membrane.

5.3. Parental RF Formation by Bacterial Enzymes

The chloramphenicol resistance of parental RF formation indicated that bacterial enzymes are sufficient for RF formation. Synthesis of M13 parental RF by a rifampicin-sensitive process has been observed in soluble extracts of uninfected *E. coli* (W. Wickner *et al.,* 1972; R. B. Wickner *et al.,* 1972). Reconstitution of this reaction has been achieved recently with purified bacterial enzymes (Geider and Kornberg, 1974).

The RF formed *in vitro* contains an intact circular viral strand and a unit-length linear complementary strand. This conversion takes place by a two-stage process. Enzymes, ribonucleoside triphosphates, and single-stranded DNA are required in the first stage and the reaction is rifampicin sensitive. The macromolecular product of this reaction supports DNA synthesis in the presence of only deoxyribonucleoside triphosphates and a fresh addition of enzymes. This second stage of the reaction neither requires ribonucleoside triphosphates nor is sensitive to rifampicin. Thus it appears that an RNA chain formed during the first stage of the reaction primes the synthesis of the complete DNA chain. The *in vitro* synthesized RF contains a single $5' \rightarrow 3'$ phosphodiester link of a deoxyribonucleotide to a ribonucleotide. Alkaline hydrolysis of the RF II synthesized with all four [α-³²P]deoxyribonucleoside triphosphates yielded approximately 1 mol of labeled ribonucleotide per mole of RF (Schekman *et al.*, 1972; W. Wickner *et al.*, 1972). The mixtures of 2′- and 3′-ribonucleotides to which ³²P was transferred contained 84% of the label in AMP.

Both intact cells and soluble extracts of *E. coli* are rifampicin sensitive in the conversion of Ff SS to RF but not in that of φX174. Upon reconstitution of the M13 reaction with purified proteins, it was found that both M13 and φX174 DNAs were converted to RF by a rifampicin-sensitive process (W. Wickner *et al.*, 1973; Geider and Kornberg, 1974). This nonphysiological conversion of φX174 SS to RF led to the identification and purification of a novel form of RNA polymerase (W. Wickner and Kornberg, 1974a). This new form of RNA polymerase, called RNA polymerase III, appears to contain a small subunit which confers on the enzyme the ability to discriminate between M13 and φX174 templates. Unlike RNA polymerase I, RNA polymerase III has only a feeble capability for transcription of duplex DNA.

In addition to RNA polymerase III, the reconstituted M13 reaction requires the *E. coli* DNA unwinding protein and a holoenzyme form of DNA polymerase III (W. Wickner and Kornberg, 1974b). The ability of RNA polymerase III to discriminate between M13 and φX174 templates depends on the coating of the template single strand with unwinding protein. In its absence, both are capable of being primed by RNA polymerase III. One function of the unwinding protein may be to facilitate the correct selection of the initiation site, perhaps by masking other possible initiation sites. A model of the *in vitro* SS→RF replication process is shown in Fig. 12.

The DNA polymerase III holoenzyme is a new form of polymerase III containing a 140,000 dalton polypeptide polymerase and a 77,000 dalton polypeptide copolymerase. The "core" polymerase activity of this enzyme was isolated initially as an oligomer of

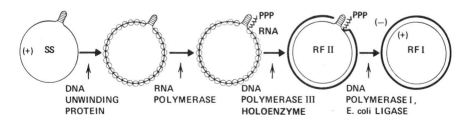

Fig. 12.   Model of the *in vitro* SS → RF reaction (Schekman *et al.*, 1974).

polymerase III called polymerase III* which required a copolymerase called copolymerase III* for the replication of long single-stranded templates (W. Wickner *et al.,* 1973). The use of the term "holoenzyme" is in analogy with the RNA polymerase holoenzyme, where the σ subunit is no longer required after a chain has been initiated. Similarly, copolymerase III* appears to be required for formation of the initiation complex but not for replication. Formation of the initiation complex requires ATP, which is cleaved to ADP and inorganic phosphate upon addition of deoxynucleotides. This need for ATP in the polymerase III* system and its participation in the synthesis of an RNA primer account for two functions that ATP performs in M13 DNA synthesis.

A further requirement for the polymerase III holoenzyme is for phospholipid (W. Wickner and Kornberg, 1974*b*). This requirement can be met by *E. coli* lipid extract, *E. coli* phosphatidylethanolamine, or ox brain diphosphatidylglycerol.

Extracts of *dna*E mutants can perform the *in vitro* conversion of SS to RF when supplemented with polymerase III* but not with polymerase I, II, or III (W. Wickner *et al.,* 1973). This result is in contrast to *in vivo* experiments showing at most only a twofold reduction in the amount of parental RF formed at nonpermissive temperature in a *dna*E mutant (Staudenbauer, 1974). Yet in a *pol*A mutant with a wild-type *dna*E gene the amount of parental RF formed is reduced still further, and in a *pol*A *dna*E double mutant under the same conditions the amount of parental RF formed is reduced more than twentyfold. This striking effect of a mutation in the *pol*A gene suggests that polymerase I may play an essential role in SS→RF synthesis *in vivo.* Whatever role polymerase I might play in this process, it would appear to be more than just a gap filling upon termination of a complete round of synthesis since formation of both RF II and RF I is reduced as a result of the *pol*A mutation.

The apparent lack of a requirement for polymerase I in the *in vitro* system sharply contrasts with the *in vivo* results and underscores the importance of *in vivo* experiments in establishing the validity and relevance of systems constructed by reconstitution of purified enzymes. However, the eventual resolution of the detailed mechanism of replication will depend largely on the successful reconstitution of the replication apparatus from the purified components. The problem is complicated, unfortunately, by the multitude of bacterial enzymes capable of participating in the replicative process *in vitro.* This point is clearly seen in the widely different requirements for host functions in SS→RF synthesis for bacteriophage M13 compared to φX174 and the related phage G4 (Schekman *et al.,* 1974). These systems differ, as far as is known, only in the requirements for specific components in the process of chain initiation. The unique initiation of a DNA chain on an M13 template requires the unwinding protein and the usual rifampicin-sensitive RNA polymerase. The rifampicin-resistant initiation on a ϕX174 or G4 template strand is more complex. The *dna*G protein and the unwinding protein are required for the RNA-primed initiation at a unique site on the G4 viral strand, and an additional four proteins, including the *dna*B and *dna*C proteins, are required for initiation on a ϕX174 template.

5.4. A Unique Gap in the Parental Complementary Strand of M13 DNA

A single and unique origin of replication has been suggested for the *in vitro* SS→RF conversion (Tabak *et al.*, 1974). The RF II molecules formed in this reaction contain a gap at a unique site in the complementary strand. This conclusion is based on the following properties of RF II molecules formed in this reaction: (1) A restriction endonuclease from *Haemophilus influenzae* cuts the RF II molecule near the site of the discontinuity, cleaving the complementary strand into a large and a small fragment. (2) A restriction enzyme from *Haemophilus parain-fluenzae* cleaves RF I molecules into at least nine fragments, one of which is missing from the RF II but is observed after filling in the gap in the complementary strand by DNA polymerase; the newly added nucleotides are contained largely in the small complementary strand fragment produced by treatment of the RF II with the *H. influenzae* restriction endonuclease, establishing the proximity of the 3′-terminus of the complementary strand to this restriction site. (3) Pyrimidine tract analysis of the repaired region shows a simple and distinct pattern compared to that of the entire strand. (4) Cleavage of the RF II within the gap by the single-strand-specific endonuclease S1 yields linear duplex molecules which, after denaturation and reannealing, form linear double-stranded molecules rather than circular duplexes; this indicates that the gap occurs at a unique site in the molecule.

5.5 Location of the RNA Primer at the 5′-Terminus of the Complementary Strand

Conversion of this gapped form of RF II to an alkali-resistant RF I has been accomplished through the joint action of the *E. coli* polymerase I and ligase (Westergaard *et al.*, 1973; Geider and Kornberg, 1974). However, substitution of the T4 DNA polymerase for the *E. coli* enzyme proved ineffective, presumably because of the unique capacity of DNA polymerase I to excise RNA at the 5′-terminus of a DNA strand. Use of both the T4 polymerase and T4 ligase, an enzyme capable of joining RNA and DNA strands, was effective in forming RF I, although in this case the supercoils were sensitive to alkali. These results further support the existence of an RNA primer for the complementary strand. The RNA can be localized at the 5′-end of the complementary strand since a DNA-RNA ligation is required for the production of an alkali-labile RF I and a 5′→3′-nuclease excision activity appears necessary for the formation of an alkali-stable RF I.

6. RF REPLICATION (RF→RF)

6.1. Requirement for a Phage Function

A single viral gene function, that of gene 2, is required for the replication of Ff RF (Pratt and Erdahl, 1968). Infection of nonpermissive host cells by amber mutants in gene 2 leads to the formation of parental RF molecules, although replication of these parental RFs is inhibited. This result is clearly seen in [^{32}P]Ff *am*2 infection of nonpermissive cells in the presence of [^{3}H]thymidine. The RF molecules formed under these conditions contain tritium label only in the complementary strand of the RF (Fidanián and Ray, 1972). Similar results are obtained in wild-type infections in the presence of chloramphenicol. The inability of the parental RF to replicate even a single time in the absence of a functional gene 2 product indicates an essential role for the gene 2 protein in RF→RF replication.

An additional effect seen in such experiments (Fidanián and Ray, 1972; Lin and Pratt, 1972; Tseng and Marvin, 1972*b*) is a significant reduction in the amount of RF II formed, suggesting an involvement of gene 2 in the formation or stabilization of RF II, as in the case of the analogous φX174 gene A function (Francke and Ray, 1971). Analysis of the circularity of the denaturation products of Ff RF II molecules formed in *rep* host cells, mutants which allow parental RF formation but not its replication, shows that the ^{3}H-labeled complementary strand is covalently closed while the ^{32}P-labeled viral strand has a single discontinuity (Fidanián and Ray, 1972).

These results suggest a direct involvement of the gene 2 protein in the stable accumulation of an RF II species which serves as the immediate precursor of replicative intermediates. As one possibility, the gene 2 protein might function as either a site-specific endonuclease or an activator of such a host enzyme. Alternatively, the gene 2 protein might play a role subsequent to the formation of RF II such as the modification of the 5′-terminus of the nicked duplex to prevent its closure by the host ligase.

6.2. Involvement of Host Functions

With the discovery that only a single viral gene is required for Ff RF replication (Pratt and Erdahl, 1968), it became evident that duplex DNA replication must also rely on bacterial functions, possibly those normally required for replication of the bacterial chromosome or those involved in repair or recombination of the host genome.

Five bacterial genes are presently known to participate in Ff RF replication, the *rep, dna*B, *dna*G, and *dna*E genes (Fidanián and Ray, 1972; Olsen *et al.*, 1972; Staudenbauer *et al.*, 1973; Staudenbauer, 1974; Ray *et al.*, 1975), and RNA polymerase (Brutlag *et al.*, 1971; Fidanián and Ray, 1974). In strains of *E. coli* carrying a thermosensitive mutation in the *dna*B gene, viral DNA synthesis is inhibited when cells are infected at the nonpermissive temperature. However, if the cells are first infected at the permissive temperature and then shifted to nonpermissive temperature after phage production has begun, the synthesis of progeny single strands and production of mature phage continue (Primrose *et al.*, 1968). This result suggests that an early stage of M13 DNA replication is inhibited by a mutation in the *dna*B gene. Experiments with *dna*B mutants infected in the presence of chloramphenicol at permissive temperature to allow formation of only the parental RF, followed by a shift to chloramphenicol-free medium at either permissive or nonpermissive temperature and [³H]thymidine pulse labeling, reveal a temperature sensitivity of RF replication (Olsen *et al.*, 1972). From these results, it appears that the semiconservative duplication, but not the synthesis of progeny single-stranded DNA, depends specifically on the *dna*B gene product.

The *dna*G protein, a rifampicin-resistant RNA polymerase (Bouché *et al.*, 1975), also appears to be required only for RF→RF replication (Ray *et al.*, 1975). Infection of an *E. coli dna*G mutant at nonpermissive temperature leads to the formation of only the parental RF. Further replication of the parental RF is inhibited under these conditions. However, if a brief period of viral DNA replication is allowed at permissive temperature prior to shifting the cells to nonpermissive temperature, viral single strands are synthesized and mature phage is released at a normal rate for at least 2 h.

The role of the *dna*G protein in RF→RF replication is unknown.

However, the recent finding that the *dna*G protein can synthesize an oligoribonucleotide primer on the single-stranded DNA of bacteriophage G4, a ϕX174-related icosahedral phage, suggests that it might function similarly in M13 RF replication. Experiments designed to detect a preferential or exclusive involvement of the *dna*G and *dna*B proteins with the initiation or synthesis of only the complementary strand during RF→RF replication indicated a requirement for these proteins for the synthesis of both strands (Ray *et al.*, 1975). Since Ff viral strand synthesis can continue in the absence of complementary strand synthesis (Fidanián and Ray, 1974) by the asymmetrical replicative mechanism by which progeny viral strands are normally synthesized, the immediate inhibition of both viral and complementary strand synthesis following a shift to nonpermissive temperature indicates that both the *dna*B and *dna*G proteins are necessary for the synthesis of both strands of the duplex replicative form. However, it should be emphasized that a selective inhibition of viral strand synthesis would also prevent the synthesis of the complementary strand since the nascent viral strand is the template for complementary strand synthesis (Tseng and Marvin, 1972a).

Pulse-labeling experiments early in Ff infection of *dna*E mutants also reveal a thermosensitivity of RF replication (Staudenbauer *et al.*, 1973). Since the *dna*E gene specifies DNA polymerase III (Gefter *et al.*, 1971; Nüsslein *et al.*, 1971), this is likely to be the enzyme responsible for polymerization of deoxynucleotides during RF duplication.

As also proposed for *E. coli* DNA replication, polymerase I may function in Ff RF→RF replication by the sealing of gaps in newly replicated DNA. The role that polymerase I might play in such a process could be the polymerization of deoxynucleotides to close any gaps and/or the removal of RNA primers (Berkower *et al.*, 1973). Although RF replication was not reduced significantly in experiments with a *pol*A mutant, there was a striking increase in the relative amount of RF II formed (Staudenbauer, 1974). Similar observations have been made for ϕX174 (Schekman *et al.*, 1971).

An important reservation about initial experiments with *pol*A mutants, however, is the finding by Lehman and Chien (1973) of a low but significant level of polymerase I in all *pol*A strains available at that time. This residual level of polymerizing activity is probably due to readthrough of the amber mutation in the original mutant. Surprisingly, all of these *pol*A mutants were found to have a near-normal level of polymerase I $5' \to 3'$-exonuclease activity. Thus the initial observation by Kluge *et al.* (1971) of a normal level of Ff phage production in a *pol*A mutant could well have been due to residual polymerase I activity and/or a normal level of the $5' \to 3'$ exonuclease.

The recent isolation of conditional lethal *pol*A mutants by Konrad and Lehman (1974) has allowed a reinvestigation of the role of polymerase I in Ff DNA replication. Initial studies with *E. coli* *pol*Aex-1, a mutant defective in the 5′→3′-exonuclease activity but not in the polymerase activity of polymerase I, have shown a striking temperature sensitivity of Ff phage production in this mutant (Chen and Ray, 1976). Further studies with this mutant may uncover a role for a polymerase I in RF→RF replication. Its role in RF→SS synthesis will be discussed later.

The specificity of Ff phage for male strains of *E. coli* raises the possibility that some sex factor genes might be involved in the replication of the viral DNA. This appears not to be the case, however, since Ff DNA is infectious to spheroplasts of female strains of *E. coli* (Ray *et al.*, 1966*a*).

6.3.   Mechanics of Ff RF Replication

Many important details of the mechanism of Ff RF replication remain to be elucidated. Currently, it appears that RF duplication may involve a replicating intermediate with some of the same structural features as in the intermediate in single-strand synthesis. As will be discussed later, single-strand synthesis occurs via a rolling circle structure (Gilbert and Dressler, 1968) in which the viral strand is "rolled off" of a circular complementary strand template while new viral strand material is being polymerized (Marvin and Hohn, 1969; Ray, 1969; Forsheit *et al.*, 1971; Staudenbauer and Hofschneider, 1972*a*; Kluge, 1974). The rolling circle model suggests that the tail of the elongated viral strand serves as a template for complementary strand synthesis. There may be one or more initiation signals for complementary strand synthesis contained on the viral strand, and, as these become exposed, complementary strand synthesis is initiated. In this model, the eventual conversion to solely viral strand synthesis is thought to result from binding of the gene 5 protein to the viral strand tail of the replicating intermediate to prevent initiation of complementary strands. An important feature of the proposed model of Ff RF replication is that the two strands of the duplex DNA are not equivalent. The model utilizes the basic asymmetry of the single-strand replication intermediate. An extension of earlier models along with the proposed involvement of viral gene functions and the sites of inhibition by several drugs is presented in Fig. 13.

A potential source of difficulty in the analysis of RF replication intermediates is the lack of a sharp division between the period of

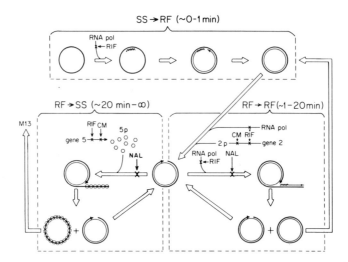

Fig. 13. Model of the M13 DNA replication process. The three stages of M13 DNA replication are indicated schematically with an indication of the approximate duration of each stage and the sites of inhibition by rifampicin (RIF), chloramphenicol (CM), and nalidixic acid (NAL). Symbols: thick line, viral strand; thin line, complementary strand; "sawtooth" line, RNA primer strand; arrowhead, 3′-OH terminus; hexagon, gene 5 protein; RNA pol, *E. coli* RNA polymerase. From Fidanián and Ray (1974).

duplex DNA replication and asymmetrical single-strand synthesis. Even very early in Ff infection, a small but readily detectable amount of single-strand synthesis is occurring (Forsheit *et al.,* 1971). This could presumably be due to a competition between complementary strand initiation and prevention of its initiation by binding of gene 5 protein to the initiation site. Thus the finding of pulse-labeled molecules having elongated viral strands could potentially be due to the presence of single-strand replication intermediates even at a time of predominant RF duplication.

This difficulty can be overcome by analyzing RF duplication in mutants carrying an amber mutation in gene 5. In this case, the switchover to asymmetrical single-strand synthesis does not occur (Pratt and Erdahl, 1968). Pulse-labeled molecules sedimenting even faster than RF I are observed in Ff *am*5-infected nonpermissive host cells (Tseng and Marvin, 1972*a*). This fast-sedimenting material contains a larger fraction of the pulse label in a 20-s pulse than in a 60-s pulse, suggesting that components sedimenting faster than RF I are enriched in replicative intermediates. Resedimentation of pulse-labeled DNA from this region in high-salt and in low-salt sucrose gradients shows that a large fraction of the presumed replicative intermediates sediment in high salt at 26 S, faster than RF I, but sediment in low salt at about 20 S, only slightly faster than RF II. This large dependence of sedimentation rate on ionic strength suggests that these molecules have partially single-stranded character. Under the same conditions, the sedimentation coefficient of viral single strands is 29 S in high salt and 13 S in low salt. Further support for a partial single strandedness of these pulse-labeled structures is the finding that these molecules have a density in CsCl of 1.704 g per ml, intermediate between that of RF (1.701 g per ml) and viral single strands (1.722 g per ml). Analysis of the denaturation products of these molecules by alkaline velocity sedimentation shows that these structures contain strands that sediment both faster and slower than unit-length circular molecules. The faster-sedimenting single strands derived from such intermediates all have the equilibrium density in alkaline CsCl of viral strands while the slower-sedimenting single strands are of both viral and complementary strand densities. These results support the proposed model of Ff RF replication, although they do not unequivocally establish the structure of the replicative intermediate. Both rolling circle and Cairns-type structures are readily visualized (Fig. 14) in Ff RF preparations (Fidanián and Ray, unpublished observations). The significance of such structures and their relationship to the replicative process remain to be determined.

An important detail of the mechanism of replication is the mechanism by which the complementary strand is initiated. The rifampicin sensitivity of Ff RF duplication (Brutlag *et al.,* 1971; Fidanián and Ray, 1974) suggests that the complementary strand may be initiated by an RNA primer just as in the formation of the parental RF (W. Wickner *et al.,* 1972). Synthesis of the complementary strand appears to be approximately tenfold more sensitive to rifampicin than is that of the viral strand (Fidanián and Ray, 1974). Since Ff complementary strand synthesis is initially stimulated by chloramphenicol (Ray, 1970; Brutlag *et al.,* 1971), its rapid inhibition by rifampicin is most probably due to a direct effect of rifampicin on an RNA polymerase mediated event in the replicative process rather than to an inhibition of gene expression. Thus, as a further elaboration of the Ff replication model, it is proposed that the viral strand contains one or more sites for the initiation of RNA primer strands for DNA chain initiation. As the viral strand is rolled off its circular complementary strand template, such sites might become exposed and lead to the formation of a new complementary strand attached to an RNA primer. In such a mechanism, the viral strand tail of the replicative intermediate would be partially single-stranded. Replicating forks showing apparent discontinuous synthesis and partial single-strandedness on one

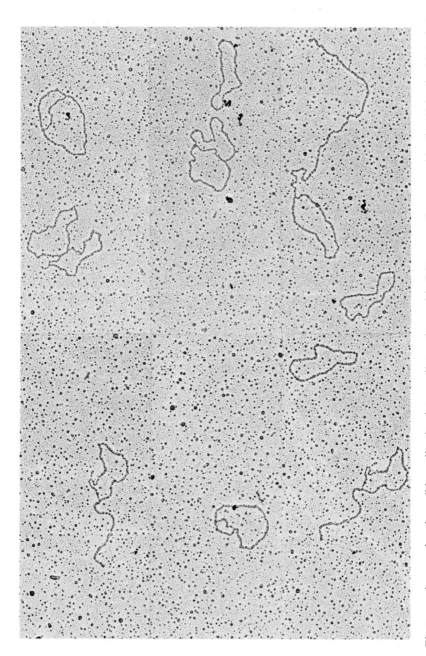

Fig. 14. Electron micrographs of possible replicating intermediates observed in RF preparations spread by the Kleinschmidt technique. RF molecules were isolated from cells in the RF → RF stage of replication. From Fidanián and Ray (unpublished observations).

side of the fork were first observed in replicating molecules of λ DNA (Inman and Schnös, 1971).

Although there is a very striking differential effect of rifampicin on the synthesis of the Ff complementary strand, rifampicin is also inhibitory to viral strand synthesis. In this case, the mechanism of inhibition appears to be an interference with the conversion of RF I to RF II, the precursor of replicative intermediates (Fidanián and Ray, 1974), rather than an inhibition of chain initiation. The relatively greater resistance to rifampicin of viral strand synthesis with respect to that of complementary strand synthesis may indicate either that the rifampicin block to viral strand synthesis is less efficient or that the rifampicin-sensitive step occurs less frequently in viral strand synthesis. As one example of the latter alternative, the formation of RF II is considered to be the rifampicin-sensitive step. Once synthesis of the viral strand has been initiated on an RF II molecule, the viral strand might be synthesized by a continuous process for several rounds of replication without the necessity of going through RF I. The complementary strand of the RF II precursor would remain circular and serve as a template for the continuous synthesis of an elongated viral strand. Sites on the growing viral strand for initiation of new complementary strands would periodically be exposed as the viral strand is "reeled off" and complementary strands would be initiated repeatedly while the viral strand is being elongated continuously. Only when the replicating molecule was converted back to RF I would viral strand synthesis again become rifampicin sensitive. A repeated utilization of the parental RF II open in the viral strand has been proposed as an explanation of the observation that in transfections with genetically heteroduplex RF molecules it is usually the complementary strand that determines the genotype of progeny phage (Enea et al., 1975).

The mechanism by which rifampicin inhibits the conversion of RF I to RF II is unknown at present. Since the function of gene 2 is required for this conversion, rifampicin might block this step through preventing expression of gene 2. This possibility seems least likely in view of the lag of some 15–20 min before exogenously added chloramphenicol starts to inhibit Ff RF duplication (Ray, 1970; Brutlag et al., 1971). In contrast, rifampicin inhibits Ff RF duplication without a lag period. Alternatively, we conjecture that RNA synthesis is directly involved in the conversion of RF I to RF II by a process perhaps similar to the transcriptional activation of the origin of λ DNA for replication (Dove et al., 1971). A rigorous test of this hypothesis may become possible upon the isolation of gene 2 protein.

6.4. Membrane Attachment of Replicating RF

During Ff RF replication, both parental ^{32}P-labeled RFs and [^{3}H]thymidine pulse-labeled RFs are found associated with a rapidly sedimenting bacterial component presumed to be membrane (Forsheit and Ray, 1971; Staudenbauer and Hofscheider, 1971; Kluge *et al.*, 1971). The relative amount of pulse-labeled RF associated with this rapidly sedimenting bacterial component increases with decreasing pulse lengths, suggesting that Ff RF is replicated in association with a cellular structure and is then released upon completion of replication. The parental ^{32}P-labeled RFs associated with this bacterial structure can be released by treatment with sarkosyl but not with Brij 58. The released molecules are heterogeneous with regard to sedimentation rate and have a range of sedimentation rates extending even beyond that of RF I in neutral high-salt sucrose gradients. Staudenbauer and Hofschneider (1971) found parental ^{32}P-labeled molecules at 15 min after infection that sedimented in alkali at rates corresponding to viral strands of 4 times unit length. These results provide further evidence for replicating intermediates containing elongated viral strands.

RF molecules have been observed in association with the cell envelope by an electron microscopic procedure (Griffith and Kornberg, 1972) in which cells in sucrose are gently lysed directly on an electron microscope grid, dehydrated, and visualized by high-resolution tungsten evaporation (Fig. 15). Many copies of Ff RF can be seen attached to the cell envelope after a 10-min infection with an amber mutant in gene 5. Under less gentle conditions of osmotic disruption of the infected cells, the circular RF molecules are found separated from the cell envelope.

6.5. Function of the RF Pool

The pool of RFs that accumulates early in Ff infections (Ray *et al.*, 1966*b*; Ray and Schekman, 1969*a*; Hohn *et al.*, 1971) appears to be utilized both for genetic transcription and for the synthesis of progeny single strands. Infection of nonpermissive host cells with amber or temperature-sensitive mutants in gene 2 prevents Ff DNA replication beyond the stage of parental RF formation and inhibits the synthesis of both the major coat protein (Smilowitz *et al.*, 1971) and the gene 5 protein (Mazur and Model, 1973). In infections with *ts*2 mutants at nonpermissive temperature, gene 5 protein synthesis is linear, as would be expected if transcription were only from the parental RF. But in a wild-

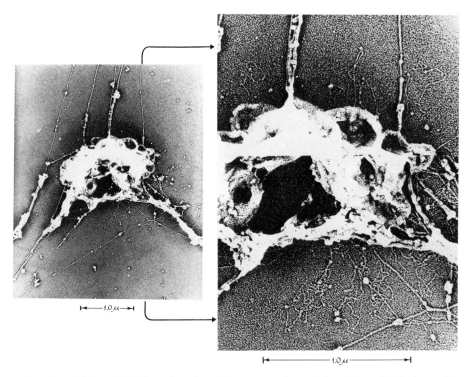

Fig. 15.   M13 *am*5 RF bound to the cell envelope of gently lysed *E. coli.* The bacterial DNA is condensed (thick fibers) and the M13 RF circles are bound to the disrupted envelope (central mass). Courtesy of J. Griffith.

type infection, gene 5 protein synthesis is exponential, indicating the participation of progeny RF molecules in transcription. Growth of infected cells containing fully labeled Ff progeny RF in an unlabeled medium chases the label out of the viral strands of the RF molecules while the label in the complementary strands is conserved (Forsheit *et al.,* 1971). This result indicates that the Ff RF pool also serves as a substrate for asymmetrical viral DNA synthesis.

7.   SINGLE-STRAND SYNTHESIS (RF→SS)

7.1.   Kinetics of Single-Strand Synthesis

Single-strand synthesis begins very early in the infectious process, although quantitatively it represents only a small fraction of the phage-specific DNA synthesis for at least the first 12 min after infection (Pratt and Erdahl, 1968; Forsheit *et al.,* 1971). During this initial period of the infectious cycle, the rate of DNA synthesis in infected cells exceeds that of uninfected bacteria by severalfold (Hohn *et al.,* 1971). This stimulation of DNA synthesis is due to the synthesis of some 100–200 RF molecules in addition to the continuing synthesis of the bacterial DNA. At approximately 10 min after infection, the rate of DNA synthesis stops increasing and remains constant for the next 50 min. This shift in rate of synthesis occurs at about the time of switchover from RF replication to SS synthesis. Analysis of the distribution of [^{3}H]thymidine between the strands of RF II molecules pulse-labeled at different times has shown that by 24–26 min after infection the pulse label is incorporated exclusively into the viral strand of the RF (Forsheit *et al.,* 1971). This pattern of labeling is characteristic of the period in which net synthesis of SS DNA is occurring. By 75 min after infection, the host cell contains approximately 200 progeny single strands (Ray *et al.,* 1966a). Encapsulation of these progeny molecules to form mature phage particles appears to occur concomitant with the release of phage through the cell wall since no intracellular phage has been observed (Watanabe *et al.,* 1967; Stegen and Hofschneider, 1970).

7.2. Requirement for Gene 5 and Gene 2 Proteins in Single-Strand Synthesis

Mutants defective in gene 5 are capable of RF replication but do not enter into SS synthesis (Pratt and Erdahl, 1968). In such mutant infections, a large pool of RF accumulates but no progeny single strands are formed. Marvin and Hohn (1969) adapted the rolling circle model of Gilbert and Dressler (1968) to Ff DNA replication, proposing that gene 5 protein acts as an inhibitor of complementary strand synthesis, presumably by binding to the nascent single strands. Recent experiments (Mazur and Model, 1973; Mazur and Zinder, 1975a) have shown that the switchover from RF→RF replication to RF→SS synthesis is regulated by the availability of free gene 5 protein. Thus the product of replication utilizing a rolling circle intermediate is either single- or double-stranded, depending on the concentration of the gene 5 protein. Intermediates in both RF replication and SS synthesis have structures compatible with this hypothesis (Ray, 1969; Tseng and Marvin, 1972a). The regulation of viral strand synthesis by the availability of gene 5 protein predicts that RF replication should resume following the inhibition of further gene 5 protein synthesis and the exhaustion of the pool of 5 protein (Mazur and Model, 1973; Mazur and Zinder, 1975a). This is, in fact, the observed result when chloramphenicol is added during the period of SS synthesis (Ray, 1970). The rate of RF synthesis is initially stimulated over that of the SS synthesis prior to the addition of the drug. This result is to be expected if replicating intermediates are switched from synthesis on only one side of the replicating fork to synthesis on both sides.

Experiments with an *E. coli dna*B mutant indicate that the shift from asymmetrical RF→SS synthesis to the symmetrical replication of both strands after the addition of chloramphenicol can occur in the absence of a functional *dna*B product (Staudenbauer and Hofschneider, 1972a). Since the *dna*B product is required for Ff RF→RF replication, these authors suggest that the symmetrical labeling of RF molecules upon adding chloramphenicol may reflect a two-stage type of synthesis in which circular single strands are synthesized and then converted to duplex forms by a *dna*B-independent mechanism. Evidence for the existence of more than a single mechanism of complementary strand synthesis has been obtained in investigations of the nalidixic acid sensitivity of complementary strand synthesis (Fidanián and Ray, 1974). The *dna*B-independent duplex DNA synthesis observed in the presence of chloramphenicol might occur by the nalidixic acid resistant mechanism used during parental RF formation.

There is not yet any direct evidence for the binding of gene 5 protein to intermediates in SS synthesis, although such an interaction would be expected. However, the results of Salstrom and Pratt (1971) indicate that the progeny single strands are held in the single-stranded state by the gene 5 protein. They observed that the pool of intracellular single strands is converted back to replicative forms following a shift to nonpermissive temperature of a culture infected with a gene 5 temperature-sensitive mutant. The ability of the gene 5 protein to inhibit complementary strand synthesis on progeny viral strands strongly suggests that the 5 protein might perform precisely the same function on replicating intermediates. In addition, the nascent viral strand might be protected from exonucleolytic degradation by the bound protein. Protection of SS DNA from exonuclease I degradation *in vitro* has been reported by Oey and Knippers (1972).

In addition to the proposed negative role of gene 5 protein in repressing complementary strand synthesis, a positive role in the production of single strands has been suggested (Staudenbauer and Hofschneider, 1973). This suggestion is based on the observation that single-strand production is temperature-sensitive in *E. coli dna*B mutant cells infected with a gene 5 temperature-sensitive phage. Since the *dna*B product is required only for RF→RF replication and not for RF→SS synthesis, it is proposed that gene 5 protein directly participates in the synthesis of the viral strand as well as repressing the synthesis of complementary strands. However, it has also been observed that viral strand synthesis is not inhibited immediately following the addition of either rifampicin or nalidixic acid to *am*5 mutant infected cells (Fidanián and Ray, 1974). In the absence of 5 protein, both strands of the RF are replicated equally. Rifampicin and nalidixic acid specifically inhibit complementary strand synthesis and inhibit viral strand synthesis only after a lag period. Thus under these conditions viral single strands are synthesized in the absence of either complementary strand synthesis or gene 5 protein. It is suggested, therefore, that 5 protein may be required for the stable accumulation of a single-stranded product rather than for the asymmetrical synthesis of viral strands. Perhaps the nascent viral strands are rapidly destroyed in the absence of the protection probably afforded by the binding of 5 protein or the synthesis of a complementary strand.

Although the accumulation of a pool of RF molecules normally precedes the synthesis of viral SS, there is no absolute requirement that it do so. Rather, the kinetics of SS synthesis appears to be determined entirely by the buildup of gene 5 protein (Mazur and Model, 1973). Cells infected at nonpermissive temperature with mutants temperature-sensitive in gene 2, a gene essential both for RF replication and for SS synthesis, form only the parental RF. When the cells are shifted down to permissive temperature at 10 min or more after infection, only single strands are synthesized immediately after the shift. By allowing sufficient gene 5 protein to accumulate in the absence of RF replication, it is possible then to totally bypass RF replication and enter directly into single-strand synthesis. In these experiments, the ^{32}P parental viral strand label transferred into the SS pool with a half-life of less than 2 min. This result is consistent with the earlier observations that the Ff parental viral strand is eventually recovered in the progeny phage (Mechler and Arber, 1969; Wirtz and Hofschneider, 1970; Boon and Zinder, 1970; Kluge *et al.*, 1971; Tseng *et al.*, 1972). These results indicate that the gene 2 protein is needed directly for SS synthesis rather than indirectly, by supplying an RF pool for SS synthesis.

In similar experiments where an excess of gene 5 protein was accumulated prior to a shift to permissive temperature in the presence of chloramphenicol, single-strand synthesis continued for a period of time rather than a switch to double-strand synthesis as in wild-type infected cells (Mazur and Zinder, 1975*a*). This continued RF→SS synthesis in the presence of chloramphenicol demonstrates that only the gene 5 protein is required to effect the switch from RF→RF replication to RF→SS synthesis.

The effect of a mutation in gene 2 is not only to prevent RF→RF replication but also to inhibit RF→SS synthesis (Lin and Pratt, 1972; Tseng and Marvin, 1972b). Since the gene 2 protein mediates the formation or stabilization of a strand-specific discontinuity in the viral strand of the RF (Fidanián and Ray, 1972), it may prove to be a strand-specific endonuclease required for the initiation of synthesis of the viral strand. The analogous protein for ϕX174 is, in fact, such a nuclease (Henry and Knippers, 1974).

The cooperative binding of gene 5 protein to DNA (Alberts *et al.*, 1972) suggests that the distribution of gene 5 protein molecules among the replicative intermediates at a time prior to the conversion of all replicating molecules to SS synthesis would be nonrandom. Once a replicating intermediate had bound some gene 5 protein molecules, it would be more likely that additional molecules would accumulate on that same intermediate rather than on one totally lacking gene 5 protein. Thus, even at early times when RF→RF replication occurs at a rapid rate, a low level of RF→SS synthesis would be expected and has been observed (Forsheit *et al.*, 1971).

7.3. Association of Gene 5 Protein with Viral Single Strands

The progeny SS DNA appears to accumulate in infected cells in the form of a DNA–protein complex (Pratt *et al.*, 1974; Webster and Cashman, 1973). These complexes can be isolated from infected cells and appear as structures 1.1 μm long and 16 nm wide by electron microscopy (Fig. 16). These structures consist of viral DNA associated with the gene 5 protein, a noncapsid protein required for single-strand synthesis (Pratt and Erdahl, 1968). Each viral DNA molecule binds approximately 1300 molecules of the gene 5 protein but little, if any, of the two known capsid proteins. Essentially all of the SS DNA and at least half to two-thirds of the gene 5 protein are contained in such complexes. The structure of complexes isolated from infected cells can be distinguished from the structure of those formed *in vitro* from purified SS DNA and gene 5 protein, suggesting that the complexes isolated from infected cells existed *in vivo* rather than having been formed in the lysate. Direct evidence for the *in vivo* association has been obtained by UV-induced cross-linking of gene 5 protein to viral SS DNA *in vivo* (Lica and Ray, 1976b). These covalently associated complexes can be purified easily from detergent lysates of the irradiated infected cells. The protein component of the complexes is identified as 5 protein on the basis of amino acid composition and chromatographic properties of both tryptic peptides and cyanogen bromide fragments.

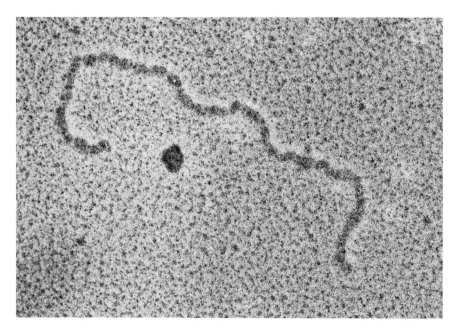

Fig. 16.   Tungsten-shadowed M13 SS complexed with gene 5 protein. The complex
was isolated from M13-infected cells during RF→SS synthesis. The length of the complex is approximately 1.1 μm. From Pratt *et al.* (1974).

Pulse-chase experiments have shown that the viral DNA can be
chased out of the complex, presumably into mature phage, while the
gene 5 protein molecules are reused to form more complex. No
turnover of the viral DNA in the complexes is observed in nonpermissive cells infected with amber mutants that do not yield progeny
phage. These results suggest that the release of gene 5 protein from the
complex is dependent on phage maturation (Webster and Cashman,
1973; Pratt *et al.*, 1974).

The gene 5 protein can be isolated from infected cells by
chromatography on DNA-cellulose and is present at a level of about
10^5 copies per cell (Oey and Knippers, 1972; Alberts *et al.*, 1972). This
enormous concentration of the gene 5 protein suggests that it plays a
structural role in DNA replication rather than an enzymatic one. In
some respects, the gene 5 protein is similar to the T4 gene 32 protein,
an unwinding protein that stimulates synthesis by the T4 DNA
polymerase (Huberman *et al.*, 1971). The gene 5 protein binds to single-
stranded but not double-stranded DNA. This property of the protein
results in a lowering of the T_m of double-stranded DNAs by about
40°C (Alberts *et al.*, 1972). This depression of the T_m is nearly inde-

pendent of GC content of the DNA, although there is a slight preferential destabilization of AT-rich DNAs.

Complexes formed *in vitro* between gene 5 protein and viral DNA are about 10 nm wide and 0.73 μm long. These structures appear by electron microscopy to be rodlike with occasional branches and are strikingly different from complexes between T4 gene 32 protein and Ff DNA which appear as open rings under identical conditions (Alberts *et al.*, 1972). The gene 5 complexes are different in that two protein-coated DNA strands coalesce to form a rod-shaped structure. Branching results whenever, by chance, two regions of the same DNA molecules are independently folded by gene 5 protein. At low concentrations of gene 5 protein, most of the complexes are un-branched. Each Ff DNA molecule binds about 1600 gene 5 protein molecules, a value slightly greater than that observed for complexes isolated from infected cells. The close resemblance of these complexes to the mature filamentous virion at first suggests that the coat protein (molecular weight 5196 daltons) might be a cleavage product of the gene 5 protein (molecular weight 9688 daltons). However, the amino acid sequences of these proteins are not compatible with this possibility. The sequence of the gene 5 protein is shown in Fig. 17.

Although there are some similarities between the T4 gene 32 protein and the Ff gene 5 protein, their *in vivo* functions may differ. While the T4 DNA polymerase is stimulated by gene 32 protein, the *in vitro* replication of *in vivo* intermediates in Ff SS synthesis by DNA polymerase II is increased in extent of synthesis but not in the rate of synthesis by gene 5 protein (Oey and Knippers, 1972). However, there is no evidence to suggest a role for polymerase II in SS synthesis. In fact, recent experiments (Mitra and Stallions, 1973; Staudenbauer,

```
                        10                                    20
Met-Ile-Lys-Val-Glu-Ile-Lys-Pro-Ser-Gln-Ala-Gln-Phe-Thr-Thr-Arg-Ser-Gly-Val-Ser-

                        30                                    40
Arg-Gln-Gly Lys-Pro-Tyr-Ser-Leu-Asn-Glu-Gln-Leu-Cys-Tyr-Val-Asp-Leu-Gly-Asn-Glu-

                        50                                    60
Tyr-Pro-Val-Leu-Val-Lys-Ile-Thr-Leu-Asp-Glu-Gly-Gln-Pro-Ala-Tyr-Ala-Pro-Gly-Leu-

                        70                                    80
Tyr-Thr-Val-His-Leu-Ser-Ser-Phe-Lys-Val-Gly-Gln-Phe-Gly-Ser-Leu-Met-Ile-Asp-Arg-

Leu-Arg-Leu-Val-Pro-Ala-Lys
```

Fig. 17.   Amino acid sequence of the M13 and fd gene 5 protein. From Cuypers *et al.* (1974) and Nakashima *et al.* (1974).

1974) have shown that the *dna*E gene product (polymerase III) is required for continuous phage production.

7.4. Requirement for Host Functions in Single-Strand Synthesis

A role for RNA polymerase in SS synthesis is suggested by the sensitivity of SS synthesis to rifampicin (Staudenbauer and Hofschneider, 1972*a,b*). However, the sensitivity of viral strand synthesis to rifampicin is approximately tenfold less than that of complementary strand synthesis (Fidanián and Ray, 1974) and appears to result from two indirect effects of the drug. The accumulation of an RF II species having a viral-strand-specific discontinuity, a step essential for single-strand synthesis, is inhibited by rifampicin. In addition, the expression of gene 5, another requirement for single-strand synthesis, is prevented by rifampicin. These indirect effects of rifampicin appear to be sufficient to account for the rifampicin sensitivity of SS synthesis without invoking a direct role for RNA polymerase in the synthetic process. Indeed, the rifampicin sensitivity of SS synthesis can be reduced by preincubation under nonreplicating conditions that allow protein synthesis and the consequent accumulation of gene 5 protein (Fidanián and Ray, 1974). Two such nonreplicating conditions are infection at nonpermissive temperature with gene 2 temperature-sensitive mutants and infection with wild-type phage in the presence of nalidixic acid.

Other host functions likely to be involved in SS synthesis are the *dna*C(D), *dna*E (polIII), and *pol*A (polI) genes. The products of each of these genes are required continuously for phage production (Mitra and Stallions, 1973; Staudenbauer, 1974; Chen and Ray, 1976). In contrast, the *dna*B and *dna*G functions are required only during RF replication. A shift of infected *dna*B or *dna*G cells to nonpermissive temperature after the onset of SS synthesis has no effect on phage production (Primrose *et al.*, 1968; Staudenbauer and Hofschneider, 1972*a*; Mitra and Stallions, 1973; Ray *et al.*, 1975). The final step in SS synthesis, ligation of the linear single strand to form a ring, might possibly be mediated by the host ligase acting on termini held in juxtaposition by base pairing within a "hairpin" region of the single-stranded DNA (Schekman and Ray, 1971).

7.5. Mechanics of Single-Strand Synthesis

Progeny viral strands appear to be synthesized by a rolling circle mechanism (Gilbert and Dressler, 1968) as outlined in the model of Ff replication presented in Fig. 13. Two lines of evidence support this model. First, a circular complementary strand serves as a conserved template for the repeated synthesis of Ff progeny viral strands (Ray, 1969; Forsheit *et al.*, 1971). The preexisting viral strands are displaced as new viral strand material is laid down. Second, pulse-labeled intermediates in SS synthesis contain elongated viral strands with lengths extending up to twice the unit length (Ray, 1969; Staudenbauer and Hofschneider, 1972*a*; Kluge, 1974). Such intermediates are readily visualized in electron microscopic examinations of RF preparations from infected cells producing progeny phage (Fig. 18).

Entry of an RF I molecule into the replication process requires specific nicking of the viral strand (Fidanián and Ray, 1972; Lin and Pratt, 1972; Tseng and Marvin, 1972*b*). The purpose of the nick may be

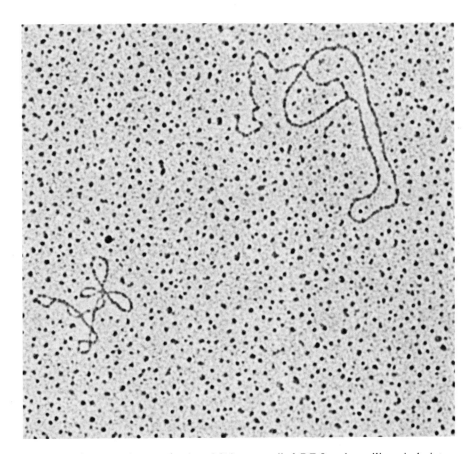

Fig. 18. Electron micrograph of an M13 supercoiled RF I and a rolling circle intermediate having a single-stranded tail. The molecules were spread by the Kleinschmidt procedure in the presence of formamide (D. S. Ray, unpublished results).

to create a 3′-OH terminus for polymerization, although this possibility has not been subjected to a critical test. Alternatively, the nick in the viral strand may serve to allow propagation of a DNA chain initiated elsewhere.

After initiation of the viral strand, synthesis probably proceeds until a unit-length piece of single-stranded DNA can be cleaved from the RF, generating a linear single strand which must be circularized and an RF II molecule that can serve as template for further synthesis or that can be repaired and joined to yield a covalently closed ring. The discontinuity in the resultant RF II molecule locates the origin of the preceding round of synthesis.

The origin of viral strand synthesis has been located by restriction enzyme mapping of the discontinuity in late life cycle RF II (Suggs and Ray, 1976). Treatment of RF II pulse-labeled during RF→SS synthesis with the *Hind*II restriction endonuclease and sedimentation in an alkaline sucrose gradient yield two discrete viral strand fragments. From the sizes of the two fragments, the gene 2 specific discontinuity has been located at approximately 10% of the genome from the *Hind*II restriction site. Further evidence for a specific location of the discontinuity in RF II was obtained by using the RF II as a template for repair synthesis with the *E. coli* polymerase I in the presence of ^{32}P-labeled triphosphates. Upon treatment of these repaired RF II molecules with the *Hpa*II restriction endonuclease and electrophoresis in an agarose gel, the discontinuity was localized in a specific restriction fragment, the F fragment (Fig. 19). Thus the origin of viral strand synthesis is contained within the intergenic region of the genome already identified as containing the origin of the complementary strand in the SS→RF reaction *in vitro* (Tabak *et al.*, 1974).

The direction of viral strand synthesis was shown to be in the opposite direction to that of the complementary strand, as expected, by determination of the gradient of pulse label in RF I molecules isolated late in infection (Suggs and Ray, 1976). The gradient of pulse label in supercoiled RF I molecules also confirmed the location of the origin of viral strand synthesis in the *Hpa*II F fragment.

The endonucleolytic cleavage of the growing tail of a rolling circle molecule to yield a linear single strand, a presumptive intermediate in ring formation, has not yet been demonstrated. The enzyme most likely to carry out such a cleavage is the Ff gene 2 protein. If the cleavage occurs within a small duplex (hairpin) region of the SS DNA, the reaction might be sufficiently similar to that involved in the nicking of RF I supercoils so that the same enzyme could reasonably catalyze both cleavages. Should the gene 2 protein be involved in cleaving the SS tail

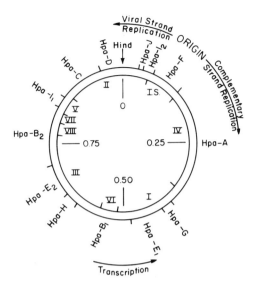

Fig. 19. Location of the M13 *in vitro* SS→RF and the *in vivo* RF→SS origins of replication (Tabak *et al.*, 1974; Suggs and Ray, 1976) on the physical and genetic maps of M13 (Edens *et al.*, 1975).

of a rolling circle molecule, the accumulation of long-tailed molecules might result after shifting cells infected by gene 2 temperature-sensitive mutants to nonpermissive temperature. Although no such accumulation has been observed (Lin and Pratt, 1972), the normal temperature sensitivity of wild-type SS synthesis (Staudenbauer *et al.*, 1973) could have interfered with the detection of these structures. Thus this enzyme still seems to be the most likely candidate for mediating the cleavage.

Pulse-labeled replicative intermediates containing viral strands of greater than unit length and having a restricted binding of propidium diiodide (Kessler-Liebscher *et al.*, 1975) may be one of the initial products of RF→SS synthesis. The exact molecular structure and the role of such molecules remain to be determined.

8. EXPRESSION OF THE Ff GENOME

8.1. Regulated Synthesis of Gene Products

Host proteins continue to be synthesized in infected cells in near-normal amounts, making detection of phage-specific proteins difficult except for those synthesized in large amounts. Minor phage proteins have been detected only by suppression of host protein synthesis by UV irradiation of the host cell prior to infection (Henry and Pratt, 1969; Lin and Pratt, 1974). The products of genes 3, 4, 5, and 8 have been detected by this procedure. At 42°C the gene 2 protein appears to be overproduced and, in this case, can also be detected in irradiated cells.

The gene 5 and gene 8 proteins, a DNA-binding protein and the major capsid protein, are synthesized in sufficiently large quantities that they are easily detected even in unirradiated cells (Webster and Cashman, 1973; Lica and Ray, 1976a). These major products of the Ff genome are synthesized in nearly equimolar amounts. The gene 5 protein has been estimated to be present in at least 10^5 copies per cell (Alberts et al., 1972). More than 10^3 copies of 5 protein are bound to the 100–200 progeny single strands per cell (Pratt et al., 1974). The gene 5 proteins are removed from the viral DNA in the process of maturation and replaced by approximately 2×10^3 copies of the gene 8 protein and one to four copies of the gene 3 protein (Henry and Pratt, 1969). This enormous differential in the synthesis of the different gene products of the Ff genome has stimulated considerable interest in the mechanisms regulating Ff gene expression.

8.2. Transcription of the Ff Genome

Phage-specific mRNA is readily detected in infected cells by hybridization of pulse-labeled RNA to M13 RF (Jacob and Hofschneider, 1969). Hybridization to viral strand DNA was found to be less than 1% of that to denatured RF, indicating that the complementary strand of the RF serves as the sole template for transcription *in vivo*. This asymmetrical copying of RF is also observed *in vitro* (Sugiura et al., 1969). Using a coupled transcription-translation system and heteroduplex RF molecules in which one strand has the coding for the premature termination of a given protein, it was shown that the information for RNA transcription of structural genes is not strongly affected by a single base change in the duplex strand not complementary to the mRNA synthesized (Pieczenik et al., 1975).

Phage-specific mRNA isolated from infected cells is heterogeneous and ranges in mass from approximately 9×10^4 up to 5×10^5 daltons, as analyzed by velocity sedimentation in denaturing dimethylsulfoxide gradients (Jacob et al., 1973). None of the hybridizable RNA corresponds to the full length of the DNA template. Such an RNA would have a molecular weight of 1.9×10^6. The physical half-lives of these RNA species were estimated to be unusually long, of the

order of 15–16 min (Jacob *et al.*, 1970). However, measurements of the
half-lives of gene 5 and gene 8 messages by determination of the decay
in the rate of synthesis of the gene 5 and gene 8 proteins following
inhibition of new RNA chain initiations with rifampicin indicates that
these messages decay at rates comparable to those of bacterial
messages (Lica and Ray, 1976*a*). This difference between the physical
and biological half-lives of phage messages may reflect an inactivation
of the mRNA as a functional messenger prior to the total degradation
of the RNA chain.

Transcription of RF I by purified RNA polymerase holoenzyme
yields at least seven RNA species ranging in size from 8 S up to 26 S
(Takanami *et al.*, 1971; Okamoto *et al.*, 1975; Chan *et al.*, 1975; Edens
et al., 1975). The larger species (23 S and 26 S) are initiated with pppA
(A-start), while five of the species (approximately 8, 11, 14, 17, and 19
S) are initiated with pppG (G-start). Three of the G-start RNAs are
synthesized in much greater quantities than the other transcripts
(Okamoto *et al.*, 1975; Edens *et al.*, 1975; Chan *et al.*, 1975). Although
there are small differences in the S values assigned to the RNA species
by different laboratories, the major G-start species are about 8–10, 13–
14, and 17–19 S. The A-start RNA is largely 26 S and corresponds to
almost a full transcript of the entire genome.

The synthesis of a small number of well-defined RNA transcripts
by RNA polymerase implies the existence of a similar number of promoter sites. On the basis of the sizes of the different transcripts and the
locations of promoter sites, it appears that there is only a single site for
RNA chain termination (Takanami *et al.*, 1971, 1975; Seeburg and
Schaller, 1975; Chan *et al.*, 1975; Edens *et al.*, 1975). In the presence of
ρ factor, the RNA transcripts are considerably truncated, indicating
the presence of sites at which ρ can terminate RNA chains (Takanami
et al., 1971). A map of the locations of promoter sites and the single ρ-
independent termination site is shown in Fig. 20. Promoter sites have
been localized by analysis of the RNA transcripts formed on individual
restriction fragments of RF and by RNA polymerase binding studies
(Okamoto *et al.*, 1975; Seeburg and Schaller, 1975; Chan *et al.*, 1975;
Edens *et al.*, 1975). It should be noted that different laboratories are in
reasonable agreement on the locations of most of the promoters,
although the precise locations of some are still uncertain. The greatest
uncertainty is with regard to whether a promoter is located between the
single ρ-independent terminator and the proximal end of gene 3 or
whether transcription of gene 3 might be due solely to a low level of
leakiness of the terminator. However, the strong polar effect of amber

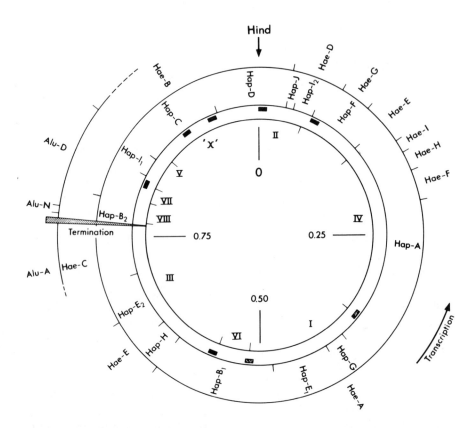

Fig. 20. Locations of G-start and A-start promoters and the single ρ-independent termination site on the M13 physical and genetic maps (Edens *et al.*, 1975). G-start promoters are indicated by solid rectangles and A-start promoters by hatched rectangles. The single ρ-independent termination site is indicated by the hatched pointer. The inner circle represents the genetic map with genes indicated by Roman numerals. The location of the "X" protein and the intergenic space between genes II and IV are also shown.

mutations in gene 3 on genes 6 and 1 suggests that these genes may be contained on a single RNA transcript (Pratt *et al.*, 1966; Lyons and Zinder, 1972).

Sequencing of the promoter having the greatest affinity for RNA polymerase has been achieved by two laboratories (Schaller *et al.*, 1975; Sugimoto *et al.*, 1975), and these results are presented in Fig. 4. This promoter is one of the G-start promoters which is contained on the *Hap-Hga*V restriction fragment of approximately 230 base pairs (Sugimoto *et al.*, 1975). A uniform RNA of 120 nucleotides length can be synthesized on this restriction fragment and this RNA has also been sequenced. This RNA chain is initiated in the center of the RNA polymerase protected fragment just following a sequence of twofold rotational symmetry.

It is of interest to note that the G-start promoters are stronger promoters than those for A-starts and that they cluster in the vicinity of the genes required in largest amounts, particularly around genes 5 and 8. Also, the weaker A-start promoters are located in the region of the genome coding for genes 3, 6, 1, and 4 all of which are expressed at a low level *in vivo*. These observations suggest that the regulation of transcription of the RF may be determined largely by the locations and strengths of the promoters and the location of the single ρ-independent terminator. Consistent with this model are the observations of Chan *et al.* (1975) that all transcripts contain information for gene 8, the last gene before the terminator. The largest RNA species (26 S) codes for all of the *in vitro* products, while the 17 S RNA has lost the ability to serve as template for gene 3 and the 13 S species codes primarily for genes 5 and 8. The smallest RNA species (8–10 S) acts as template only for gene 8 protein.

8.3. Translation of Ff Gene Transcripts

Considerable progress has been made recently on the *in vitro* translation of Ff messages. Viral proteins have been synthesized using Ff RF DNA to direct coupled transcription-translation systems (Konings, 1973; Konings *et al.*, 1973, 1975; Model and Zinder, 1974; Konings and Schoenmakers, 1974; Vovis *et al.*, 1975; van den Hondel *et al.*, 1975; Model *et al.*, 1975). The polypeptide products of such systems can be conveniently displayed on SDS-polyacrylamide gels. At least seven phage-specific polypeptides have been observed when the covalently closed RF DNA is used to program the synthetic machinery. Six of these products have been identified with known genes (genes 1–5 and 8). A seventh polypeptide (X), synthesized in substantial amounts, cannot be attributed to a known gene, and two genes (genes 6 and 7) are known to exist for which there are not yet identifiable products. The assignments of genes to specific polypeptides is based on the altered mobilities of individual bands when the synthetic machinery is programmed with RF DNAs containing amber mutations in specific genes.

These coupled systems show evidence of regulation since the ratio of gene 8 to gene 3 protein synthesized *in vitro* is approximately 10:1 (Model and Zinder, 1974; Konings *et al.*, 1975). However, some of the *in vivo* regulatory mechanisms are not functioning fully in these systems since the ratio of gene 8 to gene 3 protein formed *in vivo* is approximately 500:1–1000:1 (Henry and Pratt, 1969).

The products of genes 3 and 8, the minor and major capsid proteins, appear to be synthesized as precursor molecules having molecular weights greater than those of the *in vivo* products (Konings *et al.*, 1975). The gene 3 protein synthesized *in vitro* has a molecular weight of 59,000 daltons as compared to the *in vivo* gene 3 protein of 56,000 daltons. Similarly, the gene 8 protein formed *in vitro* has a molecular weight of 5800 daltons while that of the *in vivo* gene 8 protein is only 5196 daltons. Although there is not yet any evidence for the formation of precursor molecules in the infected cell, there is considerable precedent for precursors of functional proteins in eukaryotic systems and in the case of bacteriophage T4. Since the gene 3 and gene 8 proteins are structural components of the mature virion, it is possible that the cleavage of the precursor proteins is in some way related to the morphogenesis of the filamentous virion within the cell membrane. Both the gene 3 and gene 8 capsid proteins are found in substantial quantities in the inner membrane of infected cells (Smilowitz *et al.*, 1972; Webster and Cashman, 1973; Lin and Pratt, 1974). The fact that the products of genes 2 and 5, both required for DNA synthesis, and the product of gene 4, likely to be required for virion assembly, are also localized in the inner membrane (Lin and Pratt, 1974; Webster and Cashman, 1973) suggests that both viral DNA synthesis and phage morphogenesis occur in the inner membrane.

Restriction endonuclease fragments have been used recently to investigate the coupled transcription and translation of specific regions of the viral genome (Model *et al.*, 1975; van den Hondel *et al.*, 1975; Vovis *et al.*, 1975; Konings *et al.*, 1975). These studies have greatly aided the assignment of proteins and promoters to specific sites on the genome. Some of the restriction fragments directed the synthesis of only a single polypeptide chain. For example, the *Hap*A fragment consists of almost pure gene 4 and includes the promoter for this gene (van den Hondel *et al.*, 1975).

The major protein (X) for which no gene or function has been identified has been localized to a specific region of the genome by the use of purified restriction fragments in the coupled transcription-translation system. The X protein is encoded by RF fragment *Hap*C (van den Hondel *et al.*, 1975; Vovis *et al.*, 1975; Chan *et al.*, 1975), a region of the genome already assigned to the 3′-end of gene 2. It has been suggested that the X protein may result from the synthesis of an mRNA at an initiation site within gene 2, in analogy with the situation in ϕX174 gene A. The X protein is also unusual in that while it is a major product in the DNA-directed system it is either absent or greatly reduced when *in vitro* synthesized RNA is used as template (Chan *et al.*, 1975). When unfractionated RNA or 26 S RNA is used to direct protein synthesis, the other Ff proteins are all synthesized in amounts similar to those in the DNA-directed system.

9. FUTURE AREAS OF RESEARCH

Filamentous phage will continue to provide a powerful probe of some of the most basic questions in molecular biology. All of the genes of the Ff phage have probably been identified and located on the genetic and physical maps of the genome. It is reasonable to expect that all intergenic spaces in the viral DNA and perhaps the entire genome will be sequenced in the next few years. The amino acid sequences of two virus-coded proteins are already known and their conformations are being studied intensively. All but two of the viral proteins have been characterized to some extent, and the remaining two should be isolated and characterized soon. We are therefore drawing nearer to the time when we can describe the physiology of the growth and reproduction of these small viruses in extensive molecular detail.

Several areas of investigation will be most prominent in the future. With the enormous power recently made available to us through the use of restriction nucleases, we can expect that the most interesting nucleic acid sequences in the viral genome will soon be excised and sequenced. This work should shed some light on the mechanisms of control of replication and gene expression. It will surely have escaped the notice of few readers that the origin of replication is now sufficiently well localized that its nucleotide sequence can soon be obtained (possibly even before this work is published!). Similarly the single ρ-independent termination site and all of the promoters are equally accessible for sequence work.

Another penetrating use of restriction enzymes will be in the *in vitro* rearrangement of the viral genome. Current models of regulatory mechanisms can be subjected to critical tests by transpositions, duplications, and alterations of specific nucleotide sequences. This area of research will almost certainly yield some of the most significant advances in our understanding of the function of different regions of the genome.

Analysis of miniphage produced in Ff-infected cells may reveal something of the mechanics of DNA rearrangements and alterations occurring in cells. By applying strong selective pressure it may even be possible to reduce the size of these defective genomes to the absolute minimum required for replication. The resulting minichromosome might contain only the nucleotide sequence for the origin of replication and no portion of any of the viral genes. Such minichromosomes could shed light on the structure and function of the origin of replication.

Morphogenesis of filamentous virions still remains to be investigated in detail. This should be a most fruitful study for several reasons. The mature virion appears to be formed in the cell membrane as the virus is being extruded through the cell wall. This process involves the removal of a DNA-binding protein encoating the viral DNA and its replacement by the capsid proteins. This transaction may provide one of the best model systems for investigating the mechanism by which one protein can displace another from a chromosome. And, fortunately, both of the major proteins participating in this exchange have been completely sequenced. One of these, the major capsid protein, constitutes a significant fraction of the total membrane protein. The ability to obtain this membrane protein in large quantity and to genetically and biochemically alter the protein should provide a powerful probe of the cell membrane and the mechanism of insertion of proteins into the membrane. Other viral proteins required for phage morphogenesis but not found in the mature virion have also been localized in the cell membrane. An understanding of the roles of these proteins in virus assembly and the extrusion of the filamentous virion through the cell envelope will be of considerable relevance to the questions of how supramolecular structures are assembled within membranes and how nucleic acids are transported through membranes.

Just as the filamentous phage has aided in the dissection of the bacterial DNA replication apparatus, so will it likely prove of value in probing the host components of the cell membrane. The isolation of bacterial mutants defective in filamentous phage morphogenesis and the reconstruction of the assembly process in an *in vitro* system can be expected to yield exciting new insights into basic problems of membrane structure and function.

Our picture of the replication, transcription, and translation of the Ff genome, although considerably detailed, is still incomplete and inadequate. The recent success in reconstructing some of these processes *in vitro* has led to penetrating insights into their molecular details. Important regulatory elements still remain to be purified and characterized, and control sequences in the viral DNA and messenger RNA are only beginning to be studied in molecular detail. The study of the interactions between regulatory proteins and specific nucleic acid sequences has hardly begun.

Finally, an exciting possible use of filamentous phage is in the cloning of interesting DNA fragments from foreign sources, including eukaryotic organisms. Unlike most other phage vectors that have rigid limits on the amount of DNA that can be encapsulated, filamentous phage would probably not be limited in its capacity for accepting long DNA pieces except by the physical instability of exceedingly long filamentous virions. The ease with which Ff phage can be obtained in large quantity might also substantially reduce the biohazards associated with the cloning of potentially dangerous genetic material. Single-stranded phage vectors would be particularly valuable for studies on asymmetrical transcription because of the ability to obtain only a single strand of a cloned DNA fragment. In the case of large DNA fragments lacking any buoyant density bias between the two strands, filamentous phage would be particularly advantageous. And by inversion of the cloned sequence in the phage genome it would be possible to obtain either strand in the filamentous phage particle. In addition, the availability of the DNA in a circular single-stranded form is especially advantageous for some sequencing techniques.

Note Added in Proof

Since this review was completed Schaller *et al.* (1976, *Proc. Natl. Acad. Sci. USA* **73**:49) have isolated a specific initiation complex for the fd SS→RF reaction. A unique fragment of the viral genome is protected from nuclease digestion by the *E. coli* DNA unwinding protein and RNA polymerase. This specific fragment is about 120 nucleotides long and is located at the origin of replication. The fragment has double strand-like characteristics which prevent it from being covered by the unwinding protein and thus indirectly positions the RNA polymerase at the origin of replication.

We have also learned from K. Sugimoto, H. Sugisaki, T. Okamoto, and M. Takanami (manuscript in preparation) that they have now sequenced the precursor region of the fd major coat protein. The sequence contains the f1 ribosome binding site No. 1 of Pieczenik *et al.* (1974). AUG codons are located at the 5th and 23rd frames upstream from the first amino acid of the coat protein. The AUG codon at the 23rd frame is located in the center of the ribosome binding site. However, the size of precursor predicted is longer than the value obtained by gel electrophoresis of precursor protein synthesized *in vitro*.

ACKNOWLEDGMENTS

I wish to thank my numerous colleagues who provided original figures, reprints, and preprints of their work for this review, which was concluded in January 1976. I am particularly indebted to Dr. Jack Griffith for providing several original electron micrographs. Our own unpublished work presented here was supported by a grant from the National Institutes of Health (AI 10752).

10. REFERENCES

Alberts, B., Frey, L., and Delius, H., 1972, Isolation and characterization of gene 5 protein of filamentous bacterial viruses, *J. Mol. Biol.* **68**:139.

Arber, W., 1966, Host specificity of DNA produced by *Escherichia coli* 9: Host-controlled modification of bacteriophage fd, *J. Mol. Biol.* **20**:483.

Arber, W., and Linn, S., 1969, DNA modification and restriction, *Annu. Rev. Biochem.* **38**:467.

Arrand, J. R., and Hindley, J., 1973, Nucleotide sequence of a ribosome binding site on RNA synthesized *in vitro* from coliphage T7, *Nature (London) New Biol.* **24**:10.

Asbeck, F., Beyreuther, K., and Kohler, H., von Wettstein, G., and Braunitzer, G., 1969, Virusproteine. IV. Die Konstitution des Hullproteins des Phagen fd, *Hoppe-Seyler's Z. Physiol. Chem.* **350**:1047.

Beaudoin, J., and Pratt, D., 1974, Antiserum inactivation of electrophoretically purified M13 diploid virions: Model for the F-specific filamentous bacteriophages, *J. Virol.* **13**:466.

Beaudoin, J., Henry, T. J., and Pratt, D., 1974, Purification of single- and double-length M13 virions by polyacrylamide gel electrophoresis, *J. Virol.* **13**:470.

Benzinger, R., 1968, Restriction of infectious bacteriophage fd DNA's and an assay for *in vitro* host-controlled restriction and modification, *Proc. Natl. Acad. Sci. USA* **59**:1294.

Berg, P., Fancher, H., and Chamberlin, M., 1963, in: *Symposium on Informational Macromolecules* (H. Vogel, V. Bryson, and J. O. Lampen, eds.), Academic Press, New York.

Berkower, I., Leis, J., and Hurwitz, J., 1973, Isolation and characterization of an endonuclease from *Escherichia coli* specific for ribonucleic acid in ribonucleic acid deoxyribonucleic acid hybrid structures, *J. Biol. Chem.* **248**:5914.

Berkowitz, S. A., and Day, L. A., 1974, Molecular weight of single-stranded fd bacteriophage DNA: High speed equilibrium sedimentation and light scattering measurements, *Biochemistry* **13**:4825.

Bertsch, L. L., Marco, R., and Kornberg, A., 1974, unpublished observations cited in: Kornberg, A., *DNA Synthesis*, p. 246, Freeman, San Francisco.

Blakesley, R. W., and Wells, R. D., 1975, "Single-stranded" DNA from ϕX174 and M13 is cleaved by certain restriction endonucleases, *Nature (London)* **257**:421.

Boon, T., and Zinder, N. D., 1970, Genetic recombination in bacteriophage f1: Transfer of parental DNA to the recombinant, *Virology* **41**:444.

Boon, T., and Zinder, N. D., 1971, Genotypes produced by individual recombination events involving bacteriophage f1, *J. Mol. Biol.* **58**:133.

Bouché, J.-P., Zechel, K., and Kornberg, A., 1975, *dna* G gene product, a rifampicin-resistant RNA polymerase, initiates the conversion of a single-stranded coliphage DNA to its duplex replicative form, *J. Biol. Chem.* **250**:5995.

Boyer, H., 1971, DNA restriction and modification mechanisms in bacteria, *Annu. Rev. Microbiol.* **25**:153.

Boyer, H., Scibienski, E., Slocum, H., and Roullant-Dussoix, D., 1971, The *in vitro* restriction of the replicative form of w.t. and mutant fd phage DNA, *Virology* **46**:703.

Bradley, D. E., 1967, Ultrastructure of bacteriophages and bacteriocins, *Bacteriol. Rev.* **31**:230.

Bradley, D. E., 1973, The length of the filamentous *Pseudomonas aeruginosa* bacteriophage Pf, *J. Gen. Virol.* **20**:249.

Brinton, C. C., Jr., 1972, The properties of sex pili, the viral nature of "conjugal" genetic transfer systems, and some possible approaches to the control of bacterial drug resistance, *Crit. Rev. Microbiol.* **1**:105.

Brutlag, D., Schekman, R., and Kornberg, A., 1971, A possible role for RNA polymerase in the initiation of M13 DNA synthesis, *Proc. Natl. Acad. Sci. USA* **68**:2826.

Caro, L. G., and Schnös, M., 1966, The attachment of the male-specific bacteriophage f1 to sensitive strains of *Escherichia coli, Proc. Natl. Acad. Sci. USA* **56**:126.

Chan, T., Model, P., and Zinder, N. D., 1975, *In vitro* protein synthesis directed by separated transcripts of bacteriophage f1 DNA, *J. Mol. Biol.* **99**:369.

Chen, J., and Ray, D. S., 1976, Replication of bacteriophage M13. X. M13 replication in a mutant of *E. coli* defective in the $5' \rightarrow 3'$ exonuclease associated with DNA polymerase I, *J. Mol. Biol.,* in press.

Cuypers, T., van der Ouderaa, F. J., and de Jong, W. W., 1974, The amino acid sequence of gene 5 protein of bacteriophage M13, *Biochem. Biophys. Res. Commun.* **59(2)**:557.

Day, L. A., 1969, Conformations of single-stranded DNA and coat protein in fd bacteriophage as revealed by ultraviolet absorption spectroscopy, *J. Mol. Biol.* **39**:265.

Denhardt, D. T., 1975, The single-stranded DNA phages, in: *CRC Critical Reviews in Microbiology,* pp. 161–223, The Chemical Rubber Company, Cleveland, Ohio.

Denhardt, D. T., and Marvin, D. A., 1969, Altered coding in single-stranded DNA viruses, *Nature (London)* **221**:769.

Dove, W. F., Inokuchi, H., and Stevens, W. F., 1971, Replication control in phage lambda, in: *The Bacteriophage Lambda* (A. D. Hershey, ed.), pp. 747–771, Cold Spring Harbor Laboratory, Cold Spring Harbor, N.Y.

Dumas, B., and Miller, A., 1973, Replication of bacteriophage ϕX174 DNA in a temperature-sensitive *dna*E mutant of *Escherichia coli* C, *J. Virol.* **11**:848.

Dunker, A. K., Klausner, R. D., Marvin, D. A., and Wiseman, R. L., 1974, Filamentous bacterial viruses. X. X-ray diffraction studies of the R4 A-protein mutant, *J. Mol. Biol.* **82**:115.

Edens, L., Konings, R. N. H., and Schoenmakers, J. G. G., 1975, Physical mapping of the central terminator for transcription on the bacteriophage M13 genome, *Nucleic Acids Res.* **2**:1811.

Enea, V., and Zinder, N. D., 1975, A deletion mutant of bacteriophage f1 containing no intact cistrons, *Virology* **68**:105.

Enea, V., and Zinder, N. D., 1976, Heteroduplex DNA: A recombinational intermediate in phage f1, *J. Mol. Biol.* **101**:25.

Enea, V., Vovis, G. F., and Zinder, N. D., 1975, Genetic studies with heteroduplex DNA of bacteriophage f1: Asymmetric segregation, base correction and implications for the mechanism of genetic recombination, *J. Mol. Biol.* **96**:495.

Eskin, B., and Linn, S., 1972, The deoxyribonucleic acid modification and restriction enzymes of *Escherichia coli*. B. II. Purification, subunit structure, and catalytic properties of the restriction endonuclease, *J. Biol. Chem.* **247**:6183.

Fareed, G., Ippen, K. A., and Valentine, R. C., 1966, Active fragments of a filamentous bacteriophage, *Biochem. Biophys. Res. Commun.* **25**:275.

Fidanián, H. M., and Ray, D. S., 1972, Replication of bacteriophage M13. VII. Requirement of the gene 2 protein for the accumulation of a specific RF II species, *J. Mol. Biol.* **72**:51.

Fidanián, H. M., and Ray, D. S., 1974, Replication of bacteriophage M13. VIII. Differential effects of rifampicin and nalidixic acid on the synthesis of the two strands of M13 duplex DNA, *J. Mol. Biol.* **83**:63.

Forsheit, A. B., and Ray, D. S., 1970, Conformations of the single-stranded DNA of bacteriophage M13, *Proc. Natl. Acad. Sci. USA* **67**:1534.

Forsheit, A. B., and Ray, D. S., 1971, Replication of bacteriophage M13. VI. Attachment of M13 DNA to a fast-sedimenting host cell component, *Virology* **43**:647.

Forsheit, A. B., Ray, D. S., and Lica, L., 1971, Replication of bacteriophage M13. V. Single-strand synthesis during M13 infection, *J. Mol. Biol.* **57**:117.

Francke, B., and Ray, D. S., 1971, Fate of parental ϕX174 DNA upon infection of starved thymine-requiring cells, *Virology* **44**:168.

Francke, B., and Ray, D. S., 1972, Ultraviolet-induced cross-links in the deoxyribonucleic acid of single-stranded deoxyribonucleic acid viruses as a probe of deoxyribonucleic acid packaging, *J. Virol.* **9**:1027.

Frank, H., and Day, L. A., 1970, Electron microscopic observations on fd bacteriophage, its alkali denaturation products and its DNA, *Virology* **42**:144.

Gefter, M. L., Hirota, Y., Kornberg, T., Wechsler, J. A., and Barnoux, C., 1971, Analysis of DNA polymerases II and III in mutants of *Escherichia coli* thermosensitive for DNA synthesis, *Proc. Natl. Acad. Sci. USA* **68**:3150.

Geider, K., and Kornberg, A., 1974, Initiation of DNA synthesis. VIII. Conversion of the M13 viral single-strand to the double-stranded replicative forms by purified proteins, *J. Biol. Chem.* **249**:3999.

Gierer, A., 1966, Model for DNA and protein interactions and the function of the operator, *Nature (London)* **212**:1480.

Gilbert, W., and Dressler, D., 1968, DNA replication: The rolling circle model, *Cold Spring Harbor Symp. Quant. Biol.* **32**:473.

Grandis, A. S., and Webster, R. E., 1973*a*, Abortive infection of *Escherichia coli* with the bacteriophage f1: DNA synthesis associated with the membrane, *Virology* **55**:39.

Grandis, A. S., and Webster, R. E., 1973*b*, A new species of small covalently closed f1 DNA in *Escherichia coli* infected with an f1 amber mutant bacteriophage, *Virology* **55**:14.

Greenlee, L. L., 1973, Replication of bacteriophage ϕX174 in a mutant of *Escherichia coli* defective in the *dna*E gene, *Proc. Natl. Acad. Sci. USA* **70**:1757.

Griffith, J., and Kornberg, A., 1972, DNA-membrane associations in the development of a filamentous bacteriophage, M13, in: *Membrane Research* (C. F. Fox, ed.), pp. 281–292, Academic Press, New York.

Griffith, J., and Kornberg, A., 1974, Mini M13 bacteriophage: Circular fragments of M13 DNA are replicated and packages during normal infections, *Virology* **59**:139.

Harigai, H., Kihara, H. K., and Wantanabe, I., 1971, Specific inhibition of DNA synthesis of δA-infected *Escherichia coli* by anti-δA serum, *Virology* **43**:727.

Hattman, S., 1973, Plasmid-controlled variation in the content of methylated bases in single-stranded DNA bacteriophages M13 and fd, *J. Mol. Biol.* **74**:749.

Henry, T. J., and Brinton, C. C., Jr., 1971, Removal of the coat protein of bacteriophages M13 or fd from the exterior of the host after infection, *Virology* **46**:754.

Henry, T., and Knippers, R., 1974, Isolation and function of the gene *A* initiator protein of bacteriophage φX174: A highly specific DNA endonuclease, *Proc. Natl. Acad. Sci. USA* **71**:1549.

Henry, T. J., and Pratt, D., 1969, The proteins of bacteriophage M13, *Proc. Natl. Acad. Sci. USA* **62**:800.

Hewitt, J. A., 1975, Miniphage—A class of satellite phage to M13, *J. Gen. Virol.* **26**:87.

Heyden, B., Nusslein, C., and Schaller, H., 1972, Single RNA polymerase binding site isolated, *Nature (London) New Biol.* **240**:9.

Hoffmann-Berling, H., and Mazé, R., 1964, Release of male-specific bacteriophages from surviving host bacteria, *Virology* **22**:305.

Hoffman-Berling, H., Marvin, D., and Dürwald, H., 1963, Ein fädiger DNS-Phage (fd) und ein sphärischer RNS-Phage (fr), wirtsspezifisch für männliche Stämme von *E. coli, Z. Naturforsch.* **18b**:876.

Hofschneider, P. H., and Preuss, A., 1963, M13 bacteriophage liberation from intact bacteria as revealed by electron microscopy, *J. Mol. Biol.* **7**:450.

Hohn, B., Lechner, H., and Marvin, D. A., 1971, Filamentous bacterial viruses. I. DNA synthesis during the early stages of infection with fd, *J. Mol. Biol.* **56**:143.

Horiuchi, K., and Zinder, N. D., 1972, Cleavage of bacteriophage f1 DNA by the restriction enzyme of *Escherichia coli* B, *Proc. Natl. Acad. Sci. USA* **69**:3220.

Horiuchi, K., and Zinder, N. D., 1975, Site-specific cleavage of single-stranded DNA by a *Hemophilus* restriction endonuclease, *Proc. Natl. Acad. Sci. USA* **72**:2555.

Horiuchi, K., Vovis, G. F., Enea, V., and Zinder, N. D., 1975, Cleavage map of bacteriophage f1: Location of the *Escherichia coli* B-specific modification sites, *J. Mol. Biol.* **95**:147.

Huberman, J. A., Kornberg, A., and Alberts, B. M., 1971, Stimulation of T4 bacteriophage DNA polymerase by the protein product of T4 gene 32, *J. Mol. Biol.* **62**:39.

Ikehara, K., and Utiyama, H., 1975, Studies on the structure of filamentous bacteriophage fd. III. A stable intermediate of the 2-chloroethanol-induced disassembly, *Virology* **66**:316.

Ikehara, K., Utiyama, H., and Kurata, M., 1975, Studies on the structure of filamentous bacteriophage fd. II. All-or-none disassembly in quanidine-HCl and sodium dodecyl sulfate, *Virology* **66**:306.

Inman, R. B., and Schnös, M., 1971, Structure of branch points in replicating DNA: Presence of single-stranded connections in λ DNA Branch points, *J. Mol. Biol.* **56**:319.

Inouye, M., and Guthrie, J. P., 1969, A mutation which changes a membrane protein of *E. coli, Proc. Natl. Acad. Sci. USA* **64**:957.

Inouye, M., and Pardee, A., 1970, Changes of membrane proteins and their relation to deoxyribonucleic acid synthesis and cell division of *E. coli, J. Biol. Chem.* **245**:5813.

Iwaya, M., Eisenberg, S., Bartok, K., and Denhardt, D. T., 1973, Mechanism of replication of single-stranded φX174 DNA. VII. Circularization of the progeny viral strand, *J. Virol.* **12**:808.

Jacob, E., and Hofschneider, P. H., 1969, Replication of the single-stranded DNA bacteriophage M13: Messenger RNA synthesis directed by M13 replicative form DNA, *J. Mol. Biol.* **46**:359.

Jacob, E., Jaenisch, R., and Hofschneider, P. H., 1970, Replication of the small coliphage M13: Evidence for long-living M13 specific messenger RNA, *Nature (London)* **227**:59.

Jacob, E., Jaenisch, R., and Hofschneider, P. H., 1973, Replication of the single-stranded DNA bacteriophage M13. On the transcription *in vivo* of the M13 replicative form DNA, *Eur. J. Biochem.* **32**:432.

Jacobson, A., 1972, Role of F pili in the penetration of bacteriophage f1, *J. Virol.* **10**:835.

Jaenisch, R., Hofschneider, P. H., and Preuss, A., 1969, Isolation of circular DNA by zonal centrifugation: Separation of normal length, double length and catenated M13 replicative form DNA and of host specific "episomal" DNA, *Biochim. Biophys. Acta* **190**:88.

Jazwinski, S. M., Marco, R., and Kornberg, A., 1973, A coat protein of the bacteriophage M13 virion participates in membrane-oriented synthesis of DNA, *Proc. Natl. Acad. Sci. USA* **70**:205.

Kay, D., and Wakefield, A. E., 1972, Complementation between filamentous F-specific and I-specific bacteriophages, *J. Gen. Virol.* **14**:271.

Kessler-Liebscher, B. E., Staudenbauer, W. L., and Hofschneider, P. H., 1975, Studies on the structure of replicative intermediates in bacteriophage M13 single-stranded DNA synthesis, *Nucleic Acids Res.* **2**:131.

Khatoon, H., Iyer, R. V., and Iyer, V. N., 1972, A new filamentous bacteriophage with sex-factor specificity, *Virology* **48**:145.

Kluge, F., 1974, Replicative intermediates in bacteriophage M13: Single-stranded DNA synthesis, *Hoppe-Seyler's Z. Physiol. Chem.* **355**:410.

Kluge, F., Staudenbauer, W. L., and Hofschneider, P. H., 1971, Replication of bacteriophage M13: Detachment of the parental DNA from the host membrane and transfer to progeny phages, *Eur. J. Biochem.* **22**:350.

Knippers, R., and Hoffman-Berling, H., 1966, A coat protein from bacteriophage fd. I. Hydrodynamic measurements and biological characterization, *J. Mol. Biol.* **21**:281.

Konings, R. N. H., 1973, Synthesis of phage M13 specific proteins in a DNA-dependent cell-free system, *FEBS Lett.* **35**:155.

Konings, R. N. H., and Schoenmakers, J. G. G., 1974, Bacteriophage M13 DNA directed *in vitro* synthesis of gene 5 protein, *Mol. Biol. Rep.* **1**:251.

Konings, R. N. H., Jansen, J., Cuypers, T., and Schoenmakers, J. G. G., 1973, Synthesis of bacteriophage M13 specific proteins in a DNA-dependent cell-free System. II. *In vitro* synthesis of biologically active gene 5 protein, *J. Virol.* **12**:1466.

Konings, R. N. H., Hulsebos, T., and van den Hondel, C. A., 1975, The identification and characterization of the gene products of bacteriophage M13, *J. Virol.* **15**:570.

Konrad, E. B., and Lehman, I. R., 1974, A conditional lethal mutant of *Escherichia coli* K12 defective in the $5' \rightarrow 3'$ exonuclease associated with DNA polymerase I, *Proc. Natl. Acad. Sci. USA* **71**:2048.

Kozak, M., and Nathans, D., 1972, Translation of the genome of a ribonucleic acid bacteriophage, *Bacteriol. Rev.* **36**:109.

Kühnlein, U., and Arber, W., 1972, Host specificity of DNA produced by *Escherichia coli*. XV. The role of nucleotide methylation in *in vitro* B-specific modification, *J. Mol. Biol.* **63**:9.

Kühnlein, U., Linn, S., and Arber, W., 1969, Host specificity of DNA produced by *Escherichia coli*. XI. *In vitro* modification of phage fd replicative form, *Proc. Natl. Acad. Sci. USA* **63**:556.

Kuo, T.-T., Haung, T.-C., and Chow, T.-Y., 1969, A filamentous bacteriophage from *Xanthomonas oryzae*, *Virology* **39**:548.

Lautenberger, J. A., and Linn, S., 1972, The deoxyribonucleic acid modification and restriction enzymes of *Escherichia coli* B. I. Purification, subunit structure, and catalytic properties of the modification methylase, *J. Biol. Chem.* **247**:6176.

Lehman, I. R., and Chien, J. R., 1973, DNA polymerase I activity in polymerase I mutants of *Escherichia coli*, in: *DNA Synthesis in Vitro* (R. D. Wells and R. B. Inman, eds.), pp. 3–12, University Park Press, Baltimore.

Le Talaer, J., and Jeanteur, P., 1971, Purification and base composition analysis of phage lambda early promoters, *Proc. Natl. Acad. Sci. USA* **68**:3211.

Lica, L., and Ray, D. S., 1976*a*, The functional half-lives of bacteriophage M13 gene 5 and gene 8 messages, *J. Virol.* **18**:80.

Lica, L., and Ray, D. S., 1976*b*, Replication of bacteriophage M13. XII. *In vivo* cross-linking of M13 gene 5 protein to M13 single-stranded DNA by ultraviolet irradiation, submitted.

Lin, J.-Y., Wu, C.-C., and Kue, T.-T., 1971, Amino acid analysis of the coat protein of the filamentous bacterial virus Xf from *Xanthomonas oryzae*, *Virology* **45**:38.

Lin, N., and Pratt, D., 1972, Role of bacteriophage M13 gene 2 in viral DNA replication, *J. Mol. Biol.* **72**:37.

Lin, N., and Pratt, D., 1974, Bacteriophage M13 gene 2 protein: Increasing its yield in infected cells and identification and localization, *Virology* **61**:334.

Ling, V., 1972, Fractionation and sequences of the large pyrimidine oligonucleotides from bacteriophage fd DNA, *J. Mol. Biol.* **64**:87.

Linn, S., and Arber, W., 1968, Host specificity of DNA produced by *Escherichia coli*. X. *In vitro* restriction of phage fd replicative form, *Proc. Natl. Acad. Sci. USA* **59**:1300.

Loeb, T., 1960, Isolation of a bacteriophage specific for the F[+] and Hfr mating types of *Escherichia coli* K12, *Science* **131**:932.

Lyons, L. B., and Zinder, N. D., 1972, The genetic map of the filamentous bacteriophage fl, *Virology* **49**:45.

Marco, R., 1975, The adsorption protein in mini M13 phages, *Virology* **68**:280.

Marco, R., Jaswinski, S. M., and Kornberg, A., 1974, Binding, eclipse and penetration of the filamentous bacteriophage M13 in intact and disrupted cells, *Virology* **62**:209.

Marvin, D. A., 1966, X-ray diffraction and electron microscope studies on the structure of the small filamentous bacteriophage fd, *J. Mol. Biol.* **15**:8.

Marvin, D. A., and Hoffman-Berling, H., 1963*a*, Physical and chemical properties of two new small bacteriophages, *Nature* (*London*) **197**:517.

Marvin, D. A., and Hoffman-Berling, H., 1963*b*, A fibrous DNA phage (fd) and a spherical RNA phage (fr) specific for male strains of *E. coli*. II. Physical characteristics, *Z. Naturforsch.* **B18**:884.

Marvin, D. A., and Hohn, B., 1969, Filamentous bacterial viruses, *Bacteriol. Rev.* **33**:172.

Marvin, D. A., and Schaller, H., 1966, The topology of DNA from the small fila-
    mentous bacteriophage fd, *J. Mol. Biol.* **15**:1.
Marvin, D. A., Wiseman, R. L., and Wachtel, E. J., 1974a, Filamentous bacterial
    viruses. XI. Molecular architecture of the class II (Pf1, Xf) virion, *J. Mol. Biol.*
    82:121.
Marvin, D. A., Pigram, W. J., Wiseman, R. L., Wachtel, E. J., and Marvin, F. J.,
    1974b, Filamentous bacterial viruses. XII. Molecular architecture of the class I (fd,
    If1, IKe) virion, *J. Mol. Biol.* **88**:581.
May, M., and Hattman, S., 1975a, Deoxyribonucleic acid–cytosine methylation by
    host- and plasmid-controlled enzymes, *J. Bacteriol.* **122**:129.
May, M., and Hattman, S., 1975b, Analysis of bacteriophage deoxyribonucleic acid
    sequences methylated by Host- and R-factor-controlled enzym s, *J. Bacteriol.*
    123:768.
Mazur, B. J., and Model, P., 1973, Regulation of f1 single-stranded DNA synthesis by
    a DNA binding protein, *J. Mol. Biol.* **78**:285.
Mazur, B. J., and Zinder, N. D., 1975a, The role of gene V protein in f1 single-strand
    synthesis, *Virology* **68**:49.
Mazur, B. J., and Zinder, N. D., 1975b, Evidence that gene VII is not the distal portion
    of gene V of phage f1, *Virology* **68**:284.
Mechler, B., and Arber, W., 1969, Parental fd DNA is efficiently transferred into
    progeny bacteriophage particles even at low multiplicities of infection, *J. Mol. Biol.*
    45:443.
Meynell, G. G., and Lawn, A. M., 1968, Filamentous phages specific for the I sex fac-
    tor, *Nature (London)* **217**:1184.
Middleton, J. H., Edgell, M. H., and Hutchison, C. A., 1972, Specific fragments of
    φX174 deoxyribonucleic acid produced by a restriction enzyme from *Haemophilus
    aegyptius,* endonuclease Z, *J. Virol.* **10**:42.
Minamishima, Y., Takeya, K., Ohnishi, Y., and Amako, K., 1968, Physiochemical and
    biological properties of fibrous *Pseudomonas* bacteriophages, *J. Virol.* **2**:208.
Mitra, S., 1972, Inhibition of M13 phage synthesis by rifampicin in some rifampicin-
    resistant *Escherichia coli* mutants, *Virology* **50**:422.
Mitra, S., and Stallions, D. R., 1973, Role of *dna* genes of *Escherichia coli* in M13
    phage replication, *Virology* **52**:417.
Model, P., and Zinder, N. D., 1974, *In vitro* synthesis of bacteriophage f1 proteins, *J.
    Mol. Biol.* **83**:231.
Model, P., Horiuchi, K., McGill, C., and Zinder, N. D., 1975, Template activity of f1
    RF I cleaved with endonucleases R · Hin d, R · Eco P1 or R · Eco B, *Nature (London)*
    253:132.
Nakashima, Y., and Konigsberg, W., 1974, Reinvestigation of a region of the fd bac-
    teriophage coat protein sequence, *J. Mol. Biol.* **88**:598.
Nakashima, Y., Dunker, A. K., Marvin, D. A., and Konigsberg, W., 1974, The amino
    acid sequence of a DNA binding protein, the gene 5 product of fd filamentous bac-
    teriophage, *FEBS Lett.* **43**(1):125.
Newman, J., Swinney, H. L., Berkowitz, S. A., and Day, L. A., 1974, Hydrodynamic
    properties and molecular weight of fd bacteriophage DNA, *Biochemistry* **13**:
    4832.
Nüsslein, V., Bernd, O., Bonhoeffer, F., and Schaller, H., 1971, Function of DNA
    polymerase III in DNA replication, *Nature (London) New Biol.* **234**:285.
Oertel, W., and Schaller, H., 1972, A new approach to the sequence analysis of DNA,
    FEBS Lett. **27**:316.

Oey, J. L., and Knippers, R., 1972, Properties of the isolated gene 5 protein of bacteriophage fd, *J. Mol. Biol.* **68**:125.

Okamoto, T., Sugiura, M., and Takanami, M., 1972, RNA polymerase binding sites of phage fd replicative form DNA, *Nature (London) New Biol.* **237**:108.

Okamoto, T., Sugimoto, K., Sugisaki, H., and Takanami, M., 1975, Studies on bacteriophage fd DNA. II. Localization of RNA initiation sites on the cleavage map of the fd genome, *J. Mol. Biol.* **95**:33.

Olivera, B., and Bonhoeffer, F., 1972, Replication of ϕX174 DNA by *Escherichia coli polA in vitro, Proc. Natl. Acad. Sci. USA* **69**:25.

Olsen, W. L., Staudenbauer, W. L., and Hofschneider, P. H., 1972, Replication of bacteriophage M13: Specificity of the *Escherichia coli dna*B function for replication of double-stranded M13 *DNA, Proc. Natl. Acad. Sci. USA* **69**:2570.

Petersen, G. B., and Reeves, J. M., 1969, The occurrence of long sequences of consecutive pyrmidine deoxyribonucleotides in the DNA of bacteriophage f1, *Biochim. Biophys. Acta* **179**:510.

Pieczenik, G., Model, P., and Robertson, H. D., 1974, Sequence and symmetry in ribosome binding sites of bacteriophage f1 RNA, *J. Mol. Biol.* **90**:191.

Pieczenik, G., Horiuchi, K., Model, P., McGill, C., Mazur, B. J., Vovis, G. F., and Zinder, N. D., 1975, Is mRNA transcribed from the strand complementary to it in a DNA duplex?, *Nature (London)* **253**:131.

Pratt, D., 1969, Genetics of single-stranded DNA bacteriophages, *Annu. Rev. Genet.* **3**:343.

Pratt, D., and Erdahl, W. S., 1968, Genetic control of bacteriophage M13 DNA synthesis, *J. Mol. Biol.* **37**:181.

Pratt, D., Tzagoloff, H., and Erdahl, W. S., 1966, Conditional lethal mutants of the small filamentous coliphage M13, *Virology* **30**:397.

Pratt, D., Tzagoloff, H., Erdahl, W. S., and Henry, T. J., 1967, Conditional lethal mutants of coliphage M13, in: *The Molecular Biology of Viruses* (J. S. Colter and W. Paranchych, eds.), pp. 219–238, Academic Press, New York.

Pratt, D., Tzagoloff, H., and Beaudoin, J., 1969, Conditional lethal mutants of the small filamentous coliphage M13. II. Two genes for coat proteins, *Virology* **39**:42.

Pratt, D., Laws, P., and Griffith, J., 1974, Complex of phage M13 single-stranded DNA and gene 5 protein, *J. Mol. Biol.* **82**:425.

Primrose, S. B., Brown, L. R., and Dowell, C. E., 1968, Host cell participation in small virus replication. I. Replication of M13 in a strain of *Escherichia coli* with a temperature-sensitive lesion in deoxyribonucleic acid synthesis, *J. Virol.* **2**:1308.

Ray, D. S., 1968, The small-DNA-containing bacteriophages, in: *Molecular Basis of Virology* (H. Fraenkel-Conrat, ed.), pp. 222–254, Reinhold, New York.

Ray, D., 1969, Replication of bacteriophage M13. II. The role of replicative forms in single-strand synthesis, *J. Mol. Biol.* **43**:631.

Ray, D. S., 1970, Replication of bacteriophage M13. VI. Synthesis of M13-specific DNA in the presence of chloramphenicol, *J. Mol. Biol.* **53**:239.

Ray, D. S., and Schekman, R. W., 1969*a*, Replication of bacteriophage M13. I. Sedimentation analysis of crude lysates of M13-infected bacteria, *Biochim. Biophys. Acta* **179**:398.

Ray, D. S., and Schekman, R. W., 1969*b*, Replication of bacteriophage M13. III. Identification of the intracellular single-stranded DNA, *J. Mol. Biol.* **43**:645.

Ray, D. S., Bscheider, H. P., and Hofschneider, P. H., 1966*a*, Replication of the single-stranded DNA of the male-specific bacteriophage M13: Isolation of intracellular forms of phage-specific DNA, *J. Mol. Biol.* **21**:473.

Ray, D. S., Preuss, A., and Hofschneider, P. H., 1966*b*, Replication of the single-stranded DNA of the male-specific bacteriophage M13: Circular forms of the replicative DNA, *J. Mol. Biol.* **21**:485.

Ray, D. S., Dueber, J., and Suggs, S., 1975, Replication of bacteriophage M13. IX. Requirement of the *Escherichia coli dna*G function for M13 duplex DNA replication, *J. Virol.* **16**:348.

Robertson, H., 1975, Isolation of specific ribosome binding sites from single-stranded DNA, *J. Mol. Biol.* **92**:363.

Robertson, H. D., Barrell, B. G., Weith, H. L., and Donelson, J. E., 1973, Isolation and sequence analysis of a ribosome-protected fragment from bacteriophage φX174 DNA, *Nature (London) New Biol.* **241**:38.

Rossomando, E., 1970, Studies on the structural polarity of bacteriophage f1, *Virology* **42**:681.

Rossomando, E. F., and Bladen, H. A., 1969, Physical changes associated with heating bacteriophage f1, *Virology* **39**:921.

Rossomando, E. F., and Zinder, H. D., 1968, Studies on the bacteriophage f1. 1. Alkali-induced disassembly of the phage into DNA and protein, *J. Mol. Biol.* **36**:387.

Salivar, W. O., Tzargoloff, H., and Pratt, D., 1964, Some physical-chemical and biological properties of the rod-shaped coliphage M13, *Virology* **24**:359.

Salivar, W. O., Henry, T. J., and Pratt, D., 1967, Purification and properties of diploid particles of coliphage M13, *Virology* **32**:41.

Salser, W., Fry, K., Brunk, C., and Poon, R., 1972, Nucleotide sequencing of DNA: Preliminary characterization of the products of specific cleavages at guanine, cytosine, or adenine residues, *Proc. Natl. Acad. Sci. USA* **69**:238.

Salstrom, J. S., and Pratt, D., 1971, Role of coliphage M13 gene 5 in single-stranded DNA production, *J. Mol. Biol.* **61**:489.

Sanger, F., Donelson, J. E., Coulson, A. R., Kössel, H., and Fischer, D., 1973, Use of DNA polymerase I primed by a synthetic oligonucleotide to determine a nucleotide sequence in phage f1 DNA, *Proc. Natl. Acad. Sci. USA* **70**:1209.

Sanger, F., Donelson, J. E., Coulson, A. R., Kössel, H., and Fischer, D., 1974, Determination of a nucleotide sequence in bacteriophage f1 DNA by primed synthesis with DNA polymerase, *J. Mol. Biol.* **90**:315.

Schaller, H., 1969, Structure of the DNA of bacteriophage fd. I. Absence of non-phosphodiester linkages, *J. Mol. Biol.* **44**:435.

Schaller, H., Voss, H., and Gucker, S., 1969, Structure of the DNA of bacteriophage fd. II. Isolation and characterization of a DNA fraction with double strand-like properties, *J. Mol. Biol.* **44**:445.

Schaller, H., Gray, C., and Herrmann, K., 1975, Nucleotide sequence of an RNA polymerase binding site from the DNA of bacteriophage fd, *Proc. Natl. Acad. Sci. USA* **72**:737.

Schekman, R., and Ray, D. S., 1971, Polynucleotide ligase and φX174 single-stranded synthesis, *Nature (London) New Biol.* **231**:170.

Schekman, R. W., Iwaya, M., Bromstrup, K., and Denhardt, D. T., 1971, The mechanism of replication of φX174 single-stranded DNA. III. An enzymatic study of the structure of the replicative form II DNA, *J. Mol. Biol.* **57**:177.

Schekman, R., Wickner, W., Westergaard, O., Brutlag, D., Geider, K., Bertsch, L. L., and Kornberg, A., 1972, Initiation of DNA synthesis: Synthesis of φX174 replicative form requires RNA synthesis resistant to rifampicin, *Proc. Natl. Acad. Sci. USA* **69**:2691.

Schekman, R., Weiner, A., and Kornberg, A., 1974, Multienzyme systems of DNA replication, *Science* **186**:987.

Schott, H., Fischer, D., and Kössel, H., 1973, Synthesis of four undecanucleotides complementary to a region of the coat protein cistron of phage fd, *Biochemistry* **12**:3447.

Scott, J. R., and Zinder, N. D., 1967, Heterozygotes of phage fl, in: *The Molecular Biology of Viruses* (J. S. Colter and W. Paranchych, eds.), pp. 211–218, Academic Press, New York.

Seeburg, P. H., and Schaller, H., 1975, Mapping and characterization of promoters in phage fd, fl and M13, *J. Mol. Biol.* **92**:261.

Sheldrick, P., and Szybalski, W., 1967, Distribution of pyrimidine "clusters" between the complementary DNA strands of certain bacillus bacteriophages, *J. Mol. Biol.* **29**:217.

Shishido, K., and Ando, T., 1974, Characterization of *E. coli* RNA polymerase-binding sites on fl RF I DNA, *Biochem. Biophys. Res. Commun.* **57**:169.

Shishido, K., and Ikeda, Y., 1970*a*, Possible structure of the thymidylic acid-rich fragments obtained from bacteriophage fl DNA, *J. Biochem. (Jpn.)* **68**:873.

Shishido, K., and Ikeda, Y., 1970*b*, Preferential binding of RNA polymerase to the thymidylic acid-rich fragments obtained from bacteriophage fl DNA, *J. Biochem. (Jpn.)* **68**:881.

Shishido, K., and Ikeda, Y., 1971, Isolation of double-helical regions rich in adenine-thymine base pairing from bacteriophage fl DNA, *J. Mol. Biol.* **55**:287.

Siccardi, A. G., Shapiro, B. M., Hirota, Y., and Jacob, F., 1971, On the process of cellular division in *Escherichia coli*. IV. Altered protein composition and turnover of the membranes of thermosensitive mutants defective in chromosomal replication, *J. Mol. Biol.* **56**:475.

Smilowitz, H., 1974, Bacteriophage fl infection: Fate of the parental major coat protein, *J. Virol.* **13**:94.

Smilowitz, H., Lodish, H., and Robbins, P. W., 1971, Synthesis of the major bacteriophage fl coat protein, *J. Virol.* **7**:776.

Smilowitz, H., Carson, J., and Robbins, P. W., 1972, Association of newly synthesized major fl coat protein with infected host cell inner membrane, *J. Supramol. Struct.* **1**:8.

Smith, J. D., Arber, W., and Kuhnlein, U., 1972, Host specificity of DNA produced by *Escherichia coli*. XIV. The role of nucleotide methylation in *in vivo* B-specific modification, *J. Mol. Biol.* **63**:1.

Snell, D. T., and Offord, R. E., 1972, The amino acid sequence of the B protein of bacteriophage ZJ/2, *Biochem. J.* **127**:167.

Staudenbauer, W. L., 1974, Involvement of DNA polymerase I and III in the replication of bacteriophage M13, *Eur. J. Biochem.* **49**:249.

Staudenbauer, W. L., and Hofschneider, P. H., 1971, Membrane attachment of replicating parental DNA molecules of bacteriophage M13, *Biochem. Biophys. Res. Commun.* **42**:1035.

Staudenbauer, W. L., and Hofschneider, P. H., 1972*a*, Replication of bacteriophage M13: Mechanism of single-strand DNA synthesis in an *Escherichia coli* mutant thermosensitive in chromosomal DNA replication, *Eur. J. Biochem.* **30**:403.

Staudenbauer, W. L., and Hofschneider, P. H., 1972*b*, Replication of bacteriophage M13: Inhibition of single-strand DNA synthesis by rifampicin, *Proc. Natl. Acad. Sci. USA* **69**:1634.

Staudenbauer, W. L., and Hofschneider, P. H., 1973, Replication of bacteriophage M13: Positive role of gene 5 protein in single-strand DNA synthesis, *Eur. J. Biochem.* **34**:569.

Staudenbauer, W. L., Olsen, W. L., and Hofschneider, P. H., 1973, Analysis of bacteriophage M13 DNA replication in an *Escherichia coli* mutant thermosensitive in DNA polymerase III, *Eur. J. Biochem.* **32**:247.

Stegen, U., and Hofschneider, P. H., 1970, Replication of the single-stranded DNA bacteriophage M13: Absence of intracellular phages, *J. Mol. Biol.* **48**:361.

Suggs, S., and Ray, D. S., 1976, Replication of bacteriophage M13. XI. Localization of the origin of M13 single strand synthesis, submitted.

Sugimoto, K., Okamoto, T., Sugisaki, H., and Takanami, M., 1975, The nucleotide sequence of an RNA polymerase binding site on bacteriophage fd DNA, *Nature (London)* **253**:410.

Sugisaki, H., and Takanami, M., 1973, DNA sequence restricted by restriction endonuclease AP from *Haemophilus aphirophilus, Nature (London) New Biol.* **246**:138.

Sugiura, M., Okamoto, T., and Takanami, M., 1969, Starting nucleotide sequences of RNA synthesized on the replicative form DNA of coliphage fd, *J. Mol. Biol.* **43**:299.

Szybalski, W., 1968, Use of cesium sulfate for equilibrium density gradient centrifugation, in: *Methods in Enzymology,* Vol. 12, Part B, pp. 330–360, Academic Press, New York.

Tabak, H. F., Griffith, J., Geider, K., Schaller, H., and Kornberg, A., 1974, Initiation of deoxyribonucleic acid synthesis. VII. A unique location of the gap in the M13 replicative duplex synthesized *in vitro, J. Biol. Chem.* **249**:3049.

Takanami, M., 1973, Specific cleavage of coliphage fd DNA by five different restriction endonucleases from *Haemophilus* genus, *FEBS Lett.* **34**:318.

Takanami, M., Okamoto, T., and Sugiura, M., 1971, Termination of RNA transcription on the replicative form DNA of bacteriophage fd, *J. Mol. Biol.* **62**:81.

Takanami, M., Okamoto, T., Sugimoto, K., and Sugisaki, H., 1975, Studies on bacteriophage fd DNA. I. A cleavage map of the fd genome, *J. Mol. Biol.* **95**:21.

Tate, W. P., and Petersen, G. B., 1974*a*, A catalogue of the pyrmidine oligodeoxyribonucleotides found in bacteriophage f1 DNA, *Virology* **57**:64.

Tate, W. P., and Petersen, G. B., 1974*b*, The pyrimidine oligodeoxyribonucleotides from the DNA molecules of bacteriophages f1, fd and M13, *Virology* **57**:77.

Tate, W. P., and Petersen, G. B., 1974*c*, Structure of the filamentous bacteriophages: Orientation of the DNA molecule within the phage particle, *Virology* **62**:17.

Trenkner, E., Bonhoeffer, F., and Gierer, A., 1967, The fate of the protein component of bacteriophage fd during infection, *Biochem. Biophys. Res. Commun.* **28**:932.

Tseng, B. Y., and Marvin, D. A., 1972*a*, Filamentous bacterial viruses. V. Asymmetric replication of fd duplex deoxyribonucleic acid, *Virology* **10**:371.

Tseng, B. Y., and Marvin, D. A., 1972*b*, Filamentous bacterial viruses. VI. Role of fd gene 2 in deoxyribonucleic acid replication, *Virology* **10**:384.

Tseng, B. Y., and Marvin, D. A., 1972*c*, Filamentous bacterial viruses. VII. Inhibition of fd deoxyribonucleic acid synthesis after a temperature jump into protein synthesis inhibitors, *J. Virol.* **10**:392.

Tseng, B. Y., Hohn, B., and Marvin, D. A., 1972, Filamentous bacterial viruses. VI. Fate of the infecting parental single-stranded deoxyribonucleic acid, *Virology* **10**:362.

Tzagoloff, H., and Pratt, D., 1964, The initial steps in infection with coliphage M13, *Virology* **24**:373.

van den Hondel, C. A., and Schoenmakers, J. G. G., 1973, Cleavage of bacteriophage M13 DNA by *Haemophilus influenzae* endonuclease R, *Mol. Biol. Rep.* **1**:41.

van den Hondel, C. A., and Schoenmakers, J. G. G., 1975, Studies on bacteriophage M13 DNA. I. A cleavage map of the M13 genome, *Eur. J. Biochem.* **53**:547.

van den Hondel, C. A., and Schoenmakers, J. G. G., 1976, Cleavage maps of the filamentous bacteriophage M13, fd, f1 and ZJ/2, *J. Virol.* **18**:1024.

van den Hondel, C. A., Weijers, A., Konings, R. N. H., and Schoenmakers, J. G. G., 1975, Studies on bacteriophage M13 DNA. II. The gene order of the M13 genome, *Eur. J. Biochem.* **53**:559.

Van Ormondt, H., Lautenberger, J. A., Linn, S., and de Waard, A., 1973, Methylated oligonucleotides derived from bacteriophage fd RF-DNA modified *in vitro* by *E. coli* B modification methylase, *FEBS Lett.* **33**:177.

Vovis, G. F., and Zinder, N. D., 1975, Methylation of f1 DNA by a restriction endonuclease from *Escherichia coli* B, *J. Mol. Biol.* **95**:557.

Vovis, G. F., Horiuchi, K., Hartman, N., and Zinder, N. D., 1973, Restriction endonuclease B and f1 heteroduplex DNA, *Nature (London) New Biol.* **246**:13.

Vovis, G. F., Horiuchi, K., and Zinder, N. D., 1975, Endonuclease R *Eco* RII restriction of bacteriophage f1 DNA *in vitro*: Ordering of genes V and VII, location of a RNA promotor for gene VIII, *J. Virol.* **16**:674.

Wachtel, E. J., Wiseman, R. L., Pigram, W. J., and Marvin, D. A., 1974, Filamentous bacterial viruses. XIII. Molecular structure of the virion in projection, *J. Mol. Biol.* **88**:601.

Watanabe, I., Kihara, H. K., and Furuse, K., 1967, Formation of fibrous bacteriophage δA. I. Absence of phage particles inside the phage-producing cell, *Proc. Jpn. Acad.* **43**:768.

Webster, R. E., and Cashman, J. S., 1973, Abortive infection of *Escherichia coli* with the bacteriophage f1: Cytoplasmic membrane proteins and the f1 DNA gene 5 protein complex, *Virology* **55**:20.

Westergaard, O., Brutlag, D., and Kornberg, A., 1973, Initiation of deoxyribonucleic acid synthesis, *J. Biol. Chem.* **248**:1361.

Wheeler, F. C., Benzinger, R. H., and Bujard, H., 1974, Double-length, circular, single-stranded DNA from filamentous phage, *J. Virol.* **14**:620.

Wickner, R. B., Wright, M., Wickner, S., and Hurwitz, J., 1972, Conversion of ϕX174 and fd single-stranded DNA to replicative forms in extracts of *Escherichia coli, Proc. Natl. Acad. Sci. USA* **69**:3233.

Wickner, S., Wright, M., and Hurwitz, J., 1973, Studies on *in vitro* DNA synthesis: Purification of the *dna*G gene product from *Escherichia coli, Proc. Natl. Acad. Sci. USA* **70**:1613.

Wickner, W., 1975, Asymmetric orientation of a phage coat protein in cytoplasmic membrane of *Escherichia coli, Proc. Natl. Acad. Sci. USA* **72**:4749.

Wickner, W., and Kornberg, A., 1973, DNA Polymerase III star requires ATP to start synthesis on a primed DNA, *Proc. Natl. Acad. Sci. USA* **70**:3679.

Wickner, W., and Kornberg, A., 1974a, A novel form of RNA polymerase from *Escherichia coli, Proc. Natl. Acad. Sci. USA* **71**:4425.

Wickner, W., and Kornberg, A., 1974b, A holoenzyme form of DNA polymerase III: Isolation and properties, *J. Biol. Chem.* **249**:6244.

Wickner, W., Brutlag, D., Schekman, R., and Kornberg, A., 1972, RNA synthesis initiates *in vitro* conversion of M13 DNA to its replicative form, *Proc. Natl. Acad. Sci. USA* **69**:965.

Wickner, W., Schekman, R., Geider, K., and Kornberg, A., 1973, A new form of DNA polymerase III and a copolymerase replicative a long, single-stranded primer-template, *Proc. Natl. Acad. Sci. USA* **70**:1764.

Wirtz, A., and Hofschneider, P. H., 1970, Replication of the single-stranded DNA bacteriophage M13: Intracellular flow of parental DNA and transfer to progeny particles, *Eur. J. Biochem.* **17**:141.

Wiseman, R. L., Dunker, A. K., and Marvin, D. A., 1972, Filamentous bacterial viruses. III. Physical and chemical characterization of the IF1 virion, *Virology* **48**:230.

Zinder, N. D., Valentine, R. C., Roger, M., and Stoeckenius, W., 1963, f1, a rod shaped male-specific bacteriophage that contains DNA, *Virology* **20**:638.

CHAPTER 3

Reproduction of Large Virulent Bacteriophages

Christopher K. Mathews

Department of Biochemistry
University of Arizona
Tucson, Arizona

1. INTRODUCTION

1.1. Overview of the Field

By far the best-known representative of the large virulent bacteriophages is coliphage T4, which has been an object of intense biochemical, genetic, and morphological investigation since its original description some three decades ago (Demerec and Fano, 1945). A major reason for the popularity of T4, particularly when compared with its cousins T2 and T6, is the early availability of a relatively complete genetic map (Epstein *et al.*, 1963). Thus, at a time when biochemists were becoming aware of the value of phages as tools for study of many biological problems, a large catalogue of mutants defective in essential viral functions became available. Analysis of the molecular functions controlled by each gene product led to a productive relationship between those of primarily biochemical orientation and those of genetic persuasion. Biochemical analysis of the defect associated with a particular mutant would often suggest the existence of new types of mutants, which could then be isolated and analyzed in turn. Thus, although T4 is a large and complex virus, the ultimate goal of mapping each gene and determining the function of its product is within range. The large number of active laboratories working on T4 and the great extent to which they cooperate and communicate with one another have combined to make this a satisfying branch of science in which to work.

The closely related phages T2 and T6 have been studied less intensely than T4 because until recently the genetics of these phages had not been pursued in the same systematic fashion as that of T4. Recently, however, these three phages have been compared with respect to structure of the genetic map (Russell, 1974) and DNA base sequence homology (Cowie *et al.,* 1971; Kim and Davidson, 1974). Analysis of these closely related viruses has revealed some intriguing differences and also has provided an interesting model system for probing evolutionary mechanisms (Drake, 1974; Russell and Huskey, 1974).

Among the T-odd series of the seven coliphages described by Demerec and Fano, T7 and to a lesser extent T3 and T5 have risen to prominence in recent years. All three viruses have become attractive both because they are smaller, and presumably less complex, than T4 and because they seemed *a priori* to present better models for elucidating general mechanisms in virus replication. This latter belief derived principally from the fact that the T-even DNAs contain 5-hydroxymethylcytosine in place of the customary cytosine (Wyatt and Cohen, 1953), whereas the T-odd phages contain the same four DNA bases as do all known cellular organisms. The remaining T phage, namely T1, has continued to attract attention primarily from the standpoint of how to prevent it from contaminating one's laboratory. However, the recent discovery that T1 can transduce bacterial genes (Drexler, 1973) has aroused long-dormant interest in the molecular biology of this virus.

Phages infecting *Bacillus subtilis* have received a great deal of attention in recent years. This derived originally from the facts that (1) one could assay the biological activity of viral DNA directly by use of the transformation system available in *B. subtilis* and (2) one could use these phages as tools to study the process of sporulation. Later, when it was found that these phages have unusual properties of their own, such as substitution of uracil or 5-hydroxymethyluracil for thymine (Takahashi and Marmur, 1963; Kallen *et al.,* 1962), this class of viruses acquired considerable intrinsic interest.

Because the T-series of coliphages and the *B. subtilis* phages are best known with regard to mechanisms of reproduction, they will receive greatest emphasis in this chapter. However, unusual or interesting features of the replication of some other large virulent phages will be mentioned where appropriate.

1.2. Scope of This Chapter

A full treatment of the reproduction of large virulent phages would include consideration of the following questions: How does the virus recognize receptor sites on the surface of the host bacterium? How is viral DNA transferred from the phage head to the interior of the host cell? How does infection affect gene expression and metabolic pathways in the host? How is the host cell killed? What new metabolic capabilities does infection confer upon the cell? To what extent can interaction of the phage with the host cell membrane explain metabolic changes which occur? How does the viral DNA replicate? How do viral DNA molecules interact with one another and with the host chromosome? How is viral gene expression regulated so that components of progeny phage are produced and assembled in a coordinated fashion? How are the structural components of these complex viruses assembled? What mechanisms have these viruses evolved to protect their own genome while the genome of the host cell is being destroyed, structurally and/or functionally? How is progeny phage released from the infected cell? And, overlying all of these questions, what is the biochemical function of each known gene product?

Two of the above major topics, namely gene regulation and morphogenesis, are dealt with elsewhere in this series, in chapters by Rabussay and Geiduschek (Volume 8), and by King and Wood, respectively. To the extent that these topics are central to an understanding of phage reproduction, they must be given at least minimal coverage in this chapter, but I shall attempt throughout to emphasize those topics which are not treated elsewhere.

Because of the burgeoning literature in this field, a major objective of this chapter must be to discuss phage reproduction as we presently understand it. Various monographs are available to review the older literature and to describe historical aspects of the development of our present concepts (Adams, 1959; Stent, 1963; Cairns et al., 1966; Cohen, 1968; Mathews, 1971a). In addition, the reader is directed to various recent reviews covering some of the specific topics with which we shall be concerned: T4 DNA replication (Doermann, 1974); phage assembly (Casjens and King, 1975); physiology and genetics of T5 (McCorquodale, 1975), T7 (Studier, 1972), and Bacillus subtilis phages (Hemphill and Whiteley, 1975).

2. STRUCTURAL FEATURES OF LARGE VIRULENT PHAGES

All of the phages with which we shall be concerned are morphologically complex, with icosahedral heads and tails of varying
degrees of complexity. Some tails are much longer than the head, and
some are so short as to be almost invisible. In all cases, the tail acts as
an adsorption organ, the site of attachment to the host bacterium, and
the passageway through which the viral nucleic acid passes on its way
into the host cell. The tails of many phages, such as T2 and T4,
contract upon adsorption and thereby facilitate nucleic acid transport,
while other phages, such as T5 and T7, have noncontractile tails.

All of the known large virulent phages contain a single molecule of
linear double-stranded DNA. In fact, there is only one known phage
which contains circular double-stranded DNA—PM2, a small virus
which infects a marine pseudomonad (Espejo *et al.*, 1969). This virus is
also unique among known phages in that it contains lipid, and unique
among known double-stranded DNA phages in that it has no tail. This
small phage is discussed elsewhere in this series, together with other
lipid-containing viruses.

The DNA molecules of the tailed phages include several structural
characteristics which not only are of considerable intrinsic interest but
also provide important clues to mechanisms of replication of these nucleic acids. The earliest-known such aberration is the replacement of all
cytosine residues in T-even phage DNA by 5-hydroxymethylcytosine
(Wyatt and Cohen, 1953). Later it was found that most or all of the
hydroxymethyl groups are attached to glucose moieties (Jesaitis, 1956;
Lehman and Pratt, 1960; Lichtenstein and Cohen, 1960). Some of the
B. subtilis phages also contain bizarre substitutions, including the
replacement of thymine by 5-hydroxymethyluracil (Kallen *et al.*, 1962),
or in some temperate phages by uracil (Takahashi and Marmur, 1963),
and in a recently studied phage by 5-(4′,5′-dihydroxypentyl)uracil
(Brandon *et al.*, 1972; Neubort and Marmur, 1973). Table 1 sum-
marizes present information on base substitutions in phage DNAs.

As shown by work of Thomas and his colleagues (cf. Thomas and
MacHattie, 1967), some phages are terminally redundant with respect
to base sequence, i.e., the terminal portions of the sequence are
identical to one another. Also, some linear DNAs, such as those of the
T-even phages, have circularly permuted sequences. Molecules within a
population have different starting and ending points, even though the
nucleotide order of each molecule is identical to that of all the others.
Finally, some phage DNA molecules contain single-strand breaks,

TABLE 1
Unusual Bases in Bacteriophage[a] DNAs

Phage	Host	Unusual base	Substituted for	References[b]
T2, T4, T6	*E. coli*	5-Hydroxymethyl cytosine	Cytosine	Wyatt and Cohen (1953)
SP01, SP8, SP82, SP5c, SP01	*B. subtilis*	5-Hydroxymethyl uracil	Thymine	Kallen *et al.* (1962)
PBS1, PBS2, AR9	*B. subtilis*	Uracil	Thymine	Takahashi and Marmur (1963)
SP-15	*B. subtilis*	5-(4,5′-Dihydroxy-pentyl)uracil	Thymine	Brandon *et al.* (1972)
φW14	*Pseudomonas acidovorans*	α-Putrescinyl thymine	Thymine (partial replacement)	Kropinski *et al.* (1973)
XP-12	*Xanthomonas oryzae*	5-Methylcytosine	Cytosine	Kuo *et al.* (1968)

[a] Not all of these phages are virulent; SP-15 and all of the uracil-containing phages can establish a "pseudolysogenic" state.

[b] In each case, the reference is only to the original identification of the altered base. Other pertinent references are given in the text.

located either at specific points, as in T5 (Abelson and Thomas, 1966; Bujard and Hendrickson, 1973; Hayward, 1974), or randomly, as in SP50 (Reznikoff and Thomas, 1969). Some of these morphological features are summarized in Table 2.

By far the most extensively studied phage, with respect to structure and assembly, is coliphage T4. This complex virus contains five distinct substructures: the head, which contains DNA, its associated cations, several peptides, and three internal proteins; the head–tail connector, with a collar and attached "whiskers"; a tail, consisting of a contractile sheath surrounding an inner core or tube; a complex baseplate and attached pins containing well over a dozen proteins and a pteridine compound; and six fibers protruding from the baseplate. Powerful approaches have been developed in recent years for probing the genetic determinants of these substructures and their modes of assembly. First in this arsenal of techniques is the extensive collection of conditional lethal mutants bearing defects in practically every stage of virus assembly (Epstein *et al.*, 1963; Wood, 1974). Of the several dozen T4 genes in which conditional lethal mutations are known to exist, nearly 50 control some stage of virus assembly. One can ask whether a given gene product is actually a virion protein, and, if so, with which substructure it is associated. The discontinuous sodium dodecylsulfate–

TABLE 2

Morphological Features of Some Virulent DNA Phages[a]

Phage	Profile	Host	Head length (nm)	Tail length (nm)	DNA mol wt $\times 10^{-6}$	DNA terminally redundant?	DNA circularly permuted?	Remarks
T2, T4, T6		*E. coli*	95	110	130	Yes	Yes	HMC substituted for cytosine in DNA
T3, T7		*E. coli*	60	15	25	Yes	No	—
T5		*E. coli*	65	170	76	Yes	No	DNA contains specifically located single-strand breaks
SP01		*B. subtilis*	100	200	100	?	?	Hydroxymethyluracil substituted for thymine in DNA
SP50		*B. subtilis*	90	210	100	?	No	DNA contains randomly located single-strand breaks
SP82		*B. subtilis*	100	170	130	?	No	DNA contains HMU instead of T
φ29		*B. subtilis*	40	30	11	?	No	—
PM2		*Pseudomonas* BAL-31	60	No tail	6	—	Circular	Virion contains lipid
N1		*Nostoc moscorum* (blue-green alga)	55	110	38	?	?	—

[a] Data for this table are taken from Bradley (1967), Knight (1975), and sources cited throughout the text and in Mathews (1971a).

polyacrylamide gel electrophoresis system described by Laemmli (1970) allows extraordinarily sensitive resolution of the proteins of virions and substructures. A particular gene product can be identified as a band on an electrophoretic pattern if a corresponding pattern obtained from an amber mutant defective in that gene shows a disappearance of that band or its replacement by a lower molecular weight band. Another approach involves immunology and electron microscopy. Antiserum to purified T4 phage has long been known to consist of individual antibodies against several viral constituents. The technique of Yanagida and Ahmad-Zadeh (1970) involves incubation of T4 antiserum with a lysate of cells infected with a particular assembly-defective phage. Thus all of the antibodies are absorbed out except for that directed against the defective gene product. This can then be incubated with whole phage and the location of bound antibody be visualized electron microscopically.

By a combination of these and other techniques, nearly 30 gene products have been identified in specific substructures of the virion (Fig. 1). Several additional proteins have been identified as virion components by other methods. About half a dozen phage-specified enzymes have been implicated as structural proteins, either by direct tests for activity of purified phage or by indirect criteria. These enzymes, listed in Table 3, will be discussed at later points in this chapter.

Finally, the nonprotein constituents of T4 virions are listed in Table 4. The polyamines and most metal ions exist to neutralize the negative charge on the large DNA molecule. More will be said later about the roles of nucleotide and calcium in tail contraction and the role of a folic acid derivative in the functioning of the baseplate.

TABLE 3
T4 Enzymes Reported to Be Virion Constituents

Protein	References
Lysozyme	Emrich and Streisinger (1968), Yamazaki (1969)
Dihydrofolate reductase	Kozloff et al. (1970c)
Thymidylate synthetase	Capco and Mathews (1973)
Endonuclease V	Shames et al. (1973)
Phospholipase	Nelson and Buller (1974)
ATPase (associated with sheath)	Dukes and Kozloff (1959), Tikhonenko and Poglazov (1963)
alt gene function (responsible for alteration of α subunit of host RNA polymerase)	Horvitz (1974)

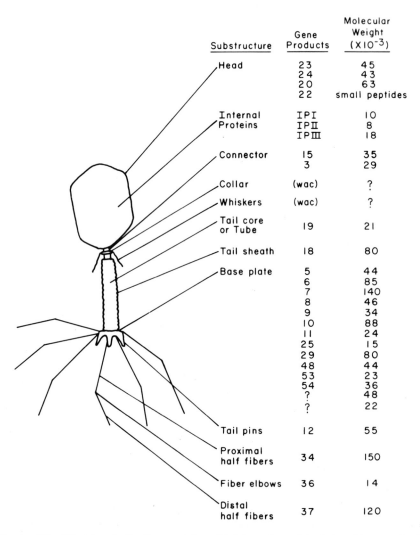

Substructure	Gene Products	Molecular Weight (×10⁻³)
Head	23	45
	24	43
	20	63
	22	small peptides
Internal Proteins	IP I	10
	IP II	8
	IP III	18
Connector	15	35
	3	29
Collar	(wac)	?
Whiskers	(wac)	?
Tail core or Tube	19	21
Tail sheath	18	80
Base plate	5	44
	6	85
	7	140
	8	46
	9	34
	10	88
	11	24
	25	15
	29	80
	48	44
	53	23
	54	36
	?	48
	?	22
Tail pins	12	55
Proximal half fibers	34	150
Fiber elbows	36	14
Distal half fibers	37	120

Fig. 1. The T4 virion, indicating proteins which have been detected and/or genetically identified through SDS-acrylamide gel electrophoresis of purified substructures. Information is taken principally from the following sources: head, Laemmli *et al.* (1974); internal proteins, Black and Ahmad-Zadeh (1971); whiskers, Dewey *et al.* (1974); tail structures, King and Mykolajewycz (1973); Casjens and King (1975); and Berget and Warner (1975); tail pins, Kells and Haselkorn (1974); tail fibers, King and Laemmli (1971) and Beckendorf (1973). Note that *wac* has not been identified as the structural gene for whisker protein or collar protein. Mutants altered in this gene lack both structures (Follansbee *et al.*, 1974; see also Conley and Wood, 1975).

TABLE 4

Nonprotein Constituents of T4 Virions[a]

Substance	Approximate number of molecules per virion	Associated with
DNA	1 (*ca.* 340,000 residues)	Head
Putrescine	60,000	DNA
Spermidine	21,000	DNA
Cadaverine	100,000[b]	DNA
Ca^{2+}	140	Sheath
ATP and dATP	140	Sheath
Mg^{2+}	136,000	DNA
Na^+	36,000	DNA
K^+	24,000	DNA
Dihydropteroylhexaglutamate	6	Baseplate

[a] Data on polyamine content are taken from Astrachan and Miller (1973). Data on metal ion content are from Ames and Dubin (1960). Other data are from sources cited in Mathews (1971a).

[b] Present at these levels only under conditions of anaerobic growth.

3. REPRODUCTION OF T-EVEN COLIPHAGES

3.1. Overview of the Phage Life Cycle

The life cycle of the T-even phages can be considered a paradigm for the modes of reproduction of all tailed virulent phages. The essential features of T-even phage growth were revealed in the classical studies of Ellis and Delbrück (1939) and of Doermann (1948). These investigations showed that there are four distinct phases in the T-even phage life cycle: (1) adsorption, during which the phages attach themselves to susceptible cells; (2) the eclipse period, during which infectious virus cannot be detected, either inside or outside the cell; (3) the remainder of the latent period, during which phage is multiplying within the cell, as determined by phage titration after artificial lysis of the cell; and (4) lysis, in which the infected cell ruptures and releases its progeny to the surrounding medium.

Subsequent study, in many laboratories (reviewed in Mathews, 1971a, and elaborated upon below), has gone far to define the molecular events occurring in each of the above phases. Adsorption, we now know, involves a recognition reaction between the tips of the tail fibers and specific receptor sites within the host cell wall. This is followed by positioning of the baseplate directly above the cell wall and its attachment via the tail pins, or short fibers. The baseplate undergoes an amazing conformational change, almost coincident with the contraction of the tail sheath. This results in forcing the tail core through the cell wall. DNA passes from the head through the cell surface and into the interior of the cell, all within less than a minute. Separation of the DNA from its head and tail signifies the start of the eclipse period, since artificial lysis of the cell will release not intact phage but noninfectious protein coats and DNA molecules.

Shortly after adsorption, the synthesis of host cell specific nucleic acids and proteins ceases, apparently by a variety of mechanisms. Phage gene expression occurs almost immediately. The earliest phage gene products are mRNA molecules and several tRNA species. The early viral messages code for a variety of proteins, most of which are involved in synthesis of phage DNA and its precursors. Some of these proteins are detectable within 1 min after infection at 37°C and all continue to accumulate until 10–15 min after infection.

The transcription of phage genes is timed by an exquisite series of control mechanisms. After several minutes, the transcription of early classes of genes slows, and later classes begin to be expressed. The transcripts of these later classes of genes code for structural proteins of the virus and other proteins which play nonstructural roles in assembly of the virion. Also, at about 6 min after infection replication of the viral DNA begins, and in fact transcription of the latest classes of phage genes requires concurrent DNA synthesis. After several minutes, pools of replicating DNA molecules and of structural proteins have accumulated, and assembly of viral substructures can be detected. DNA is packaged into heads by a still mysterious process. At the same time, two independent pathways are generating tails and tail fibers. Heads and tails are joined in a spontaneous reaction. Fibers are then joined to the baseplate in an enzyme-catalyzed reaction. This generates an infectious particle, which can first be detected at about 12 min after infection. Accumulation of infectious progeny continues until 25–30 min, or much longer under some conditions of infection. Meanwhile a series of phage-evoked changes in the structure of the host cytoplasmic membrane and cell wall culminates in rupture of the cell, with release of a few hundred mature phage particles, from a cell originally infected with as few as one viral particle. These events are schematized in Fig. 2.

Several features of the T-even phage life cycle, while not unique, present technical advantages which help explain their popularity among experimentalists. First, adsorption rates are rapid, so that infections are well synchronized in populations of cells. Second, the shutoff of host polymer synthesis is essentially complete and occurs fairly rapidly. Thus one can use isotopic precursors to specifically label phage proteins or nucleic acids. Third, the presence of an unusual base,

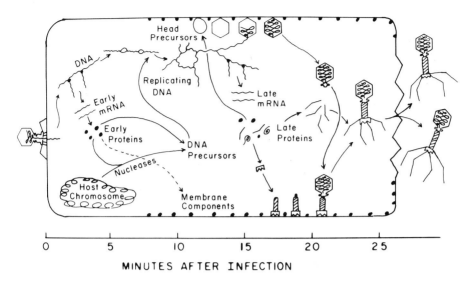

MINUTES AFTER INFECTION

Fig. 2. Life cycle of T4 (schematic). Note that host cell DNA breakdown provides some DNA precursors, that replicating DNA is much longer than virion DNA, that glucose residues are added after polymerization of DNA, that several phage-coded proteins become associated with the cytoplasmic membrane of the host, and that maturation of the head occurs at a membrane site.

hydroxymethylcytosine, provides a "handle" for specifically following phage DNA synthesis or isolating phage DNA. So does the presence of glucose. Fourth, plating efficiencies are high; i.e., under appropriate conditions virtually every infected cell releases viable progeny. Finally, T-even phages undergo genetic recombination with extremely high frequencies, making it possible to map genes with such high resolution that mutant sites in adjacent base pairs can be distinguished from each other. This leads naturally into our next topic.

3.2. Physiological Genetics of T-Even Coliphages

3.2.1. The Genetic Map

A complete understanding of the reproduction of any virus requires that one be able to identify each gene and its product and to know the physiological function of each gene product. For small viruses, with fewer than ten genes, this task is close to completion. For a virus such as T4, whose genome contains enough DNA to code for more than 150 proteins, the task assumes much greater dimensions.

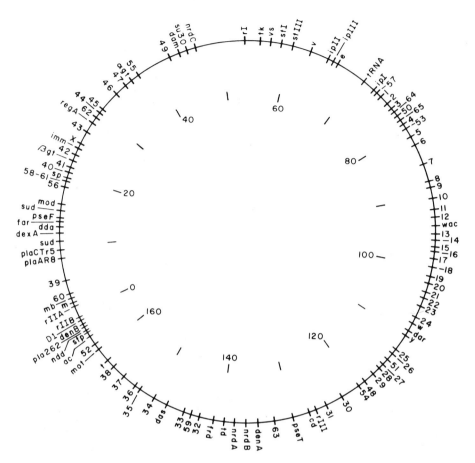

Fig. 3.   Genetic map of T4 phage, adapted from Wood (1974). The total map length is
1.66 × 10⁵ kb (kilobases, or thousand nucleotide pairs), as determined by electron
microscopy of T4 DNA (Kim and Davidson, 1974). The inner circle indicates length in
units of 10 kb, starting at the *r*IIA/*r*IIB cistron divide. The function controlled by each
gene, or the gene product, where known, is given in Table 5. In addition to the genes
shown on the map, there are five sites defined in terms of sensitivity of phage mutants
to hydroxyurea (Goscin and Hall, 1972; Goscin *et al.*, 1973). At least two of these sites
represent known genes, namely, genes 49 and *dex*A. A third site maps very close to
gene 45 and may be within that gene. The other sites are close to genes 38 and 39,
respectively. Also, an additional gene, *q*, confers sensitivity to acridine dyes. It has not
been mapped accurately, but is separated from *ac* by about half the map (cf. Silver,
1965).

The longest step toward that goal came with the development of conditional lethal mutants, first for phage λ (Campbell, 1961) and shortly
thereafter for T4 (Epstein *et al.*, 1963). This allowed one to recognize
and map mutations in genes essential to phage growth. More than 60
such genes, defined by temperature-sensitive (*ts*) or amber (*am*) muta-

tions, have been mapped in T4 (reviewed in Wood, 1974). Many other genes have been defined in terms of the existence of mutants selected in various other ways, such as resistance or sensitivity to certain chemicals, sensitivity to ultraviolet light, altered plaque morphology, inability to synthesize known phage-coded enzymes, or suppression of mutations in already known genes. Figure 3 presents a version of the T4 map, indicating the approximate position of essentially every gene which has been named and mapped; Table 5 gives some information about the function of each gene. The map shows the presence of 117 genes, but this number should not be taken too seriously, for several reasons. First, the "tRNA" gene is known to code for eight tRNA species, and thus could be considered eight separate genes. Second, at least two, and possibly three, additional unnamed genes are defined in terms of the existence of phage mutants sensitive to hydroxyurea (Goscin and Hall, 1972). Finally, mutants selected by different criteria in different laboratories may map in the same gene. For example, three classes of mutations are reported to map between genes 24 and 25. However, when the gene products have been isolated and characterized, it may turn out that these mutations actually define only one or two genes.

In addition to the mapped genes and their products, there are about ten known phage-specified enzymes and other metabolic altera-tions which are presumably under the control of phage genes, but whose genes have not been mapped. These are listed in Table 6. In some cases, such as polynucleotide kinase and RNA polymerase α-subunit alteration, mutants defective in the respective function have been isolated but not mapped. In no case has it been ruled out that the controlling gene(s) might already be on the T4 map, having been identified by some other criteria. Thus we can only estimate the total number of known genes and gene functions as a number between 110 and 130. Since the T4 genome could contain 160–170 genes with an average length of about 1000 kilobases (kb), this means that the T4 map is now about three-quarters saturated.

3.2.2. Physical Significance of the T4 Map

The map shown in Fig. 3 was constructed from data on recom-bination frequencies in genetic crosses. Because of the circularly permuted orders of bases, it generates a circle, even though T4 DNA is a linear duplex molecule. What is the physical significance of the T4 map? In other words, what is the correspondence between genetic

TABLE 5

Genes of T4 Phage[a]

Gene	Gene product, function controlled, or mutant phenotype	References
rIIA	A cistron of rII gene (rapid lysis)	
(m)	Suppresses gene 30 (DNA ligase) mutants	Chan and Ebisuzaki (1973)
(mb)	Involved in tRNA synthesis	Wilson and Abelson (1972)
60	DNA delay; DNA negative at low temperature	Mufti and Bernstein (1974)
39	DNA delay; DNA negative at low temperature	Mufti and Bernstein (1974), Huang (1975)
(placTr5x)	Unknown function; required for growth in E. coli CTr5x	Homyk and Weil (1974)
(plaAR-8)	Unknown function; required for growth in E. coli AR-8	Homyk and Weil (1974)
dexA	Exonuclease A	Warner et al. (1972)
(dda)	DNA-dependent ATPase	Behme and Ebisuzaki (1975)
(far)	Resistant to folate analogues; possibly involved in posttranscriptional regulation	Chace and Hall (1975a)
(pseF)	Polynucleotide 5′-phosphatase	Homyk and Weil (1974)
(sud)	Allows gene 32 amber mutants to grow in ochre-suppressing hosts	Little (1973)
mod	ADP-ribose addition to the α subunit of host RNA polymerase	Horvitz (1974)
56	Deoxynucleoside di- and triphosphatase (dCTPase–dUTPase)	
58–61	DNA delay; DNA negative at low temperature	Mufti and Bernstein (1974)
sp	Controls an alteration of the host cell envelope; mutants in this gene can cause lysis even when lysozyme is absent	Emrich (1968), Cornett (1974)
40	Head assembly	
41	DNA negative; required for DNA replication in vitro	Alberts et al. (1975)
βgt	DNA β-glucosyltransferase	
42	Deoxycytidylate hydroxymethylase	
(imm)	Mutants unable to develop immunity to superinfecting phages or ghosts	Vallée and Cornett (1972), Mufti (1972), Childs (1973)
(x)	Involved in DNA repair synthesis	Maynard-Smith and Symonds (1973)
43	DNA polymerase	
regA	Posttranscriptional regulation; may stabilize T4 early mRNAs	Wiberg et al. (1973), Karam and Bowles (1974)
62	DNA negative ⎫	
44	DNA negative ⎬ Required for DNA replication in vitro	Alberts et al. (1975)
45	DNA negative ⎭ Protein subunit of modified RNA polymerase	Ratner (1974b)
46, 47	DNA arrest phenotype; (?) cytosine-specific nuclease; mutants are defective in host cell DNA degradation	Hosoda et al. (1971), Shah and Berger (1971), Shalitin and Naot (1971)
αgt	DNA α-glucosyltransferase	

TABLE 5—Continued

Gene	Gene product, function controlled, or mutant phenotype	References
55	Maturation-defective phenotype; gene product becomes associated with host RNA polymerase	Ratner (1974*a*)
49	DNA maturation and/or packaging	Frankel *et al.* (1971), Luftig and Lundh (1973)
(*dam*)	DNA-adenine methylase (mapped in T2 only)	Brooks and Hattman (1973)
(*su*30)	Enhances *r*II suppression of gene 30 (DNA ligase) mutants	Krylov (1972)
nrd C	Thioredoxin	
*r*I	Rapid lysis	
tk	Thymidine kinase	Chace and Hall (1975*b*)
v	Endonuclease V	
(*vs*)	Modification of host cell valyl tRNA synthetase	Müller and Marchin (1975)
(*st*I)	Involved in lysis (demonstrated in T4B)	Krylov and Yankofsky (1975)
(*st*III)	Involved in lysis (suppresses *e* and *t* defects; demonstrated in T4B)	Krylov and Yankofsky (1975)
(*far*)	Involved in posttranscriptional regulation	Chace and Hall (1975*a*)
*ip*II	Internal protein II	Black (1974)
*ip*III	Internal protein III	Black (1974)
e	Lysozyme	
tRNA	Eight transfer RNAs.	McClain *et al.* (1972), Wilson *et al.* (1972), Abelson *et al.* (1975)
*ip*I	Internal protein I	Black (1974)
57	Tail fiber assembly	
1	Deoxynucleoside monophosphate kinase	
2	Head assembly	
3	Head–tail connector	
64	Head assembly	
50	Head assembly	
65	Head assembly	
4	Head assembly	
53	Baseplate component	
5	Baseplate component	
6	Baseplate component	
7	Baseplate component	
8	Baseplate component	
9	Baseplate component	
10	Baseplate component	
11	Baseplate component	
12	Short tail fibers	
wac	Controls collar and whisker formation	Dewey *et al.* (1974), Follansbee *et al.* (1974)
13	Head assembly	
14	Head assembly	
15	Head–tail connector	
16	Head assembly	

TABLE 5—Continued

Gene	Gene product, function controlled, or mutant phenotype	References
17	Head assembly	
18	Tail sheath protein	
19	Tail tube protein	
20	Head assembly	
21	Head assembly; necessary for cleavage of head precursors	Onorato and Showe (1975)
22	Precursor, via proteolytic cleavage, of head peptides	
23	Major head protein	
24	Head component	
(*w*)	Involved in DNA repair and recombination	Hamlett and Berger (1975)
(*dar*)	Suppresses DNA arrest phenotype of gene 59 mutants	Wu and Yeh (1974)
(*y*)	Essential for growth in *su*⁻ hosts and involved in DNA repair synthesis	Symonds *et al.* (1973)
25	Baseplate component	
26	Baseplate assembly	
51	Baseplate assembly	
27	Baseplate assembly	
28	Dihydropteroylpolyglutamate synthesis (cleavage to hexaglutamate)	Kozloff and Lute (1973)
29	Baseplate component	
48	Baseplate component	
54	Baseplate component	
30	DNA ligase	
31	Head assembly	
*r*III	Rapid lysis	
cd	Deoxycytidylate deaminase	
*pse*T	DNA and deoxynucleotide 3′-phosphatase	Depew and Cozzarelli (1974)
63	Catalyzes attachment of tail fibers to baseplates	
*den*A	Endonuclease II	
*nrd*B, *nrd*A	Subunits of ribonucleoside diphosphate reductase	
td	Thymidylate synthetase	
frd	Dihydrofolate reductase	
32	DNA unwinding protein	
59	DNA arrest	Wu and Yeh (1974)
33	Maturation-defective phenotype; gene product becomes associated with host RNA polymerase	Horvitz (1973)
das	Suppresses mutations in genes 46 or 47	Hercules and Wiberg (1971), Krylov and Plotnikova (1971)
34	Proximal tail fiber protein	
35	Tail fiber assembly	
36	Tail fiber "elbows"	
37	Distal tail fiber protein	
38	Tail fiber assembly	

TABLE 5—Continued

Gene	Gene product, function controlled, or mutant phenotype	References
t	Lysis-defective; may control synthesis of a viral phospholipase	Josslin (1971a), Nelson and Buller (1974)
mot	Regulates expression of early genes, possibly by controlling promoter recognition	Mattson *et al.* (1974), Chace and Hall (1975a)
52	DNA delay; DNA negative at low temperature; membrane protein	Mufti and Bernstein (1974), Naot and Shalitin (1973), Huang (1975)
ac	Mutants are resistant to acridine dyes	
stp	Suppresses DNA 3′-phosphatase (*pse*T) mutant phenotype	Depew and Cozzarelli (1974)
ndd	Controls disruption of the bacterial nucleoid	Snustad and Conroy (1974)
*pla*262	Unknown function; required for T4 growth in *E. coli* CT262	Depew *et al.* (1975)
*den*B	Endonuclease IV	Vetter and Sadowski (1974)
D1	Function unknown; existence defined only by deletions	Depew *et al.* (1975)
*r*IIB	B cistron of rII gene; rapid lysis	

[a] Genes whose precise locations are unknown are indicated by parentheses surrounding the name of the gene. References are given only for genes not identified on Wood's map, or for gene products on which there is important new information. Further references are given in the text and in Casjens and King (1975) or Mathews (1971a).

TABLE 6

T4 Phage Functions for Which Controlling Genes Have Not Been Mapped

Enzyme or function	References
Thymine dimer excision exonuclease	Oshima and Sekiguchi (1972), Friedberg *et al.* (1974)
Endonuclease III	Sadowski and Bakyta (1972)
Endonuclease VI	Kemper and Hurwitz (1973)
Polynucleotide kinase	Chan and Ebisuzaki (1970)
RNA ligase	Cranston *et al.* (1974)
Inactivation of a host cell leucine tRNA	Kano-Sueoka and Sueoka (1969), Yudelevich (1971)
"Alteration" of subunit of host cell RNA polymerase (distinct from "modification")	Horvitz (1974)
Modification of host ribosomes, including synthesis of two to four new ribosomal proteins	Rahmsdorf *et al.* (1973), Hsu (1973), Singer and Conway (1975)
Alteration of translational initiation factors (?)	For discussion, see Schiff *et al.* (1974), and also chapter by Geiduschek and Rabussay, this series
Inactivation of host cell ATP-dependent DNase (*rec*BC nuclease)	Tanner and Oishi (1971), Sakaki (1974)
Synthesis of dihydropteroylpolyglutamates	Kozloff and Lute (1973)

distances, in map units, and physical distances, in kilobases? The correspondence is remarkably good, as shown by several approaches. In one such approach, Goldberg (1966) asked how far he could fragment T4 DNA and still have it contribute two markers in a transformation system. In this system, genetically marked DNA is introduced into spheroplasts infected with urea-disrupted phage, which serves as a helper. Goldberg found that one genetic map unit (i.e., a distance corresponding to 1% recombination frequency) corresponded to a physical distance of 140 base pairs, in good agreement with genetic data. Although transformation frequencies were low in Goldberg's study, the system has recently been improved (Baltz and Drake, 1972) and has several potentially useful applications.

Another approach, developed by Mosig (1968) and modified by Childs (1971), uses petit phage particles. These are defective particles, produced with low frequency in normal infection but with much higher frequency in infection by certain mutants in gene 23. These particles contain, on the average, one-third less DNA than whole phages (Doermann et al., 1973). These short DNA molecules contain circularly permuted random segments of the entire genome. The basic principle of this approach is that the closer together two genes are, the greater the frequency with which both will be carried on the genome of a single petit particle. Again, this technique generates a map quite similar to the linkage map, with some difference in the area near genes 34 and 35.

An extremely informative approach, both for physically mapping genes and for determining homology relationships among the T-even phages, is DNA-DNA hybridization (Cowie et al., 1971), and, in particular, heteroduplex mapping in the electron microscope (Bujard et al., 1970; Kim and Davidson, 1974; Homyk and Weil, 1974; Depew et al., 1975). Kim and Davidson examined T2/T4, T2/T6, and T4/T6 heteroduplexes, and oriented them with respect to the genetic map by comparing them with T4 heteroduplexes in which one strand comes from a strain bearing a deletion in gene e (lysozyme) or rII (a membrane protein which controls lysis but is not essential for growth). The heteroduplexes all show more than 85% homology, as expected for organisms which are serologically related and which can recombine with one another. The heteroduplexes are circular, as expected from the permuted nucleotide orders. Measurements of the lengths of the circles show that the total genome length of T2 (160 kb) is less than that of T4 or T6, even though all three DNA molecules are equal in length. Differences in molecular weights are accounted for in terms of varying degrees of glucosylation and varying lengths of terminally redundant ends. Similar close relationships between T-even phages have been shown in an extensive comparative study of the genetics of these three viruses (Russell, 1974).*

A final approach involves analysis of a series of amber mutants in gene 23, the major head protein (Celis *et al.,* 1973). Since an amber mutation leads to premature termination of translation at the site of the mutation, each mutant should synthesize an "amber polypeptide" P23 (the product of gene 23) whose molecular weight is related to its map position. When molecular weights were determined by SDS-polyacrylamide gel electrophoresis and plotted against map position, a straight line was obtained. This indicates that map distances correspond to physical distances and that recombination frequencies are constant throughout this gene. The slope of the line yields an average recombination frequency of 0.012 map unit per amino acid residue.

3.2.3. "Nonessential" Genes in T4

More than half of the known genes in T4 are defined by the existence of conditional lethal mutations; inactivation of the gene product blocks an essential stage of virus multiplication. For example, mutational inactivation of gene 43 abolishes DNA replication, because P43 is a virus-coded DNA polymerase, and inactivation of gene 23 blocks phage assembly at the stage of head formation. Since many hundreds of *ts* and *am* mutations have been isolated, one might suppose that all genes essential to T4 growth have been identified. Does it follow, then, that all other genes, whether identified or undiscovered, are "nonessential"? And, if so, why have they been conserved through evolutionary processes, particularly when much smaller viruses are capable of reproduction in the same hosts?

To answer these questions, one must recognize first that many genes, while not "essential," do confer a selective advantage in terms of quantitative growth characteristics, and second that the term

---

* An interesting aspect of relations among T-even and related phages is the phenomenon of exclusion. For example, in mixed infection with T2 and T4 very few T2 particles appear among the progeny; T2 is excluded by T4, even though T2 markers can appear in the progeny as a result of recombination (cf. Mahmood and Lunt, 1972; Russell and Huskey, 1974). The mechanism of exclusion is unknown. It apparently does not involve breakdown of the excluded DNA, for 85% of the T2 DNA in a T2-T4 mixed infection remains intact, as shown by sucrose gradient centrifugation (Okker, 1974); nor, apparently, are DNA glucosylation patterns determinants of exclusion (Russell and Huskey, 1974). T4 mutants unable to exclude T2 map in several different loci (Pees and deGroot, 1975).

"essential" is operationally defined. Conferral of a selective advantage can be seen if we consider the several enzymes of DNA precursor synthesis for which T4 codes, including a number which duplicate preexisting activities of the host cell. For example, gene *td* codes for thymidylate synthetase, and mutants defective in this gene are viable (Mathews, 1971*a*; Krauss *et al.,* 1973). However, such mutants can synthesize DNA at only about half the wild-type rate, and phage yields are correspondingly decreased. Regarding the significance of the term "essential," one must recall that laboratory strains of *Escherichia coli,* such as strain B, were selected for their ability to grow rapidly in chemically defined media. They may not be representative of host strains in the wild. Moreover, growth conditions, whether in liquid media or on agar plates, certainly differ from natural environments for *E. coli.*

Workers at the California Institute of Technology (Cal Tech) have developed a useful tool for analysis of the functions controlled by "nonessential" genes (cf. Wilson, 1973). This arose from questions about the physiological roles of phage-coded tRNA species. Phage strains deleting as much as all eight of the known tRNA species can still plate on laboratory strains of *E. coli,* with reductions in burst size of less than 50%. Accordingly, several hundred wild *E. coli* strains were isolated from patients at Los Angeles County Hospital, and a number were found to restrict the growth of tRNA deletion mutants. This provides a "handle" for analysis of the functions in which phage-coded tRNAs participate. Twenty-seven of the Cal Tech strains are now available as a set and have been used by several laboratories to define restrictive conditions for growth of mutants in "nonessential" genes. In my laboratory, for example, we are interested in the functions of the phage-coded enzymes dihydrofolate reductase and thymidylate synthetase. While point mutants in the *frd* or *td* gene plate on all the Cal Tech strains, deletions extending into these genes are restricted by several of them. Of course, we must now identify the gene included in each deletion whose absence is responsible for restriction. These and other restrictions by representatives of the Cal Tech strains are summarized in Table 7.

3.3. Early Steps in Infection

3.3.1. Overview

In this section, we shall be concerned generally with those events occurring early in infection which are not directly concerned with the

TABLE 7
T4 Mutants Restricted by Hospital Strains[a]

tRNA	CT439	Wilson (1973), Guthrie and McClain (1973)
DNA and deoxynucleoside 3′-phosphatase	CT196	Depew and Cozzarelli (1974)
Internal protein I	CT596	Black and Abremski (1974)
ndd (involved in host nuclear disruption)	CT447	D. P. Snustad et al. (1976a)
pla262	CT262	Depew et al. (1975)
plaCTr5x	CTr5x	Homyk and Weil (1974)
plaAR-8	AR-8	Homyk and Weil (1974)
del(63-32)1, a deletion including denA, nrdA, nrdB, and td	CT196, CT271, CT312, CT511, CT526, CT569	C. Mathews (unpublished data)
del(63-32)9, a deletion including frd, td, and probably nrdA	CT89, CT196, CT271, CT312, CT511, CT526, CT569	C. Mathews (unpublished data)

[a] The genes pla262, plaCTr5x, and plaAR-8 are defined only in terms of the existence of deletions unable to plate on the respective hosts. Nothing is known about the functions they control.

synthesis of phage components—either nucleic acid or protein. Many of these events do not require phage gene expression. In such cases, a useful experimental tool is the phage ghost. Ghosts are prepared by osmotic rupture of phage heads as they are rapidly diluted from a medium of high ionic strength into distilled water. The contents of the head are lost during this process, but the rest of the virion remains intact. As we shall see, effects of ghosts are often quite different from those of phages, but they do allow investigators to study virus–host interactions in the known absence of phage gene expression. For an excellent review of the literature on T-even ghosts through 1970, see Duckworth (1970a).

Our discussion of early events is divided into the following general areas: (1) Attachment of phage and injection of DNA. How does the phage recognize sites for adsorption to the host cell, and how do components of the virion function to deliver parental phage DNA to the cytoplasm of the host? (2) Interactions of phage with the host cell envelope. How does infection change the structure and function of the host membrane? What virus-specified components become associated with the membrane, and what are the roles of these components? Obviously this topic overlies much of what we shall say both about early steps in infection and synthesis and assembly of viral components. (3) Arrest of host cell gene expression. How does the infecting phage inhibit cell division and the synthesis of host-specific nucleic acids and proteins? (4) Inhibition of other functions of the host cell, including the catabolism of deoxyribonucleosides, the degradation of bacterial DNA by colicin E2, and the ability of the cell to support the growth of small DNA or RNA phages. What is the mechanism and biological significance of each effect? (5) Unfolding of the host cell chromosome. What are the mechanism and significance of this event?

3.3.2. Phage Attachment and DNA Injection

An excellent review of the status of the study of phage attachment and DNA injection some 8 years ago is presented by Kozloff (1968). As is discussed in that review, receptor sites for adsorption by the T-series of coliphages are located in the outer membrane of the cell, which surrounds the rigid peptidoglycan layer of the *E. coli* cell wall. T2 and T6 bind to sites in the lipoprotein component of the outer membrane, while a common receptor for T3, T4, and T7 is located in the lipopolysaccharide component. The T5 receptor, a relatively easily isolated particle, contains both lipoprotein and lipopolysaccharide. Recently it has been found that this site also binds ferrichrome, and hence is probably involved in the transport of iron compounds (Luckey *et al.*, 1975). However, relatively little is known about the structures and possible other functions of the other T-phage receptors. Dawes (1975) has described a simple approach to probing the structure of the T4 receptor. She tested the ability of several mono-, di-, and trisaccharides to inhibit T4 adsorption to cells, on the assumption that sugars most closely related to the carbohydrate portion of the receptor would be the most effective inhibitors. Although high concentrations (0.2–0.6 M) are required to inhibit, the effects seen are specific. For example, glucose inhibits adsorption to 100%, while galactose has no discernible effect.

Early work on the kinetics of T-even phage adsorption (reviewed in Stent, 1963) suggested that this process occurs in two stages, an early reversible stage and then an irreversible stage. This was confirmed by the elegant morphological studies of Simon and Anderson (1967a). The earliest step in adsorption is attachment of the phage via the tips of the tail fibers. Following this, the fiber tips probably remain attached, but the phage can still move about on the cell surface, until it encounters a site at which it becomes "pinned," through the short tail fibers (the product of gene 12, Kells and Haselkorn, 1974). These sites seem to occur at points where the cell wall adheres to the inner or cytoplasmic membrane (Bayer, 1968). This probably represents the irreversible step, for isolation of outer membranes from infected cells, by standard procedures, results in a preparation still containing attached phage particles (DePamphilis, 1971).

The requirement for fibers and receptor sites can be circumvented if pinning sites are made accessible. For example, urea-treated phage, in which the tail has contracted as a result of the treatment, can infect spheroplasts (Wais and Goldberg, 1969; Benz and Goldberg, 1973) or intact cells of an actinomycin-permeable mutant (Iida and Sekiguchi, 1971). The infection of spheroplasts forms the basis of the transformation assay in T4, which we mentioned earlier, since intact cells cannot take up free DNA.

Following the positioning of the phage at the membrane, there occurs an amazing series of conformational changes involving the baseplate and associated structures (Simon and Anderson, 1967b; Simon et al., 1970; Benz and Goldberg, 1973) (see Fig. 4). The tail sheath contracts, becoming shorter and thicker, and pulling the baseplate away from the wall. The pins, which remain attached, elongate, and the baseplate undergoes a change from a hexagonal shape to that of a six-pointed star. A central hole in the baseplate enlarges, allowing the core to pass through.

Contraction of the tail forces the tail core through the cell wall. Early work in Kozloff's laboratory (cf. Kozloff, 1968) indicated that cell wall material is hydrolyzed during this process. For some time it

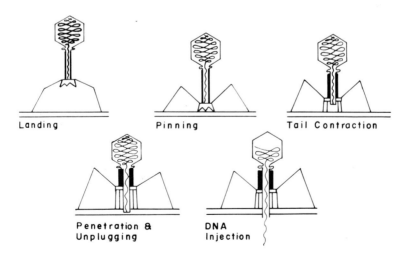

Fig. 4. Stages of T4 phage attachment and DNA injection as modified from Simon and Anderson (1967a) and Benz and Goldberg (1973). Descriptions of each stage are given in the text.

was thought that phage lysozyme (the *e* gene product) is responsible for this cleavage. This enzyme has long been known to participate in lysis, for *e* gene mutants cannot lyse their hosts spontaneously. It was felt that this protein may be a virion constituent as well, for purified T-even phages possess lysozyme activity. However, *e* mutant phages are indistinguishable from wild type in their ability to initiate infection (Emrich and Streisinger, 1968). Such phages do have a second lytic activity, whose role is as yet undefined (Emrich and Streisinger, 1968; Yamazaki, 1969). In any event, as the core is traversing the envelope, its tip apparently interacts with a phospholipid component of the membrane, and this triggers an "unplugging," which allows DNA to be released (Benz and Goldberg, 1973) through the core.

The mechanism of tail contraction has attracted considerable attention because it seems in some ways similar to the contraction of muscle. Indeed, as discussed by Kozloff (1968), purified T-even phages contain bound ATP and calcium, and ATPase activity can be detected in purified sheaths. However, it is not clear from available evidence that these constituents must be present for contraction to occur. Whatever the mechanism, the end result of the above changes is the insertion of the tail core into the interior of the cell, such that DNA can now be injected out of the phage head. The mechanism of this process remains quite obscure. We do know that the DNA must pass through the core "single file," since the opening is barely wider than the width of a double helix. Moreover, we know that the energy for this process must somehow be stored in the virion. Injection does not require metabolic energy, for phages can inject DNA into killed cells or even into purified cell wall fragments. However, the process is temperature dependent, and this was used in an ingenious experiment to verify the cyclic permutations of gene orders in T4 chromosomes (Mekshenkov and Guseinov, 1970). At low temperatures, DNA injection could be interrupted by shearing the infected cells in a blender. Cells which were multiply infected and then subjected to incomplete chromosome transfer could still produce progeny. This can only be explained if different phages introduce different genes, such that the infected cell receives at least one whole complement of phage genes.

Most of what we have learned recently about phage attachment has involved not biochemical experimentation but morphological investigations and physiological studies on phages structurally altered by mutation or by experimental manipulation. An exception to this statement is the extensive research, primarily by Kozloff and his colleagues, on the roles of pteridine compounds in T-even phage virions. This arose originally in an attempt to understand why some phages require adsorption cofactors such as tryptophan (Anderson, 1945). For example, T4B (the so-called Benzer strain) requires tryptophan in the medium in order to adsorb to its host, while T4D (the Doermann strain) does not. An additional type of interaction is seen with T2H (the Hershey strain), which does not itself require tryptophan for adsorption but is inhibited by indole. Cummings (1964) has found that these indole compounds affect the configuration of the tail fibers. T4B in the absence of tryptophan has its fibers extended upward along the tail, but upon addition of tryptophan the fibers become extended distally as the phage becomes activated for adsorption. Similarly the addition of indole to T2H causes the fibers to align themselves along the tail as they become inactivated. Moreover, indole activates the addition of fibers to fiberless T4D particles *in vitro* (Nashimoto and Uchida, 1969). These interactions have some of the characteristics of the formation of π–electron complexes, and Kozloff and Lute (1965) examined purified phages for the presence of heterocyclic compounds which might serve as electron donors in such charge transfer complexes. Tests for nicotinamide nucleotides and flavin nucleotides were negative, but the presence of a folate compound was established. Later Kozloff *et al.* (1970*b*) identified the viral folate as dihydropteroylhexaglutamate, present in the baseplate. This is an unusual compound, since most of the folates in uninfected bacteria contain three, not six, glutamate residues. Moreover, the requirement for six glutamates is specific, for Kozloff *et al.* (1970*a*) found that baseplate assembly *in vitro* could be inhibited by charcoal treatment of the complementing extracts. Addition of synthetic hexaglutamate, but not the corresponding penta- or heptaglutamate, restored complementing activity. In addition, phage infectivity is sensitive to treatment with conjugase, an enzyme which cleaves glutamate residues from pteroyl polyglutamates. This is one of the very few instances known in which the number of glutamate residues on a folate cofactor molecule materially affects its biological activity.

The viral folate was originally sought as a component of the "hinge" between fibers and baseplates. If this indeed is its role, then one might expect to find six, or a multiple thereof, folates per virion. The actual number seems somewhat less, although it has been difficult to measure accurately. In any event, this seems to suggest a different role for the viral folate. In support of this is the recent finding of Kozloff *et al.* (1975*c*) that a folate-specific antibody blocks the addition of P11 to the baseplate, but does not affect the binding of fibers to fiberless particles. Thus the folate seems more centrally located within the baseplate.

The synthesis of the phage folate requires the action of at least two phage gene products. One, whose controlling gene has not been identified, converts the preexisting folates (primarily triglutamate) to polyglutamates with 9 to 12 residues per molecule (Kozloff and Lute, 1973; Kozloff *et al.,* 1973), while the other, which has been identified as the gene 28 product, cleaves these higher polyglutamates to the hexaglutamate form. P28 is thus the first nonvirion protein of known biochemical role in phage maturation.

Phage-bound folates were originally sought on the basis of the assumption that they interact with exogenous indole compounds. Do such interactions occur? Gamow and Kozloff (1968) carried out an intriguing experiment which, while not providing an unequivocal answer, did point to the existence of such interactions. T4D, which does not require tryptophan and is not inhibited by indole, was treated with 2-hydroxy-5-nitrobenzylbromide, an alkylating agent specific for tryptophan residues in proteins. The surviving phage resembled T4B, in that it required tryptophan for adsorption and was inhibited by indole. One interpretation of this result is that a T4D virion protein contains an endogenous tryptophan residue which forms the putative charge transfer complex, while T4B lacks this residue, and tryptophan must be supplied exogenously.

What virion protein might contain this tryptophan residue, or, to phrase the question more broadly, what protein binds the viral folate? Since the folate is at the dihydro oxidation level and since T-even phages code for a dihydrofolate reductase (Mathews, 1967; Hall, 1967), Kozloff *et al.* (1970c) assayed purified T4 virions for this enzyme activity. Although activity was very low, it was detectable in partially disrupted ghosts, and it seemed to be localized in the baseplate. One reason for the low activity may be that the enzyme is buried within the baseplate, under the gene 11 protein (Kozloff *et al.,* 1975b).

What is the evidence that dihydrofolate reductase is a functional element of the baseplate and not an adventitious component? First, phage is inactivated by treatment with NADPH, a cofactor for dihydrofolate reductase (Kozloff *et al.,* 1970c). It was thought for some time that the NADPH was reducing the bound dihydropteridine *in situ.* However, *frd* mutants, which make inactive dihydrofolate reductase, are also inactivated by NADPH, and it would appear that the bound enzyme need not function catalytically (Dawes and Goldberg, 1973a; Male and Kozloff, 1973), but perhaps need only undergo a conformational change, possibly as a result of interaction with something released from the cell surface. However, dihydrofolate reductase has not been unequivocally identified as the target site for inactivation by NADPH. Second, dihydrofolate reductase is a determinant of the heat stability of the virion (Mathews, 1971*b*; Kozloff *et al.*, 1975*b*). In this context, it is of interest that thermolabile mutants of T4 (as distinct from temperature-sensitive mutants)* map in at least five other genes coding for proteins of the baseplate (Dawes and Goldberg, 1973*b*; Arscott and Goldberg, 1975; Yamamoto and Uchida, 1975). This is consistent with the idea that cooperative interactions must occur among baseplate components as a correlate of the conformational changes taking place. Third, phage infectivity is neutralized by antiserum prepared against homogeneous T4D dihydrofolate reductase (Mathews *et al.*, 1973), and there is evidence that bound dihydrofolate reductase is the target site for inactivation.

It is appealing to propose dihydrofolate reductase as a candidate for the virion protein with the critical tryptophan residue whose inactivation makes T4D cofactor dependent. First, the dihydrofolate reductases of T4D and T4B are different from each other, as shown by heat sensitivity of partially purified enzyme (C. Mathews, unpublished results). Moreover, T4D and T4B differ in heat lability of the virion and in rate of inactivation by dihydrofolate reductase antiserum (C. Mathews, unpublished results). Second, T4D contains four or five tryptophan residues per mole of enzyme, and at least some of this tryptophan interacts with pteridines, as shown by quenching of tryptophan fluorescence upon binding pteridine compounds in solution (Erickson and Mathews, 1973). This evidence is, of course, quite circumstantial, and it will be of interest to purify the T4B enzyme and ask whether tryptophan residues in this protein can interact with pteridines.

Somewhat unexpectedly, evidence is accumulating in favor of another phage-coded enzyme of intermediary metabolism as a baseplate protein, namely thymidylate synthetase (Capco and Mathews, 1973; Kozloff *et al.*, 1975*a*). Although enzymatic activity has not been detected in purified phage, persuasive indirect evidence has been obtained. First, antiserum against T4 thymidylate synthetase neutralizes phage infectivity and also blocks a step in baseplate morphogenesis *in vitro*. Second, the *td* gene, which codes for thymidylate synthetase, is a determinant of the heat lability of T4 virions.

Although there seems little question that dihydropteridines and two related enzymes are present in T-even phage baseplates, several disturbing questions remain. First, no specific roles have yet been identified for any of these components beyond the catchall designation

---

* A thermolabile mutant is one in which the infectivity of the virion is heat labile, while a temperature-sensitive mutant is one which cannot grow at high temperature (typically 42°C). The virion of a temperature-sensitive mutant is almost always no more heat labile than that of wild-type phage.

of "conformational changes." Second, both enzymes are synthesized early in infection, yet we have been unable to detect early proteins of the appropriate size among the T4 tail proteins, as resolved by poly-acrylamide gel electrophoresis (R. Mosher and C. Mathews, unpublished results). Third, of the several hundred conditional lethal mutants of T4 which have been isolated, none maps in the *td* or *frd* gene. Finally, Homyk and Weil (1974) have isolated T4D deletions which extend into, and possibly through, both the *td* and *frd* genes. Although these mutants grow poorly, they are viable, suggesting that the two enzymes are dispensable as baseplate elements. Although *ad hoc* explanations can be advanced to explain all of these data, it is clear that these questions must be resolved by unambiguous experiments.

3.3.3.   Interactions with the Host Cell Envelope

Potentially one of the most informative areas of phage research is the use of phages as tools for understanding how metabolic and mor-phogenetic events are controlled by interactions with the cell membrane. It has long been known from physiological studies that T-even phage infection drastically alters the properties of the cell membrane. More recently it has become clear that sites of phage DNA replication and assembly of heads and tails all occur in association with the membrane. At the same time, studies on the synthesis and metabolism of membrane components have revealed changes in membrane protein and lipid synthetic patterns. So far, few of the biochemical changes have been correlated with specific aspects of membrane function. However, knowledge of the numerous biochemical and functional changes wrought in membranes by phage infection, plus the availability of many appropriate mutants, combines to present one of the most attractive experimental systems available for analysis of membrane structure and function.

Pointing to the existence of phage-induced alterations are several well-recognized phenomena, including the following:

1.   Lysis from without. Infection of cells at very high multiplicity causes them to rupture immediately, with no production of progeny phage.
2.   Lysis inhibition. The latent period is greatly prolonged (i.e., lysis is delayed) and the burst size correspondingly increased when an infected cell is superinfected under appropriate conditions.

3. Superinfection exclusion. A superinfecting phage is restricted in its growth under certain conditions, and its DNA breaks down near the cell surface, probably through action of endonuclease I in the "periplasmic space" between the cell wall and the membrane (Sauri and Earhart, 1971; Anderson and Eigner, 1971; Anderson *et al.*, 1971).

4. Development of tolerance to superinfection by ghosts. This suggests that the membrane has "toughened" to exclude ghosts, which almost certainly act through the membrane (Duckworth, 1971*a*).

Another similar phenomenon has been described (Hewlett and Mathews, 1975). It has long been known that nonglucosylated T-even phage DNA is restricted by most common *E. coli* strains, and that the restricted DNA is degraded at the cell surface. We have recently learned that infection rapidly abolishes the ability of the host to restrict nonglucosylated DNA.

In addition to the above physiological evidence for phage-induced changes in the host membrane, there is abundant evidence from the existence of phage mutants in genes which apparently control aspects of membrane function. Some examples include the following:

1. The *ac* gene. Mutations in this gene or the unlinked *q* gene lead to decreased permeability of the infected cell membrane to various substances, including acridine dyes (Silver, 1965, 1967), and hence mutant-infected cells are more resistant to the lethal effects of acridines than are normal cells.

2. The *r*II gene. Mutations in any of the three *r* genes lead to loss of lysis inhibition, and infected cells have a "rapid-lysis" phenotype. The polypeptide products of both the *r*IIA and *r*IIB cistrons constituting this gene have been shown to be tightly associated with the host membrane after infection (Weintraub and Frankel, 1972; Ennis and Kievitt, 1973; Boikov and Gumanov, 1972).

3. The *imm* gene. Mutants in this gene cannot develop immunity to either superinfecting phages or ghosts (Mufti, 1972; Vallée and Cornett, 1972, 1973; Cornett, 1974).

4. The *t* gene. Mutants cannot lyse their hosts, even though ample phage lysozyme is present (Josslin, 1970), perhaps because lysozyme cannot pass the inner membrane to get to sites of action on the cell wall.

5. The DNA delay (DD) genes. Mutants in these genes are slow to turn on DNA synthesis after infection.

Although there is no direct evidence that these genes control membrane function, this is one reasonable interpretation of published data on these mutants (Yegian *et al.,* 1971; Naot and Shalitin, 1973; Mufti and Bernstein, 1974). Recently the gene 39 and 52 products have been identified as membrane proteins (Huang, 1975).

Several laboratories have investigated changes in membrane function directly. In an early study, Puck and Lee (1955) showed that the permeability of *E. coli* increases after infection, as monitored by the leakage of intracellular contents, but that a "sealing reaction" occurs a few minutes later to restore the original permeability. Many substances leak out of infected cells, but the apparent leakage of macromolecules reported by Puck and Lee is probably due to lysis from without of a significant fraction of the cells (Israeli and Artman, 1970). Ghosts also cause leakage of cellular metabolites, but there is no repair (cf. Duckworth, 1970*a*), suggesting that phage gene expression is necessary for restoring the integrity of the membrane. This has been confirmed in extensive studies on cation fluxes—both into and out of the infected cell (Silver *et al.,* 1968; Shapira *et al.,* 1974).

If membrane permeability is increased after infection, one might expect osmotic effects to cause swelling of the cells. Indeed, significant cell enlargement does occur, although some of it is caused by continued cell growth coupled with blocked cell division (Freedman and Krisch, 1971*a,b*).

The concept of reversible membrane damage after T4 infection is borne out if one examines another facet of bacterial membrane function—oxidative metabolism. Although extensive studies have not been carried out, it is known that intracellular levels of reduced pyridine nucleotides transiently increase after infection (Mathews, 1966). Moreover, as we shall see later, the pattern of phospholipid metabolism after infection resembles that seen in anaerobic bacteria. It would appear, therefore, that the cell goes temporarily anaerobic, even in the presence of vigorous aeration.

Several major processes in phage assembly occur in association with the membrane. Following the original suggestion of Jacob *et al.* (1963) that bacterial DNA replication occurs at membrane attachment sites, several laboratories have provided evidence that T4 DNA replication also occurs at the membrane (Earhart, 1970; Miller, 1972*a*; Siegel and Schaechter, 1973; Earhart *et al.,* 1973). The basic type of observation is that after gentle lysis of infected cells labeled parental or replicating DNA is found in a large complex which is sensitive to the action of detergents and which requires for its formation normal energy metabolism and phage gene expression. The functional significance of such complex formation is indicated by the fact that mutants defective in DNA synthesis are also defective in their ability to form stable DNA–membrane complexes (Shalitin and Naot, 1971; Naot and Shalitin, 1973; Shah and Berger, 1971). Although little is known about the specific mode of attachment between DNA and the membrane, the internal proteins may be important, for Bachrach *et al.* (1974) have shown that these proteins are bound to the membrane throughout infection and that they are highly conserved (i.e., transferred quantitatively from parental to progeny phages).

Late gene expression is essential for DNA to become detached from the membrane as it matures. However, Siegel and Schaechter (1973) found that only certain genes involved in head assembly must act for detachment to occur. Formation of tails and tail fibers is not necessary. This is of interest because head assembly also occurs on the membrane (Simon, 1972). Finally, it appears that steps in tail assembly may also occur at the membrane, for Simon (1969) has observed many intracellular phages in which the baseplate is attached via short fibers to the inner side of the membrane, possibly in similar fashion as they are attached to the outside early in infection. This association probably occurs in an earlier stage of infection, for sheathless tails are observed in the same configuration.

Does the bacterial membrane play an active role in any of these processes, or is it analogous to a ribosome, a more or less nonspecific workbench which can serve as the site of assembly for many types of structures? If the former supposition is true, then one would expect mutational alterations of membrane structure to affect processes in phage assembly. Several laboratories have described "host-defective" (*hd*) *E. coli* mutants, i.e., mutants which can adsorb T-even phages and be killed but cannot support the production of viable progeny (Takano and Kakefuda, 1972; Georgopoulos *et al.*, 1972; Coppo *et al.*, 1973; Simon *et al.*, 1974, 1975; H. R. Revel, personal communication). Most such mutants are defective in head formation, and in an exciting recent paper Simon *et al.* (1975) have shown that one of these mutants has extensive alterations in both the phospholipid and fatty acid composition of its inner membrane. The host-defective phenotype and altered lipid apparently derive from the same mutation, as shown by studies on revertants and transductants. The importance of membrane lipid synthesis in general had been demonstrated earlier when Cronan and Vagelos (1971) found that a mutant temperature-sensitive for phospholipid synthesis was also temperature-sensitive for phage production.

The other evidence that *hd* mutants have altered membranes is more indirect. In most host-defective mutants, abortive infection results

in the accumulation of "lumps," or early intermediates in head formation, on the membrane. A few *hd* mutants are defective in their ability
to support DNA replication (Simon *et al.*, 1974; H. R. Revel, personal
communication). Although there is no evidence for membrane involvement here, T4 mutants able to grow on these strains have been isolated.
These map in gene 39, a DNA delay gene which may control some
aspect of membrane function.

Although few physiological events in phage infection have been
correlated with changes in the metabolism of membrane components,
many such changes have been described. Several laboratories have
used polyacrylamide gel electrophoresis in the presence of sodium
dodecylsulfate (SDS) to analyze the protein composition of membranes
before and after infection (Frankel *et al.*, 1968; Pollock and Duckworth, 1973; Fletcher *et al.*, 1974; Beckey *et al.*, 1974; Huang, 1975).
Several newly synthesized, and apparently phage specific, proteins are
found in membrane proteins isolated from infected cells. Pollock and
Duckworth (1973) have detected five new proteins associated with the
outer membrane, none of which is a phage structural protein. We have
already mentioned that the *r*II gene product is associated with the
membrane, although few if any of the other virus-coded membrane proteins have been identified. At least one known bacterial protein, namely
DNA polymerase I, becomes associated with the membrane after infection (Majumdar *et al.*, 1972), although the functional significance of
this event is not clear, since *pol*A mutants of *E. coli* seem normal in
their ability to support T4 growth. Another interesting aspect of
membrane protein metabolism is that the synthesis of host cell
membrane proteins is shut off after T4 infection much more slowly
than the synthesis of soluble proteins (Pollock and Duckworth, 1973;
Beckey *et al.*, 1974). Another fate of cell envelope material—and not
only protein—is its release into the medium (Loeb, 1974). This material
is not extensively degraded, for it is released in nondialyzable form.
Loeb feels that this may represent lytic damage as a result of the initiation of infection, for the rate of release is dependent on multiplicity of
infection, even when the major phage lysozyme is not present.

Late in infection, the membrane is modified further, probably as
the result of its association with structural proteins which are beginning
to accumulate at membrane sites. Fletcher and Earhart (1975)
described a lipopolysaccharide structure, of density intermediate
between those of inner and outer membranes, which accumulates late in
infection and which contains structural proteins of the T4 head.

Several changes in phospholipid metabolism have been reported to accompany T4 infection, but the functional significance of most of these changes is unclear at present. Furrow and Pizer (1968), Buller and Astrachan (1968), and Peterson and Buller (1969) reported that the total rate of phospholipid synthesis decreases after infection and the proportion of labeled phosphate incorporated into phosphatidyl-ethanolamine decreases. However, the changes observed may be a non-specific effect of the apparent transient anaerobiosis in infected cells, for similar effects are seen with cyanide-treated cells. Cronan and Wulff (1969) reported that phospholipids in the *E. coli* membrane are hydrolyzed late in infection, and they hypothesized that this triggers lysis by effecting the functional destruction of the membrane, which both inhibits most metabolic events and allows passage of lysozyme to sites of action in the cell wall. This idea received impetus when Josslin (1970) identified the *t* gene. Mutants in this gene cannot lyse their hosts even though they synthesize ample quantities of *e* gene lysozyme, and one could speculate that the *t* gene controls the breakdown of the membrane. However, Josslin himself (1971*b*) challenged this idea when he showed that many treatments other than phage infection evoke free fatty acid release, probably by activation of a latent bacterial phospholipase, and that lysis can occur even when phospholipid hydrolysis is inhibited. However, the *t* gene product is required for free fatty acid release in infected cells, in accord with an idea that the *t* gene product is itself a phospholipase. In keeping with this hypothesis, Buller and colleagues (Vander Maten *et al.,* 1974; Nelson and Buller, 1974; Buller *et al.,* 1975) have described a phospholipase activity which is associated with T4 virions and is present in reduced amounts in the virions of *t* gene mutants. The virion phospholipase apparently stimu-lates the activity of bacterial phospholipase, although this seems to be a dispensable step, for phospholipase-deficient *E. coli* mutants are killed normally by ghosts, and their membranes become sensitive to lysis by SDS, just as do normal cells. We are left, therefore, with the somewhat unsatisfying situation that none of the known phage-evoked alterations in phospholipid metabolism has been characterized with regard to specific function.

3.3.4 Arrest of Host Cell Gene Expression

T-even phages are rather unusual among known viruses in being able to effect complete arrest of the synthesis of nucleic acids and pro-teins specific to the host cell. This has greatly facilitated biochemical work on replication of these phages, for one can use labeled nucleic acid or protein precursors with the expectation that only phage-specific polymers will become labeled (although there are some exceptions).

How do phages turn off gene expression in the cells they infect? This is a difficult question to answer, because, contrary to earlier expectations, there is not a single event leading to arrest of replication, transcription, and translation. Moreover, there are many known events which could conceivably participate in host cell arrest—such as changes in the structure of RNA polymerase—but few which have yet been assigned a specific role in this process. In the shutoff of host protein synthesis, for example, one can conclude that at least two mechanisms are in operation, since, as already mentioned, synthesis of envelope proteins is arrested much more slowly than that of soluble proteins.

One of the earliest events in T-even phage infection is disruption of the host chromosome, or nucleoid. This can be easily detected cytologically (cf. Kellenberger, 1960), and for some time it was thought that this event was responsible for cessation of all host gene expression. Since bacterial DNA is ultimately degraded, with reutilization of the nucleotides for phage DNA synthesis, it was certainly clear that host genes could not be expressed later in infection simply because they did not exist. However, Nomura et al. (1962) challenged the idea that bacterial DNA degradation is responsible for the early arrest of host gene functions. Their data indicated that 5 min after T4 infection the host chromosome was still intact, as shown by sucrose gradient centrifugation. Moreover, regions of the chromosome remained functional for some time after infection, because cells infected while in the midst of conjugation could continue to transfer markers for several minutes. Subsequent analysis of chromosome breakdown, using gentler DNA extraction techniques, revealed that the chromosome had undergone partial degradation by 5 min after infection (Warner et al., 1970; Snustad et al., 1974), but the fragments were still quite large, comparable in size to the T4 chromosome itself.

It seems clear that degradation of host DNA occurs too late for this to be assigned the primary role in arrest of host cell transcription and translation. Synthesis of host proteins, for example, is undetectable by 3 min after infection at 37°C (Hosoda and Levinthal, 1968). However, it does seem reasonable to propose that destruction of the chromosome is responsible for arrest of host DNA replication. For some time it was thought that arrest of replication occurs almost immediately after infection. However, Scofield et al. (1974) showed that host DNA synthesis continues at substantial rates for at least 10 min at 37°C. By making infected cells totally dependent on exogenous thymidine for DNA synthesis, by pulse labeling to measure DNA synthesis instead of following accumulation of isotopic precursor into (rapidly turning over) DNA, and by using DNA-DNA hybridization to detect bacterial DNA, we could measure host DNA synthesis with greater sensitivity than previous workers. At 9 min after infection, we found that host DNA synthesis was occurring at 40–80% of the preinfection rate, depending on conditions. This is primarily a nonconservative synthesis, which presumably represents attempted repair of damage being inflicted by phage-coded nucleases. Earlier in infection, replicative host DNA synthesis can be detected.

The conclusion that host DNA arrest is caused primarily by DNA fragmentation is in accord with the findings of Baker and Hattman (1970), who studied the effects of T4 superinfection on replication of the small DNA phage M13. Degradation of this small DNA can be followed without concern for artifactual breakdown during extraction, and the results of Baker and Hattman are compatible with the conclusion that degradation is responsible for shutoff of replication. This, of course, involves the assumption that T4 infection affects *E. coli* and M13 DNA replication by similar mechanisms.

Because phage ghosts can arrest host DNA synthesis (cf. Duckworth, 1970*a*), one could argue that the ghost effect—whatever it is—participates in arrest of bacterial DNA synthesis. This may well be true, but Duckworth (1971*b*) has shown that protein synthesis is required for maximal arrest of host DNA synthesis. Moreover, as we shall see shortly, the effects of ghosts seem to be quite different from those of intact phages.

What is the effect of ghost infection on bacterial macromolecular synthesis? In general, ghost-evoked shutoff is more rapid than that caused by phages. This is to be expected if phage-evoked arrest depends on phage gene expression, as indicated by many studies, and ghost effects occur by a different mechanism. Moreover, ghost effects are multiplicity dependent; the more phages infect a cell, the more immediate and complete the inhibition. Since ghosts also do not inject anything into cells but remain bound at the cell surface, it seems that the effect of ghosts is mediated through the membrane. One could propose that ghosts abolish the selective permeability of the membrane, with loss of nucleic acid and protein precursor pools, and indeed many of the cell's low molecular weight substances leak out of the cell following ghost infection (Duckworth, 1970*b*). However, there is not a complete loss of selective permeability, indicating that the effect of ghosts is more complex than simply "punching holes" in the membrane (Duckworth and Winkler, 1972). Surprisingly, Takeishi and Kaji (1975) have found that, in cells infected by ghosts in high magnesium, polyribosomes remain intact and functional *in vitro,* even though protein synthesis is abruptly halted. Pools of amino acids and aminoacyl tRNAs are not depleted by ghost infection, and Takeishi and Kaji propose the rapid leakage of a critical low molecular weight substance, such as GTP, to account for inhibition of protein synthesis. This specific possibility has not been tested, but Duckworth (1970*b*) found that maximal loss of nucleotide pools is not attained until 5 min after ghost infection.

Understanding ghost effects is complicated by the fact that there seem to be two modes of ghost attachment to cells, one which is irreversible and kills the cell and one which is reversible (Fabricant and Kennell, 1970). The biochemical consequences of each type of binding are different, and the proportion of ghosts infecting each way depends in some undefined way on the composition of the growth medium.

Ghost infection was originally studied as a model for early events in phage infection, where phage gene expression could be completely blocked. Although the model is a poor one in many respects, it has been useful. In turn, some workers have used colicin K as a model for understanding ghost effects (cf. Plate *et al.,* 1974). This single bactericidal protein, elaborated by a bacterial plasmid, binds to *E. coli* at the same site as phage T6 and shuts off the synthesis of DNA, RNA, and protein. Extensive experiments, primarily by Luria and his colleagues, have shown that this protein profoundly affects the energy metabolism of cells to which it binds. Studies of comparable depth have not been conducted on phage ghosts, but this would seem a fruitful line of investigation for understanding how ghosts kill bacteria.

With respect to the effects of phage infection on transcription, early studies indicated that the synthesis of all bacterial RNAs was abruptly halted upon infection. Careful attention to the design of DNA-RNA hybridization experiments, however, led Kennell (1968, 1970) to detect host transcription occurring until 7 min after T4 infection, with about half of all transcription at 4 min being host specific. This included ribosomal, transfer, and messenger RNAs in about the same proportion as found in uninfected cells. However, mRNAs synthesized during this period do not become associated with ribosomes, and it seems that some event immediately after infection is responsible for this ribosomal exclusion of host messages.

Although the precise mechanism of arrest of host transcription is not known, two possible effects come to mind: (1) modification of RNA polymerase so that it initiates transcription preferentially at phage, rather than host, promoters, and (2) reduced availability of templates as host DNA is degraded, coupled with increased availability of phage templates as T4 DNA begins to replicate. Regarding the first mechanism, RNA polymerase certainly undergoes many structural changes after infection (see chapter by Geiduschek and Rabussay, this series), but these changes have not been assigned roles in shutoff. Snyder (1973) has reported important circumstantial evidence; a phage mutant defective in arrest of host transcription is also delayed in undergoing a change in sedimentation behavior of RNA polymerase. Regarding relative template abundances, there is little support for this mechanism, beyond the fact that the kinetics of arrest of host transcription roughly parallels the degradation of the chromosome. It would be of interest to examine host cell transcription in infection by mutants defective in their ability to degrade the bacterial chromosome.

With regard to protein synthesis, several changes in the translational apparatus occur after T4 infection, but none has been unequivocally identified as responsible for the cessation of host translation. Changes in tRNA populations were studied extensively in the 1960s in Sueoka's laboratory. One species of leucine tRNA is cleaved within 1 min after infection, and Kano-Sueoka and Sueoka (1969) reported that the codon to which this tRNA corresponds, CUG, is abundant in host messages and rare in phage messages. However, the suggestion that this codon limitation is responsible for arrest of host translation has not been critically tested in other laboratories.

T4 superinfection inhibits phage protein synthesis in cells infected with RNA phages, such as f2 and M12 (Hattman, 1970a; Goldman and Lodish, 1971, 1973), and several laboratories have studied this as a model for understanding how bacterial protein synthesis is abolished by infection. Ribosomes from T4-infected cells cannot translate RNA phage RNA *in vitro* (Klem *et al.,* 1970; Dube and Rudland, 1970; Schedl *et al.,* 1970). What alterations in the ribosomes are responsible for this template specificity? Several new proteins are associated with ribosomes after infection (Smith and Haselkorn, 1969; Rahmsdorf *et al.,* 1973), but their functions have not been identified. There were indications that the factor determining template specificity is contained in the high-salt wash of the ribosomes, which contain the initiation factors. However, there is now some doubt that phage infection alters these factors (discussed in Schiff *et al.,* 1974, and by Rabussay and Geiduschek, in Vol. 8 of this series). More recently, Singer and Conway (1975) have found that treatment of uninfected *E. coli* ribosomes with *N*-ethylmaleimide confers changes in translational specificity almost exactly the same as those brought about by infection, and they speculate that intracellular oxidation of sulfhydryl groups in ribosomal proteins is responsible for the changes seen in infection.

3.3.5. Inhibition of Other Host Cell Activities

In addition to the arrest of bacterial nucleic acid and protein synthesis, T-even phage infection brings about several other known inhibitions of host cell activities, including inhibition of the restriction activity against nonglucosylated DNA, which we have mentioned. T4 phages or ghosts inhibit the degradation of exogenous deoxyribonucleosides in the growth medium (Munch-Petersen and Schwartz, 1972). Normal catabolism of these compounds involves cleavage by the appropriate nucleoside phosphorylase to give a free base plus deoxyribose 1-phosphate, which then goes to deoxyribose 5-phosphate via deoxyribomutase and thence to acetaldehyde and glyceraldehyde 3-phosphate via deoxyriboaldolase. All three activities are membrane bound, and none of the individual activities is changed by infection. However, their functional interactions seem to be altered, since large pools of deoxyribose 1-phosphate accumulate in infected cells. This is almost certainly responsible for the finding of Kammen and Strand (1967) that thymine is incorporated into DNA far more efficiently after infection than before. Uninfected *E. coli,* prototrophic for thymine, does not contain enough deoxyribose 1-phosphate to react with thymine and form thymidine.

Another activity is an inhibition of breakdown of bacterial DNA by colicin E2 (Swift and Wiberg, 1971, 1973*a,b*). This protein attaches at the cell membrane and brings about, through a yet unknown mechanism, the degradation of DNA to acid-soluble products. This process can be interrupted by T4 infection. Like the inhibition of macromolecular synthesis, there appear to be at least two different effects, one of which requires phage gene expression and one which does not. Since one theory of colicin E2 action is that it somehow "activates" endonuclease I, an envelope-specific enzyme, one can speculate that interaction of phage with the membrane simply reverses this activation, but the mechanism of the effect is not yet known.

Finally, infection by T4 or other double-stranded DNA phages inactivates the "*rec*BC" nuclease, the ATP-dependent DNase coded for by the *E. coli rec*B and *rec*C genes (Tanner and Oishi, 1971; Sakaki, 1974). The physiological significance of this effect is unknown, but it apparently does require phage gene expression.

3.3.6. Disruption of the Host Chromosome

It has long been known from cytological observations that the bacterial chromosome becomes disrupted soon after infection, and instead of occupying a central position within the cell becomes associated with the membrane at numerous points. Superimposed on this process, and beginning slightly earlier, is an "unfolding" of the chromosome, i.e., a relaxation of the superhelical twists which give the chromosome, or nucleoid, its cohesiveness (Tutas *et al.*, 1974). Both processes—disruption and unfolding—are apparently independent of each other and of DNA degradation, which begins later. Snustad and Conroy (1974) have described mutants unable to bring about nuclear disruption. These *ndd* mutants seem unaltered from wild type with respect to most physiological parameters, but they are restricted by one of the Cal Tech hospital strains of *E. coli* (Table 7). Nuclear disruption is not directly related to host DNA breakdown, although it may facilitate this process. Nuclear disruption occurs normally in infection by *den*A mutants, which cannot degrade host DNA (Snustad *et al.*, 1972). Conversely, the nucleoid can unfold, and DNA be broken down, in infection by *ndd* mutants (Snustad *et al.*, 1974). It seems that the *ndd* gene product, whatever its biochemical function, brings about attachment of chromosomal DNA to the membrane at multiple points. The concurrent binding of DNA polymerase I to the membrane may be involved in this step (Parson *et al.*, 1973). In this context, it would be interesting to know whether DNA polymerase I becomes membrane bound in *ndd*-infected cells.

Quite recently, Snustad *et al.* (1976*b*) have described T4 mutants defective in unfolding of the host cell nucleoid. The gene involved, termed *unf*, maps near gene 63. Consistent with the idea that unfolding, disruption, and degradation are independent processes, these mutations have little effect on either the rate of host cell DNA degradation or the arrest of host gene expression.

3.4. Physiological Roles of T-Even Phage-Coded Enzymes

3.4.1. Early Enzymes and Their Structural Genes

A germinal concept in our understanding of how viruses reproduce themselves arose from the discovery by S. S. Cohen and his colleagues that T-even phages can direct the synthesis of new enzyme activities in the cells they infect (reviewed in Cohen, 1968). This concept derived primarily from studies on biosynthesis of the unique viral pyrimidine, 5-hydroxymethylcytosine. This substance arises at the nucleotide level, via a tetrahydrofolate-dependent reaction from dCMP. Cohen and his colleagues realized early that a related enzyme, thymidylate synthetase, is also synthesized in response to phage infection. This enzyme, however, also exists in uninfected *E. coli.* Infection augments the activity, by synthesis of a distinct form of the enzyme, which acts to help the cell increase its rate of synthesis of DNA precursors. Since the total rate of DNA synthesis increases severalfold after infection, while the rate of RNA synthesis decreases greatly (recall that rRNA and host tRNA syntheses are shut off), it is clearly to the advantage of the infected cell to be able to funnel its nucleotides into DNA precursor pools.

The development of conditional lethal T4 mutants made it possible to identify genes coding for particular phage enzymes and greatly facilitated studies on their physiological roles. For example, mutants defective in gene 42 have a DNA-negative phenotype, and dCMP hydroxymethylase activity is undetectable under restrictive conditions of infection. Thus this enzyme can be definitely assigned a role in synthesis of HMC nucleotides. Moreover, as shown in Buchanan's laboratory, *ts* gene 42 mutants direct synthesis of a heat-labile form of dCMP hydroxymethylase, and the enzyme in suppressed amber gene 42 mutants can be distinguished from the wild-type enzyme. Thus gene 42 is identified as the structural gene for dCMP hydroxymethylase, and the presumed physiological role of the enzyme is confirmed.

By approaches such as these, the genes coding for about two dozen enzymes of nucleic acid metabolism have been identified, as was shown in Fig. 2 and previously reviewed (Mathews, 1971*a*). These "early enzymes" can be roughly subdivided into three classes: enzymes of DNA precursor synthesis, nucleases, and enzymes of nucleic acid synthesis. We shall consider their physiological roles in that order.

3.4.2. Enzymes of DNA Precursor Synthesis

Pathways in the T4-infected cell for DNA precursor synthesis are shown in Fig. 5. Inspection of this figure reveals several novel aspects of DNA precursor synthesis in this system. First, the breakdown of host DNA provides an important source of deoxyribonucleotides. This complex process requires the action of at least five phage gene products. Second, there are several multifunctional enzymes involved, such as the gene 1 deoxynucleoside monophosphate (dNMP) kinase,

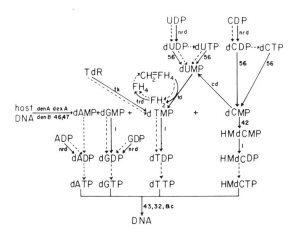

Fig. 5. Pathways of DNA precursor synthesis in T4 phage infected cells. Each reaction known to be catalyzed by a phage-coded enzyme is indicated with a solid arrow and the name or number of the controlling gene(s). Reactions catalyzed by host enzymes are indicated with dashed arrows.

which phosphorylates HM-dCMP, dGMP, and dTMP, and the gene 56 nucleoside di- and triphosphatase, which catalyzes the breakdown of dCTP, dCDP, dUTP, and dCDP to the respective monophosphates. In light of the large amounts of information in T-even phage genomes, it is perhaps surprising that evolutionary mechanisms have selected for these and other proteins with multiple functions. Third, the ultimate step in DNA precursor synthesis, namely the synthesis of deoxynucleoside triphosphates (dNTPs) from diphosphates (dNDPs), seems not to be catalyzed by virus-specific enzymes.

While the pathway involving P42 and P1 is involved in synthesis of HMC nucleotides, the reaction catalyzed by P56 is essential to assure exclusion of cytosine from phage DNA (and also as a biosynthetic route to dCMP, Price and Warner, 1969). One might ask what is the advantage to a virus of maintaining elaborate mechanisms to synthesize DNA of unique base composition, particularly when the base substitution does not affect the coding properties of the DNA molecule. An obvious answer is that since these phages degrade bacterial DNA to provide viral precursors, there must be some mechanism to protect phage DNA from the same fate. Indeed, multiple mutants in which both P56 and nucleases specific for cytosine-containing DNA are inactivated can accumulate cytosine-containing T4 DNA. However, this DNA is defective, because genes normally expressed late in infection cannot be transcribed (Bolle *et al.*, 1968; Kutter and Wiberg, 1969; Kutter *et al.*, 1975), nor can the small amount of late RNA be translated (Wu *et al.,* 1975*a*). Thus HMC plays an additional role in determining the ability of DNA to serve as a template for transcription, although we do not yet understand the nature of this effect. Finally, the hydroxymethyl groups in HMC serve as the site for glucosylation, a reaction essential for protection of HMC-containing DNA against host-controlled restriction, which we shall discuss later.

In eukaryotic cells, enzymes of DNA precursor metabolism are subject to elaborate feedback control mechanisms, usually involving dNTPs. Have such mechanisms survived in phage-coded enzymes, which are designed to operate continuously until the host cell has lysed? Apparently so, judging from work on dCMP deaminase (Scocca *et al.,* 1969; Maley *et al.,* 1972) and on ribonucleoside diphosphate (rNDP) reductase (Berglund, 1972; Yeh and Tessman, 1972). However, T4-induced thymidine kinase seems to be insensitive to feedback inhibition and activation by dNTPs (Ritchie *et al.,* 1974).

Do feedback regulatory effects seen *in vitro* actually operate to control metabolism in the infected cell? This question has not been answered for dCMP deaminase, but it does now appear that rNDP reductase is subject to the same control mechanisms *in vivo* and *in vitro*. Mathews (1972) reported that the intracellular concentrations of nucleoside triphosphates in *E. coli* B are within the range known to activate or inhibit either the cellular or virus-coded rNDP reductase. However, the pools of dNTPs expand manyfold when DNA synthesis is blocked genetically, suggesting that the phage enzyme activity is poorly regulated, if at all. On the other hand, about half of the pool expansion is derived from nucleotides released by bacterial DNA breakdown (Mathews, 1976), and not from synthesis *de novo*. Moreover, dATP, which acts as a general inhibitor of the *E. coli* enzyme, inhibits only the reduction of GDP by the T4 enzyme (Berglund, 1972), and in my studies the dGTP ·pool was the only one which did not expand when DNA synthesis was blocked.

Ribonucleotide reductase utilizes a small protein, thioredoxin, as electron donor in reducing rNDPs. The enzymes are species specific in that the T4-specified thioredoxin (the *nrd*C gene product) cannot interact with the host enzyme and *vice versa*. Berglund and Holmgren (1975) have reported that *E. coli* thioredoxin preferentially reduces T4 thioredoxin. They speculate that this would tend to leave *E. coli* thioredoxin oxidized, and hence inactive, in the infected cell, so that only the phage enzyme functions. However, the electrons for reduction of both thioredoxins derive ultimately from TPNH, and levels of this nucleotide are far higher in infected cells than those of TPN (Mathews,

1966). Hence it would appear that both enzymes should be capable of functioning.

Several lines of evidence indicate that the physiological roles of some early enzymes are much more complex than simply participation in DNA precursor biosynthesis. We have already mentioned that thymidylate synthetase and dihydrofolate reductase apparently play additional roles as structural elements of the baseplate. An equally intriguing story pertains to the role of dCMP hydroxymethylase. A particular gene 42 *ts* mutant was found to synthesize significant quantities of hydroxymethylase as measured in extracts of cells infected at a restrictive temperature, even though no DNA was made *in vivo*. Chiu and Greenberg (1968) interpreted this as evidence that P42 plays an additional role, possibly in DNA synthesis, and that this second function is more heat labile than the hydroxymethylase step. However, these cells do not accumulate pools of HMC nucleotides (Mathews, 1972; Tomich and Greenberg, 1973), indicating that the enzyme is not functioning *in vivo*, even though activity can be detected in extracts. This point was further investigated by Tomich *et al.* (1974), who devised an ingenious assay for hydroxymethylase activity *in vivo*, based on the release of tritium from [^{3}H]deoxyuridine provided to infected cells as a pyrimidine precursor. They found that even in normal infection the activity of this enzyme in extracts is detectable for several minutes before it begins to function intracellularly. The same is true for thymidylate synthetase, and Greenberg and colleagues feel that these and other early enzymes become active *in vivo* only after they have been incorporated into a complex of enzymes of dNTP and DNA synthesis. In this context, Karam and Chao (1975) have presented genetic evidence for interaction between dCMP hydroxymethylase and DNA polymerase.

Certainly it is attractive to visualize such a complex, because in general DNA chain growth is very rapid and occurs at a limited number of sites within a cell (even though this limited number in a T4-infected cell may be as high as 60, Werner, 1968). Complex formation could provide a "funnel" to ensure that precursors are available where needed and in sufficient quantity. However, there is evidence that the enzyme must be functional even when it is not needed to supply precursors. Cells infected with gene 42 amber mutants cannot synthesize DNA *in situ* in the presence of added dNTPs, in either toluene-treated or sucrose-plasmolyzed cell systems (Wovcha *et al.*, 1973; Dicou and Cozzarelli, 1973; Collinsworth and Mathews, 1974). Wovcha and colleagues interpreted this as evidence for direct participation of hydroxymethylase in replication. However, since DNA synthesis *in situ* represents extension of chains which were growing *in vivo* before cell harvesting, Dicou and Cozzarelli reasoned that the failure of 42 mutants to direct DNA synthesis *in situ* merely reflects a failure of growing points to have been formed *in vivo*. In a test of this idea, we found that cells infected at permissive temperature with gene 42 *ts* mutants still display a DNA-defective phenotype *in situ* at restrictive temperature (North *et al.*, 1976). Thus an active P42 is required *in situ*, even when precursors and replication forks are present. The nature of this requirement is not clear, particularly in light of the fact that six purified T4 proteins, not including P42, can carry out extensive DNA replication *in vitro* (Alberts *et al.*, 1975).

An additional facet of regulation of dNTP synthesis has come to light in recent studies on DNA precursor pool dynamics when DNA synthesis is inhibited (Mathews, 1976). As shown previously, dNTP pools expand manyfold, but in the more recent study we found that dNDPs accumulate almost as rapidly and to comparable extents. Bello and Bessman (1963) reported that uninfected *E. coli* contains a highly active dNDP kinase which, even after full synthesis of the gene 1 dNMP kinase, is some thirtyfold more active than the phage-induced enzyme. If the same ratio of activities were maintained *in vivo*, one would not expect dNDPs to accumulate. The fact that they do suggests that dNDP kinase is regulated *in vivo*, perhaps by interaction with virus-specific components. Evidence for this has recently been obtained in our laboratory (Mathews *et al.*, to be published).

3.4.3. Nucleases

We treat nucleases in a separate subsection of our discussion because of the large number of known phage-specific nucleases and the difficulty of assigning physiological roles to each. Many processes in the T-even phage life cycle are known or presumed to require the action of nucleases, including DNA replication, DNA repair, genetic recombination, host DNA degradation, and DNA maturation, in which a giant replicative intermediate is cut into genome-length pieces and packaged into heads. Against this panoply of functions are arrayed a battery of nine known nucleases and about four others whose existence is presumed but not yet demonstrated.

Properties of the six known T4-specified endonucleases and three exonucleases are summarized in Table 8. Endonucleases II through VI create 5′-P- and 3′-OH-terminated breaks. Endonuclease II functions

TABLE 8

Nucleases Induced in T4 Infection

Enzyme	Time of synthesis	Preferred substrate	Divalent cation activator	Action on T4 DNA?	Function	References
Endonuclease II	Early	Native DNA	Mg^{2+}	No	Host DNA degradation	Sadowski and Hurwitz (1969)
Endonuclease III	Early	Single-stranded DNA	Mg^{2+}	A little	?	Sadowski and Bakyta (1972)
Endonuclease IV	Early	Single-stranded DNA	Mg^{2+}	No	Host DNA degradation (alternate pathway)	Sadowski and Bakyta (1972), Parson and Snustad (1975)
Endonuclease V	Early	UV-irradiated DNA	None	Yes	Excision repair	Yasuda and Sekiguchi (1970), Minton et al. (1975)
Endonuclease VI	Late	Single- or double-stranded DNA	Mn^{2+}	Yes	?	Kemper and Hurwitz (1973)
Unnamed endonuclease	Late	Native T4 DNA	Mg^{2+}	Yes	?	Altman and Meselson (1970), Ando et al. (1970)
Exonuclease A	Early	3'-OH-termini in oligonucleotides	Mg^{2+}	A little	?	Short and Koerner (1969)
Exonuclease B	Early	5'-side of thymine dimers in UV-irradiated, endonuclease V treated DNA	Mg^{2+}	Yes	Excision repair	Ohshima and Sekiguchi (1972), Friedberg et al. (1974)
Polymerase-associated exonuclease	Early	Unpaired 3'-OH-termini in double-stranded DNA	Mg^{2+}	Yes	Error erasure in replication	Hershfield and Nossal (1972), Muzyczka et al. (1972)

in host DNA degradation, for *den*A mutants, defective in this enzyme, cannot degrade the DNA of their host. In a mutant lacking both endonuclease II and the *ndd* function, some breakdown catalyzed by endonuclease IV is observed. Neither endonuclease is required for phage growth under most conditions, for the nucleotides released by DNA breakdown can also be supplied by *de novo* synthesis. An additional activity, controlled by genes 46 and 47, is necessary to complete the degradation of host DNA fragments to acid-soluble material (Kutter and Wiberg, 1968). Presumably this activity is an exonuclease, but since the gene products have not been isolated in active form, this has not been tested directly. Unlike the *den*A or *den*B mutation, however, inactivation of either gene 46 or 47 is lethal to the phage, for these functions are involved in DNA replication as well as in host DNA degradation (Shalitin and Naot, 1971; Shah and Berger, 1971; Hosoda *et al.*, 1971).

Endonuclease V is involved in excision repair of DNA, for *v* gene mutants, which cannot synthesize this enzyme, are abnormally sensitive to ultraviolet light. In an intriguing report, Shames *et al.* (1973) presented evidence that endonuclease V is a virion protein, which is injected into cells with viral DNA and can repair UV-damaged parental phage DNA in previously irradiated phage, even when new protein synthesis after infection is prevented by chloramphenicol treatment. They also reported that "phenotypic mixing" can occur in a v^+ × v^- mixed infection, i.e., the formation of genotypically v^- phage which carries the v^+ enzyme and hence is phenotypically normal. However, these conclusions were challenged by Chiang and Harm (1974), who examined 300 phenotypically v^+ phages from a v^+ × v^- mixed infection. None of these was genotypically v^-, indicating that phenotypic mixing had not occurred. Chiang and Harm explain the results of Shames and colleagues in terms of a small amount of protein synthesis occurring even in cells infected in the presence of chloramphenicol. Thus a small but significant amount of endonuclease V could have been synthesized after infection in the experiments of Shames and colleagues. To this observer, it seems that the arguments of Chiang and Harm have considerable merit, particularly since biological expression of the *v* function should require very little enzyme.

The polymerase-associated exonuclease is an activity of the T4 DNA polymerase coded for by gene 43. Indeed, some unsuppressed amber mutants in gene 43 specify an incomplete gene product which has nuclease activity but no polymerase activity (Nossal, 1969; O'Donnell and Karam, 1972). Involvement of this activity in replication is inferred from studies on *ts* gene 43 mutations which are either mutagenic or antimutagenic (Speyer and Rosenberg, 1968; Drake, 1974). It was presumed that the exonuclease activity could function as an error-correcting mechanism during replication; when a mispaired base was erroneously inserted by polymerase action, it could be removed by the exonuclease activity. In accord with this prediction, Muzyczka *et al.* (1972) found that mutator forms of P43 have low ratios of exonuclease-to-polymerase activity when compared to wild-type enzyme, while antimutator forms have a high exonuclease-to-polymerase ratio. Presumably the ratio found in wild type represents an evolutionary balance reflecting the adaptive value to an organism of being able to undergo mutation at a particular rate.

Physiological functions for the remaining four nucleases are unknown. In the case of exonuclease A, mutants lacking this enzyme are largely indistinguishable from wild type (Warner *et al.,* 1972), and mutants altered in synthesis of the other enzymes have not been described. An additional nuclease function may be associated with the *r*II gene product. *r*II mutations suppress the DNA-defective phenotype of gene 30 (DNA ligase) mutations (Karam and Barker, 1971; Krisch *et al.,* 1971). One possible explanation for this phenomenon is that *r*II controls, either directly or indirectly, a nuclease which attacks nicked DNA, which could accumulate if the phage ligase were defective.

3.4.4. Enzymes of Nucleic Acid Synthesis

Figure 6 indicates the reactions catalyzed by several T4-specified enzymes which act upon DNA, including polymerase, ligase, glucosyltransferases, methyltransferase, kinase, and phosphatases. The properties of these enzymes have been reviewed in some detail (Mathews, 1971*a*; Kornberg, 1974), and here we shall be concerned primarily with their physiological functions.

3.4.4a. DNA Polymerase

DNA polymerase, the product of gene 43, is a single polypeptide chain of molecular weight 112,000, containing both a template-directed nucleotidyltransferase activity and a 3′-exonuclease activity. Although gene 43 mutants have a DNA-negative phenotype under restrictive conditions, there was some resistance to the idea that this enzyme catalyzes the major chain elongation step in replication. First, this enzyme, like most other purified DNA polymerases, has a V_{max} *in vitro* which is far lower than necessary *in vivo,* as calculated from DNA chain growth

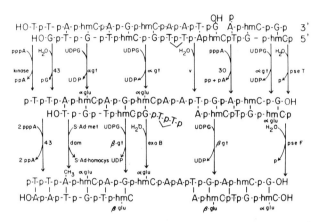

Fig. 6. Reactions of DNA metabolism in T4 phage infected bacteria. Each reaction is indicated by the name or number of the controlling gene, or the name of the enzyme involved. Note the removal of a mismatched base by P43, followed by incorporation of correct nucleotides.

rates. Second, and again like other polymerases, P43 catalyzes a repair-type process *in vitro* and not extensive synthesis (even though the enzyme is apparently not involved in repair *in vivo*, Schnitzlein *et al.*, 1974). Third, the enzyme can only elongate chains at 3′-termini, whereas we known that both chains are elongated simultaneously within a replication fork. The discontinuous replication model of Okazaki *et al.* (1968) provided a mechanism for simultaneous elongation of both growing strands in a fork, and, as we shall see later, the evidence supporting this mechanism in T4 seems overwhelming. With regard to the rate of reaction and the type of reaction catalyzed, one must consider interactions with other proteins in reaching conclusions about the role of P43. The activity of this enzyme *in vitro* is stimulated about tenfold in the presence of P32, the DNA-unwinding protein (Huberman *et al.*, 1971). Moreover, P32 allows T4 DNA polymerase to replicate nicked duplex DNA, a reaction the polymerase cannot catalyze by itself (Nossal, 1974). Even more convincingly, Alberts *et al.* (1975) have described a system containing purified P43, P32, and four other T4 proteins—P41, P44, P45, and P62. This system, in the presence of dNTPs, catalyzes extensive DNA synthesis at essentially the rate of *in vivo* replication, although this system does not initiate replication.

The finding that some gene 43 mutations are mutagenic or anti-mutagenic at other loci strongly supported a major role in replication for this enzyme. Presumably, an altered enzyme would permit insertion of an incorrect base with greater or lesser frequency. In support of this interpretation, Drake and Greening (1970) found that antimutagenic gene 43 mutations suppressed the mutagenic effects of agents such as bromodeoxyuridine, which must be incorporated into DNA during replication in order to act as mutagens. As mentioned in our discussion of nucleases, the frequency of mutation is dependent on the activity of the associated 3′-exonuclease activity (Goodman *et al.,* 1974). This activity serves an "editing" function, to eliminate mispaired nucleotides. Obviously, the higher the exonuclease activity, the higher the probability that an incorrect nucleotide will be removed. Consistent with this interpretation, Lo and Bessman (1976) have described an anti-mutagenic *ts* gene 43 mutant which cannot synthesize DNA at the restrictive temperature even though ample polymerase is present. DNA is, in fact, synthesized but is just as rapidly degraded because the higher temperature (43°C) renders the DNA susceptible to attack by the highly active 3′ exonuclease.

Two additional factors have been proposed to account for the extemely high fidelity of DNA replication. Gillin and Nossal (1975) have reported that K_m values for mispaired dNTPs in a homopolymer system with T4 DNA polymerase are orders of magnitude higher than those for the appropriate substrates. Also, Hopfield (1974) has proposed a "kinetic proofreading" process in which the incorrect substrate is selected against by inclusion of an energy-requiring preincorporation step, such as the DNA-dependent hydrolysis of ATP. Alberts *et al.* (1975) have proposed that the apparent interactions between DNA precursor enzymes and the replication apparatus may be important in such a scheme.

3.4.4b. DNA Ligase

The properties of both bacterial and T4 phage-induced ligases have been extensively reviewed by Lehman (1974). The T4 enzyme is a single polypeptide chain of molecular weight around 65,000, coded for by gene 30. It catalyzes an ATP-dependent phosphodiester bond formation at single-strand breaks in DNA duplexes which have 5′-phosphate and 3′-hydroxyl termini. Gene 30 mutants are defective in replication, and the small amount of DNA which accumulates is of low molecular weight, as expected if it represents replicative intermediates which have not been attached to high molecular weight DNA. DNA ligase is also involved in genetic recombination and ultraviolet repair, for gene 30 mutants show defects in both of these processes (reviewed in Hamlett and Berger, 1975).

Koch (1973) has found that gene 30 defects can be rescued in infection of cells previously infected with phage T7, which codes for a DNA ligase and also does not exclude the replication of superinfecting T-even phages. T7 ligase-negative phage cannot similarly rescue gene 30 T4 mutants, indicating that function of the T7 ligase is the essential element in rescue. In my laboratory, Mr. P. V. Reddy has confirmed this observation (unpublished results), but he finds that T7 preinfection cannot similarly correct the defects associated with mutations in gene 41, 44, 45, or 62. Thus the structural requirements for DNA ligase seem less species specific than those for other proteins of DNA synthesis.

3.4.4c. Polynucleotide Kinase

Polynucleotide kinase, originally described by Richardson (1965), transfers phosphate from ATP to 5´-hydroxyl termini of DNA, RNA, or polynucleotides. The enzyme has been enormously useful as a reagent for end-group analysis. Recent studies have described the purification and mechanism of this enzyme in some detail (Panet *et al.,* 1973; Lillehaug and Kleppe, 1975). However, we still have no information about its role in the infective process. Chan and Ebisuzaki (1970) isolated kinase-negative T4 mutants but found them indistinguishable from wild type with regard to every parameter investigated. Further analysis of these mutants might be fruitful if a restrictive host could be found, perhaps among the Cal Tech strains.

3.4.4d. DNA Phosphatases

The DNA phosphatases were described by Becker and Hurwitz (1967). They include a 3´-deoxynucleotidase which can cleave phosphate from 3´-deoxynucleotides or from 3´-termini in DNA, and a 5´-phosphatase which can cleave 5´-phosphoryl termini from either DNA or RNA. Mutants unable to synthesize the 3´-phosphatase are restricted by one of the Cal Tech hospital strains of *E. coli* (Depew and Cozzarelli, 1974). Under restrictive conditions, DNA synthesis and packaging are defective, and Depew and Cozzarelli conclude that in that strain 3´-phosphate termini are somehow generated in DNA and that these must be removed if replication is to occur normally. Depew and Cozzarelli (cited in Homyk and Weil, 1974) have also found that certain deletions between genes 39 and 56 are defective in 5′-phosphatase synthesis, but to date studies on the function of this enzyme have not been reported.

3.4.4e. DNA-Dependent ATPases

Ebisuzaki *et al.* (1972) purified two DNA-dependent ATPases from T4-infected *E. coli.* Mutants deficient in this activity map between genes 39 and 56 (Behme and Ebisuzaki, 1975). These mutants are identical to wild type with respect to burst size, recombination, and UV repair. Thus the function of the gene remains unknown. Alberts *et al.* (1975) have described a DNA-dependent ATPase activity associated with a complex of the purified protein products of genes 44 and 62. Since these gene products are essential to DNA replication, it is presumed that this activity is involved in this process, perhaps as suggested by Hopfield (1974). One wonders whether this activity might represent the second of the two activities described by Ebisuzaki and colleagues.

3.4.4f. RNA Ligase

RNA ligase activity was originally described by Silber *et al.* (1972) as one which catalyzed the ATP-dependent circularization of polyadenylate, and has since been described as capable of carrying out a variety of phosphodiester bond formations involving 5′-phosphate and 3′-hydroxyl termini of RNA (Cranston *et al.,* 1974; Linné *et al.,* 1974). Although DNA ligase can function as an RNA ligase under certain conditions (Sano and Feix, 1974), it is clear that the RNA ligase of Silber and colleagues is a different enzyme, for gene 30 mutants synthesize normal levels of RNA ligase. Mutants deficient in RNA ligase have not been described, and nothing is known at present about the physiological role of this enzyme.

3.4.4g. DNA Glucosyltransferases

The DNA glucosyltransferases are responsible for synthesis of the glucosylated HMC residues unique to T-even phage DNA. In each case, the sugar is transferred via uridine diphosphoglucose to the hydroxymethyl group of an HMC residue in nascent DNA, or, in the case of diglucosylated residues in T2 or T6 DNA, to the 6-position of glucose already attached. A major question about the action of these enzymes, which has not been pursued in recent years, is how their activities are controlled *in vivo* to generate the patterns of glucosylation seen in phage DNA. For example, 25% of the HMC residues in T2 or T6 DNA are not glucosylated. What keeps these positions free *in vivo*? Also, in T4 DNA 70% of the glucosyl residues are attached in α linkage, and 30% in β. Yet these enzymes can transfer glucosyl residues to unglucosylated DNA *in vitro* to greater than 70% and 30%, respectively, and DNA from αgt mutants contains DNA which is 100% β-glucosylated. DeWaard *et al.* (1967) proposed that the intracellular magnesium level regulates the activities of these two enzymes, but to my knowledge the question of intracellular control of these activities has not been pursued since then.

What is the function of DNA glucosylation? Most of what we know pertains to glucosylation as a mechanism to protect HMC-containing DNA from host-induced restriction (cf. Revel and Luria, 1970). However, it seems that glucosylation plays an additional direct role in phage replication. Montgomery and Snyder (1973) described a bacterial mutant with an altered RNA polymerase, which poorly supports T4 replication. Phage mutants which grow well in this strain are defective in β-glucosyltransferase. One interpretation of these data is that particular DNA base sequences containing β-glucosylated HMC residues are recognition signals for initiation of transcription.

Just as HMC residues protect phage DNA from attack by phage-coded nucleases, glucosylation of some or all of these residues protects phage from restriction by a host enzyme system. Phage containing nonglucosylated DNA can be prepared either by growth in a host strain unable to synthesize UDP-glucose or by growth of a glucosyl-transferase-negative mutant in a host strain which permits its growth. Such a phage cannot grow in most wild-type hosts. Upon infection, the phage DNA is rapidly degraded at the cell surface by a still unidentified enzyme system. Two genes in common *E. coli* strains control this restriction; the $r6$ gene product restricts all nonglucosylated T-even phages, while $r2,4$ controls restriction of T2 and T4. Presumably at least one of these genes controls a nuclease specific for HMC residues, but this enzyme has proven an elusive target. Fleischman and Richardson (1971) devised a means for assaying restriction by *E. coli* K12 *in vitro*. Toluenized cells of wild-type K12 strains cannot synthesize DNA in the presence of hydroxymethyl-dCTP as a DNA precursor, presumably because any DNA synthesized is rapidly degraded by the restriction system. When such experiments are done with host strains permissive for nonglucosylated phages, DNA accumulation is seen. The idea that DNA breakdown is occurring in this system has been confirmed by Fleischman *et al.* (1975), who prepared phage fd replicative form DNA containing either cytosine or HMC in one strand. The HMC-containing DNA is rapidly broken down *in vitro,* while the cytosine-containing DNA remains intact. This can be used as an assay for purification of the restriction activity.

A somewhat different mechanism for restriction of nonglu-cosylated T6 phage in *E. coli* B has been advanced by Hewlett and Mathews (1975). We found a difference in the protein composition of virions of wild-type T6 and *αgt* mutants. If the altered protein leads to abnormal interaction with the host cell, the DNA could fail to be transported into the cytoplasm, but could instead accumulate in a com-partment where it is attacked by an enzyme, such as one of the peri-plasmic nucleases, which need not be specific for HMC-containing DNA. Our study also showed that host cell restriction activity is rapidly abolished after infection in a process which does not require phage gene expression. This may be important to permit nascent repli-cating DNA to exist within the cell for the approximate 2-min interval before it becomes glucosylated (Erikson and Szybalski, 1964).

Kaplan and Nierlich (1975) have found that nonglucosylated T4 DNA can be attacked *in vitro* by the *Eco*R1 restriction endonuclease to give about 40 specific fragments of molecular weight $0.3–10.5 \times 10^6$. Glucosylated DNA was not attacked. The availability of restriction enzyme fragments of the T4 chromosome should allow multiple advances in our knowledge of the structure and expression of phage genes.

3.4.4h. DNA Methylase

DNA methylase, discovered by Hausmann and Gold (1966) in T2- and T4-infected cells, but not T6-infected cells, also acts to help protect phage DNA against restriction. Prophages of P1, a generalized transducing phage, can restrict nonglucosylated T2 or T4 (Revel and Georgopoulos, 1969). Phage mutants which can overcome this restric-tion contain abnormally high levels of 6-methyladenine residues (the product of DNA methylation) and induce the formation of an altered DNA methylase (Hattman, 1970*b*; Revel and Hattman, 1971).

3.5. DNA Replication

A general picture of T-even phage DNA replication can be painted as follows. Replication commences at about 6 min after infection at 37°C, as judged either by incorporation of isotopic precursors into

DNA or by the detection of replicative hybrids. Newly synthesized DNA accumulates at an ever-increasing rate until a maximal rate is achieved at 10–12 min, by which time some 40–80 phage-equivalent units of DNA have accumulated per cell. Apparently all of this is present as one megamolecular replicative intermediate (Huberman, 1968). Maturation of DNA from this intermediate involves concomitant cleavage and packaging into phage heads. Once maturation has begun, the rate of DNA synthesis is constant for some time, usually until lysis. Thus a constant excess of unpackaged DNA remains in the replicating pool and is released when the cells lyse.

T4 represents an excellent system for analyzing the mechanism and control of double-stranded DNA replication. Many proteins are required for replication in any system, and in the case of T4 virtually all of them are phage coded, and many of them have been purified. We shall explore the functions of those gene products not already discussed, and we shall also ask how replicative intermediates are generated from single molecules of parental DNA.

3.5.1. Proteins Involved in Replication

We have already discussed the functions of DNA polymerase and ligase and alluded to other activities, such as the DNA-dependent ATPase activity of the P44-P62 complex. Many other proteins are involved in this complex process.

3.5.1a. DNA-Binding Proteins

One of the real success stories in furthering our understanding of DNA replication is the work of Alberts and colleagues on the structure and function of the T4 DNA-binding protein specified by gene 32 (Alberts and Frey, 1970). Reasoning that at least some proteins involved in replication should bind to DNA, Alberts devised DNA-cellulose chromatography as a means to isolate such proteins. P32 proved quite abundant (approximately 10^4 molecules per infected cell) and easy to purify. The gene product is required for recombination and repair, as well as for replication. The purified protein binds preferentially, and cooperatively, to single-stranded DNA, and hence promotes both denaturation and renaturation. The significance of cooperativity is that P32 is bound more tightly to DNA at high than low protein concentrations. Thus the protein must bind preferentially when protein–protein interactions occur as well, and these have been extensively analyzed by Carroll *et al.* (1973, 1975). This leads it to bind to DNA in clusters. P32 is unlike other early enzymes of DNA metabolism in that it is required in stoichiometric, not catalytic, amounts for replication (Sinha and Snustad, 1971). All available evidence is consistent with the idea that P32 facilitates the unwinding of DNA during replication and that it "coats" DNA in the replicating fork. This simultaneously maintains a single-stranded template for replication and protects that template from nuclease attack. Consistent with this interpretation, DNA-binding proteins of similar properties have been found in many other biological systems.

Hosoda *et al.* (1974) have described a cleavage product of P32, P32*, which has a molecular weight of 27,000, as compared to 35,000 for the native protein. Only P32* can denature T4 DNA *in vitro*. More recently Moise and Hosoda (1976) have described several forms of P32 and have presented persuasive evidence supporting the idea that different forms of the protein facilitate DNA unwinding, ahead of the replication fork, and renaturation, behind the fork.

Mosig and Breschkin (1975) have presented genetic evidence for interaction between P32 and ligase, which is not surprising if both proteins participate in replication, recombination, and repair. We conclude our discussion of P32 by observing that it apparently regulates its own synthesis, since mutants which make an inactive gene product overproduce that product by at least tenfold (Krisch *et al.,* 1974). The economy to a cell of using a DNA-binding protein to regulate its own synthesis is appealing, and Russel (1973) has made similar observations *vis à vis* another T4 DNA-binding protein, namely DNA polymerase.

Other early-synthesized proteins bind to DNA, as determined by disc gel electrophoretic analysis either of DNA–protein complexes isolated from infected cells (Miller and Buckley, 1970) or of the total proteins bound to DNA-cellulose (Huang and Buchanan, 1974). In the latter study, 19 DNA-binding proteins were identified, although the binding of some of these was dependent on the presence of other proteins. At any rate, those DNA-binding proteins which were identified included the products of genes 32, 43, *r*IIA, 30, 39, 46, 52, *gt,* and IPIII.

3.5.1b. Other Products of DNA Genes

Of the 64 numbered T4 genes in which conditional lethal mutants are known to exist, mutations in 18 genes generate a pattern of defective DNA synthesis. Through studies on uracil incorporation into DNA and RNA, Warner and Hobbs (1967) were able to classify DNA-defective mutants as DNA-zero (D0: genes 1, 42, 43, 44, and 45), some DNA synthesis (DS: genes 30, 32, 41, 56, and 62), DNA-delay (DD: genes 39, 52, 58–61, 60, and 63), and DNA-arrest (DA: genes 46, 47, and 59). Warner and Hobbs showed that uracil incorporation into RNA is severely inhibited in infection by D0 mutants, and later Mathews (1968, 1972) showed that this represents a true decrease in the rate of RNA synthesis. It is well known that the transcription of *late* genes is coupled to DNA replication (Riva *et al.,* 1970), but these findings show that total transcription is coupled to replication as well.

One approach to identifying the function controlled by each gene is to carry out studies on DNA metabolism in cells infected under restrictive conditions. We have already discussed, for example, evidence that the action of DD gene products occurs at the membrane, that P46 and P47 are essential both for host DNA breakdown and for maintenance of DNA in a membrane complex, and that P52 and P59 are similarly involved in maintaining the structural integrity of replicating DNA. A more direct approach involves development of *in vitro* assays for the gene products. Barry and Alberts (1972) showed that extracts of cells containing a particular gene product could "complement" the defective DNA synthesis seen in lysates of cells infected with mutants defective in the same gene. This has now been used as the basis for purification to near-homogeneity of P41, P45, and a tight complex of P44 and P62 (Alberts *et al.,* 1975). These purified proteins, plus P32 and P43, catalyze extensive replication, in the presence of rNTPs, at essentially *in vivo* rates. Although this system does not contain added DNA ligase, Alberts believes that it is present as a contaminant of P41. The system does not initiate replication of duplex molecules *de novo,* but apparently begins replication of a duplex by strand displacement at a nick. In addition, the system will replicate virtually any template offered it *in vitro.* Thus the determinants of template specificity and initiation are lost in this system, probably because they are controlled in part by some of the other DNA genes. Nonetheless, the proteins in this complex undoubtedly represent the heart of the chain elongation machinery, and further analysis of this system should teach us a great deal about the mechanism of duplex DNA replication.

3.5.1c.   Host Proteins in Replication

Whereas smaller viruses use genetic functions of the host cell extensively in replicating their own nucleic acids, there is little evidence for such host functions in T4 DNA replication. As mentioned earlier,

Simon *et al.* (1974) have described a mutant of *E. coli* which is defective in its ability to support DNA synthesis after T4 infection. It seems likely that the cause of defective DNA synthesis is indirect, perhaps through the membrane, since (1) the genetic block is not complete, (2) some DNA synthesis can be restored by EDTA, and (3) some mutations which overcome host defectiveness map in gene 31, which controls an early step of head assembly at the membrane. Finally, in my laboratory we have found (M. E. Stafford, unpublished) that plasmolyzed infected cells of this mutant are capable of substantial DNA synthesis in the presence of added dNTPs. Other evidence for involvement of a host function comes from Mosig *et al.* (1972), who found that the ability of host strains to support an initial round of T4 replication was reduced by about 30% in infection of a strain lacking DNA polymerase I. The *pol*A strains used by these authors were not isogenic with the wild-type control, a factor which is important in interpreting these kinds of experiments (cf. Mortelmans and Friedberg, 1972).

3.5.2. Origin and Direction of Replication

The most direct way to analyze the origin and direction of replication of a DNA molecule is denaturation mapping (Schnös and Inman, 1970), in which AT-rich regions of partially replicated DNA are analyzed electron microscopically under partially denaturing conditions. To get useful information, however, one must be able to orient these molecules with respect to points of reference, such as ends. Since the ends are variable with respect to the genome in T-even phage DNAs because of circular permutation, this technique is inapplicable. As a result, it has taken much effort to clarify this question for T4. The earliest approaches utilized petit phage particles, which, it will be recalled, contain random DNA segments with an average of two-thirds of a complete DNA molecule. By density labeling experiments, Mosig and Werner (1969) found that in single infection only one-third of parental DNA was replicated. This was interpreted in terms of unidirectional replication from a fixed origin (missing in one-third of the molecules) and obligatory circularization of the molecule for travel of the fork back to the origin. Since these molecules lack terminal redundancy and hence cannot circularize, DNA distal to the origin could not replicate. Another approach involved attempts to establish a gradient of marker frequency in replicating DNA (Mosig, 1970; Marsh *et al.*, 1971). This was measured either by incorporation of markers into viable progeny in mixed infection with whole and petit phage or by genetic transformation. Both of these studies suggested unidirectional clockwise replication from a fixed origin near gene 43.

These studies have been criticized on various grounds (cf. Doermann, 1974). For example, most two-thirds length segments of the T4 genome would lack one or more of the genes essential to replication, and the failure of an incomplete chromosome to replicate could be explained on this basis alone. Moreover, analyzing marker frequencies from the genotypes of progeny phage gives information not about the initial round of replication following initiation but rather about the entire replicative process. Finally, the mechanism of transformation in the T4 system is poorly understood, and there is considerable variation in efficiencies of transformation for different markers which, even when corrected for, provide a source of uncertainty. In the meantime, Kozinski and his colleagues have published an extensive series of papers which seem to establish that, at least for the first round of replication, initiation occurs at multiple specific origins and is bidirectional.

Delius *et al.* (1971) isolated partially replicated DNA early in the first round of replication. Electron microscopic analysis showed multiple loops in each replicating molecule, suggesting multiple origins of replication. These structures could not have arisen from recombination, for infection was at single multiplicity. At each fork in each loop was a single-stranded tail with a 3′-hydroxyl terminus. Delius and colleagues suggested that this represented collapse of replicating structures once P32, which coats single-stranded molecules, is removed during phenol extraction. The 3′-terminated tail, by this scheme, represents the "leading" progeny strand (cf. Alberts *et al.*, 1975), which judging from its length contains about 900 nucleotide residues (Fig. 7).

The above experiment can be criticized on two grounds: (1) electron microscopic analysis is not necessarily representative of a population of molecules, and (2) isolation of the hybrid involved incorporation of the "unphysiological" density label, 5-bromodeoxyuridine. Kozinski's group has satisfactorily met both criticisms. Howe *et al.* (1973) examined the density distribution of the products of controlled shear of partially replicated, density-labeled DNA. For example, in molecules which had replicated 18 μm of DNA (out of a total of about 50), shear analysis showed that this was present in three to six separate regions, each of 3–6 μm in length. Incidentally, Werner (1968) had earlier carried out similar experiments to examine the distribution of growing points in replicating T4 DNA, but since he started from the premise that replication is unidirectional from a fixed origin, he reached conclusions which may not be correct (see also Emanuel, 1973).

The experiments of Howe and colleagues established that the

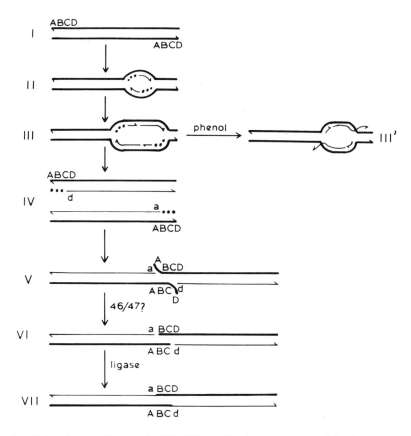

Fig. 7. Role of recombination in T4 DNA replication, as suggested by Broker (1973). I, Linear duplex DNA; II, formation of a bidirectional replicating loop (a single origin is shown for simplicity); ——, parental DNA; ——, newly replicated DNA; →, 3′-terminus; ●, gene 32 protein; III, further replicated DNA, showing discontinuous synthesis; III′, structure of III after deproteinization by phenol extraction, as suggested by Delius *et al.* (1971); IV, two replicated DNA molecules; V, recombination at the incompletely replicated ends; VI, presumed trimming of single-stranded ends by gene 46 and 47 products; VII, covalently sealed recombinant molecule.

visual inspection of partially replicated DNA did indeed give results representative of the entire population of molecules. Carlson (1973), by careful application of Cs_2SO_4 gradients, was able to separate partially replicated T4 DNA from *E. coli* DNA without using BUdR as a density label, and electron microscopic analysis of these molecules gave results identical to those observed by Delius *et al.* (1971). Finally, Kozinski and Doermann (1975) have shown that incomplete T4 chromosomes, about 0.86 phage equivalent in length, can replicate repeatedly. This contradicts the finding of Mosig and Werner (1969) that terminally deficient chromosomes cannot complete a round of replication.

The gradient of marker frequency established by Mosig (1970) suggests that rounds of replication subsequent to the first might be different from the first round, but present data indicate that the first round of replication is bidirectional with multiple, specifically located origins (although the relative rates of synthesis in each direction have not been established). In this respect, T4 resembles eukaryotes more than microbes, in that no other bacterium or virus has been found to replicate normally from more than one origin. Howe *et al.* (1973) speculate that T4, which is a large virus, might have evolved through a series of recombinational events involving smaller viral genomes, plasmids, and chromosomal fragments, and that it was to the selective advantage of the virus to retain all of the replicative origins which were incorporated thereby into the evolving genome.

One final comment: although published evidence supports the existence of multiple origins, Mosig (personal communication) has pointed out that loops of the type observed can be generated either by replication or by recombination. She has observed that loops generated by replication have but one single-stranded tail when viewed in the electron microscope, indicative of unidirectional replication, while recombination loops have two tails. This seems to conflict with the results of Delius *et al.* (1971), where two-tailed loops were seen in single infection. One hopes for an early and final resolution of this important question.

3.5.3. Structure of Replicating DNA

The first analysis of T4 DNA trapped in the midst of replication was carried out by Frankel (1966, 1968), who gently lysed cells and subjected labeled intracellular phage DNA to sedimentation analysis through neutral and alkaline sucrose gradients. This showed that the strands of replicating DNA are far longer than those of mature DNA, a finding which was in concert with the electron microscopic analysis of Huberman (1968). Recently, Curtis and Alberts (1976) have shown that concatemeric intermediates contain regions of single-stranded DNA, spaced about one genome length apart and stabilized by gene 32 protein. This finding is important for understanding how replicating DNA is folded, and also how it matures into genome-sized molecules.

How are long strands generated? Several workers at the 1968 Cold Spring Harbor Symposium suggested that they arise through a "rolling circle" mechanism, whereby T4 DNA first circularizes and then one or more forks traverse the circle, as often as necessary to generate molecules of the length observed. However, the fact that T4 DNA need not circularize to replicate puts a crimp in this model. Moreover, a prediction of the rolling circle model is that DNA strand lengths would increase during the first round of replication, whereas Miller *et al.* (1970) showed that long strands cannot be detected until after several rounds of replication have occurred. Bernstein and Bernstein (1973, 1974) have observed a variety of branched and unbranched circular structures through autoradiography of ^{3}H-labeled replicating DNA, and, while their observations are consistent with the idea that late stages of replication occur *via* a rolling circle model, one cannot rule out the possibility that the Bernstein structures have been created largely by recombination. As discussed later, there is good reason to expect *a priori* that a recombination step is essential for T4 DNA replication. On the other hand, it is entirely possible that late rounds of replication occur by a rolling circle mechanism, as has been shown for phage λ (Skalka *et al.,* 1972).

What is the structure of replicating DNA in the vicinity of a fork? We have already mentioned, in connection with our discussion of ligase, that both strands of DNA are almost certainly replicated discontinuously, in a 5′ to 3′ direction. Even in very short pulses (5 s or less), labeled DNA precursors are incorporated into chains which sediment in alkaline sucrose gradients as though they were approximately 1100 nucleotides long and which hybridize with either separated strand of T4 DNA. By pulse labeling at low temperatures, Sugino and Okazaki (1972) were able to selectively label the growing ends of these fragments. Isolation of the 5′-ends showed that they were unlabeled, indicating that both strands grow from the 3′-end. Also, by considering the length of pulses which would fully label the 5′-ends of Okazaki fragments, these workers could estimate the DNA chain growth rate of such pieces: approximately 20 nucleotides per second at 8°C and 100 nucleotides per second at 14°C (compare with a rate of 250 nucleotides per second for the rate of fork movement at 25°C, Werner, 1968).

Finally, is there any evidence that synthesis of Okazaki fragments is initiated with RNA primers, as has been shown in many other systems? Since known DNA polymerases can only extend chains from preexisting termini (either DNA or RNA), while RNA polymerase can initiate chain growth *de novo,* various workers sought, and found, evidence that each step in replication commences with synthesis of a short RNA primer, which is then elongated by a DNA polymerase, followed by a repair-type reaction which erases the primer and replaces it with

DNA. Confirmation of a similar mechanism in T4 DNA replication has proven difficult, possibly because RNA primers, if present, are exceptionally short and/or quickly erased. Although direct evidence for RNA primer involvement has not yet been presented, three reports are suggestive of an involvement of RNA in T4 DNA metabolism. Buckley *et al.* (1972) described an RNA-DNA copolymer, synthesized early in infection by a chloramphenicol-resistant process, which hybridizes preferentially to the *l* strand of T4 DNA. The material consists of about 95% RNA, and no information has been presented about its size or physiological role. Similarly Speyer *et al.* (1972) reported that [5-^{3}H]uridine labels T4 phage to a small extent. Since conversion of uridine to dTMP or HM-dCMP would involve removal of the 5-H, Speyer and colleagues conclude that the incorporated label represents RNA (terminally located, since alkaline denaturation does not shorten T4 DNA strands). However, only about 40% of this material is sensitive to alkali or ribonuclease, and Speyer and colleagues give little indication of how much of the material is present or what its physiological role is. Of considerable interest is the report of Ratner (1974*b*), who identified P45 among the proteins which bind to an affinity column containing immobilized T4-modified RNA polymerase. One interpretation of this is that the modified enzyme containing P45 may participate in the synthesis of RNA priming fragments. However, the lack of requirement for RNA polymerase in the system of Alberts *et al.* (1975) must render this interpretation speculative. Finally, the reported resistance of T4 DNA synthesis to rifampicin (Rosenthal and Reid, 1973) could signify either the involvement of a modified or different RNA polymerase in forming primers, or else a lack of involvement of RNA in phage DNA synthesis.

3.5.4. DNA Maturation

The final step in T4 DNA metabolism is its packaging into partially completed phage heads and cleavage from the replicating pool. Little is known about the biochemistry of this process, but we do know that the products of genes 16 and 17 are essential for encapsulation of DNA, and P49 is involved in a cleavage step, possibly the step at which a "headful" of DNA is cleaved from the replicating pool. Frankel *et al.* (1971) have demonstrated a nuclease activity in P49, but so far the packaging and cleavage of DNA have not been reproduced *in vitro*. P22 and IPIII, proteins in the head precursor particle, are cleaved concurrently with DNA encapsulation (Laemmli and Favre,

1973), and Luftig and Lundh (1973) have argued persuasively that concurrent DNA replication must occur as well. In this context, Hulick-Bursch and Snustad (1975) have shown that under conditions where host DNA is not degraded it is still not packaged. Is this because it is not replicating or because the maturing head has specificity for HMC-containing DNA? To answer this question, one would need to ask whether replicating, cytosine-containing T4 DNA can be packaged—no mean feat, since cytosine-containing DNA cannot serve as a template for late gene transcription (Kutter *et al.*, 1975).

Most available evidence favors the idea that DNA is encapsulated within a head precursor whose size and shape are already determined and thus that the amount of DNA packaged is a dependent variable of the size of the head (cf. Casjens and King, 1975). Certainly the fact that phages bearing long deletions have commensurately lengthened terminally redundant regions (Streisinger *et al.*, 1967) supports this idea. However, an influence of DNA metabolism on head morphogenesis was suggested by Chao *et al.*, (1974), who reported that infection of a host strain lacking DNA polymerase I and endonuclease I generates progeny with a greatly increased abundance of petit phage. This surprising finding has not yet been reconciled with the idea that head size is the determinant of DNA length, although various *ad hoc* explanations can be entertained.

3.5.5. DNA Repair and Recombination

We mention DNA repair and recombination in a subsection of our discussion of replication because of the extensive involvement of replicative functions in both processes. Since additional functions can be used interchangeably in recombination and repair, and since there is evidence that host functions can also participate in these processes, it has been difficult to unambiguously identify reaction pathways for either process.

As discussed by many authors (cf. Mortelmans and Friedberg, 1972; Hamlett and Berger, 1975), T4 controls two separate pathways for DNA repair, formally analogous to the excision repair and postreplication repair systems in *E. coli*. The excision repair system is specific for ultraviolet-damaged DNA, while the postreplication system will repair damage caused by UV, X-ray, alkylating agents, or cross-linking agents such as mitomycin C. Excision repair involves nicking of damaged DNA by endonuclease V on the 5′-side of a thymine dimer. The dimer is excised, probably by exonuclease B, and the gap is filled by the combined action of DNA polymerase and ligase. The function controlled by genes 46 and 47 may be important, also, because gene 47 mutants, as well as gene 30 or 43 mutants, are defective in this pathway (Baldy, 1968). This pathway is analogous to that controlled by the *uvr* genes in *E. coli,* and indeed Taketo *et al.* (1972) have devised an *in vitro* system in which T4 endonuclease V can replace the initial step in the *uvr*-controlled pathway of *E. coli.*

The biochemistry of postreplication repair is less well understood. The process apparently involves chromosome replication after the infliction of damage, with the damaged portions not being replicated. The resultant gaps are then filled by exchanges with sister strands. As one might expect, genes which control this process are involved in recombination as well. This points up the analogy between this system and that controlled by the *rec* genes of *E. coli,* which are also involved both in recombination and in postreplication repair. Genes involved in this pathway include 30, 43, *x, y, w,* 58, 59, and the gene(s) controlled by a mutant called 1206 (Symonds *et al.,* 1973; Hamlett and Berger, 1975; Wu *et al.,* 1975*b*). As a starting point for biochemical analysis of this pathway, Hamlett and Berger have pointed out that the controlling genes of endonucleases III and VI and the endonuclease of Altman and Meselson (1970) have not yet been identified, and they may be included among the several uncharacterized genes involved in this pathway.

The involvement of host gene products in repair synthesis is still not completely resolved. Several authors have described an involvement of DNA polymerase I in either or both repair pathways, based on increased UV sensitivity of T4 growth in *pol*A strains lacking this enzyme. However, such differences were not seen when the *pol*A$^+$ and *pol*A$^-$ mutations tested were in otherwise isogenic strains (Mortelmans and Friedberg, 1972).

Although various T4 genes have been implicated in recombination, there are no truly recombination-defective mutants. A triple mutant containing lesions in *w, x,* and *y* exhibits a fifteenfold reduction in recombination frequency relative to wild type, but this is apparently the most severely recombination-defective strain known (Hamlett and Berger, 1975). One might conclude from this that recombination is essential for growth of the phage and that truly "*rec*-zero" mutations would have to be sought among conditional lethal mutants. Broker (1973) has suggested a plausible reason that recombination might be essential in DNA replication (see Fig. 7). If T4 DNA initially replicates bidirectionally as a linear molecule, the 5′-ends of the daughter molecules might not be filled in because 3′-termini to extend are not available, either from primers or from the endless replication available in a circle. If the resultant gaps are not repaired, a little bit of DNA will be lost in each succeeding round of replication. To prevent this, Broker suggested that the daughter molecules can recombine at the redundant termini to generate a double-length concatemer. Broker also suggested that the 46/47 function might be necessary to trim single-stranded ends prior to the sealing of each nick or gap by polymerase and ligase. This inspired proposal, which was also made by Watson (1972) for T7 DNA replication, explains many unusual facets of the T4 life style. It provides a *raison d'être* for concatemers and terminal redundancies; it provides a specific function for the putative 46/47 nuclease, one which need not be present *in vitro,* where recombination should not be required (Alberts *et al.,* 1975); and it explains why recombination is so active in T-even phage infection and is evidently an essential function.

The most penetrating biochemical analysis of recombination in T4 has been carried out by Lehman and his colleagues, as represented by the contribution of Broker (1973). The general approach involves electron microscopic analysis of branched molecules accumulating in cells infected with various T4 multiple mutants, all containing a polymerase defect (gene 43) to prevent replication (although P43 is necessary to complete recombination, Miller, 1975). A pathway of recombination, as suggested from this work, is shown in Fig. 8. The lack of indicated involvement of genes *w, x,* and *y,* despite the fact that they participate in recombination (Hamlett and Berger, 1975), suggests the existence of more than one pathway for recombination.

3.6. Control of Gene Expression

The control of gene expression is reviewed in detail elsewhere in this series by Geiduschek and Rabussay, and also it has been capably reviewed by Witmer (1974). Therefore, only a cursory treatment is presented here, emphasizing principal experimental approaches and unanswered questions.

The fact that T-even phage genes are expressed sequentially during the viral life cycle was put into focus by Hershey and his colleagues when they showed that proteins synthesized early in infection are for the most part not incorporated into virions, whereas structural proteins predominate among those synthesized late. Workers in Spiegelman's laboratory first showed that transcriptional regulation is responsible in large part for this temporal pattern of gene expression, and this has been elaborated upon subsequently in many laboratories. Whether

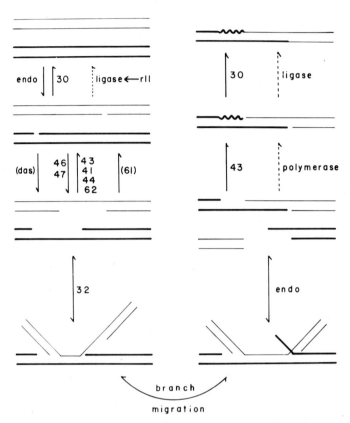

Fig. 8. A pathway for recombination in T4, as suggested by Broker (1973). Involvement of T4 gene products is indicated with solid arrows and, where possible, the names or numbers of the genes involved. Steps which can be catalyzed by host enzymes are indicated with dashed arrows.

translational, or posttranscriptional, regulation occurs as well has proven a more elusive question. Certainly numerous phage-evoked changes occur in the cell's translational machinery, notably the synthesis of virus-coded tRNA, and evidence abounds that specific untranslated mRNA molecules exist at different times in the infectious cycle (for a recent treatment, see Zetter and Cohen, 1974). Moreover, specific T4 genes, such as *reg*A, seem to affect the functional stability of phage messages (Wiberg *et al.*, 1973; Karam and Bowles, 1974). However, it has been difficult to correlate alterations of translational machinery with specific regulatory events or with the physiology of the infected cell.

Analysis of transcriptional regulation, on the other hand, has benefited from several powerful techniques for analyzing the synthesis of specific messenger molecules or classes of messages. First among these was competitive DNA-RNA hybridization, which allowed demonstration that there is more than one temporal class of early transcripts (Salser *et al.,* 1970) and that both DNA replication and the action of the maturation genes 33 and 55 are essential for transcription of late genes (Bolle *et al.,* 1968). Hybridization analysis could be extended to follow the transcription of individual genes where the existence of deletions (notably in the *r*II region or the *e* gene) presented opportunities for analysis of gene-specific RNAs (Kasai and Bautz, 1969). The availability of specific fragments of the T4 genome in restriction endonuclease digests of unglucosylated DNA (Kaplan and Nierlich, 1975) should greatly extend the utility of this approach. Hybridization analysis, coupled with the ability to separate strands of T4 DNA, has permitted the demonstration that early messages are transcribed predominantly from the *l* strand of DNA, while late mRNA classes are *r* strand specific (Guha *et al.,* 1971).

Three other techniques have allowed investigators to analyze the expression of individual genes. First, disc gel electrophoresis of labeled intracellular proteins or RNA molecules, followed by autoradiography, allows one to identify and quantitate the synthesis of individual gene products (Hosoda and Levinthal, 1968; O'Farrell *et al.,* 1973). This approach is more successful for analyzing specific protein synthesis rather than transcription, since the rapid decay of mRNA molecules prevents their accumulation in discrete size classes. Second, either DNA or RNA can be tested for its ability to serve as template for the *in vitro* synthesis of specific proteins, which can be either assayed biologically or quantitated by gel electrophoresis (reviewed in Schweiger and Herrlich, 1974). Finally, Hercules and Sauerbier (1973, 1974) have described an ingenious approach for mapping transcription units and determining the direction of transcription of individual genes. One simply assays for the expression of individual genes in cells infected by phages irradiated with varying UV doses. Since transcription is terminated at sites of UV damage, the sensitivity of expression of a particular gene increases in proportion of its distance from its promoter. This technique has allowed determination of the lengths of blocks of cotranscribed genes as well as the direction of transcription.

Applications of the above approaches have led to identification of four temporal classes of T4 mRNA: immediate early (IE), delayed early (DE), quasi-late (QL), and true late (TL). Differentiating characteristics of each of these classes are summarized in Table 9. Note, for example, that QL messages are distinguished from early classes in that

TABLE 9

Characteristics of T4 mRNA Classes

Class	Template DNA strand	Synthesis is chloramphenicol sensitive?	Synthesis requires DNA replication and MD gene expression?	Change in rate of synthesis between 5 and 20 min (30°C)
IE	*l*	No	No	↓
DE	*l*	Yes	No	↓
QL	*l* and *r*	Yes	Yes (*r*), no (*l*)	↑
TL	*r*	Yes	Yes	↑↑↑

their rates of synthesis increase late in infection, and but by a much smaller factor than that seen with TL messages.

A major unsettled question relates to the relations between IE and DE messages. These were originally distinguished from the observation that DE genes are not transcribed in the presence of chloramphenicol. This suggested a role for phage protein synthesis in effecting transition from IE to DE gene transcription, e.g., through modification of bacterial RNA polymerase, so that it could recognize new promoters. However, inhibition of protein synthesis by other means does allow transcription of DE genes both *in vivo* and *in vitro* (O'Farrell and Gold, 1973; Morse and Cohen, 1975; Witmer *et al.*, 1975). In the meantime, transcription mapping and other approaches have shown that many known DE genes are adjacent to IE genes on the linkage map and that they are farther from early-recognized promoters than the IE genes. Seen in this context, the inhibition of DE transcription by chloramphenicol is a manifestation of the polarity, or premature termination of transcription, which this drug has been shown to bring about in other systems. The interval between IE and DE transcription represents the time needed to transcribe IE genes, which is significant because the RNA chain growth rate in T4-infected *E. coli* is about half that seen in uninfected cells (Bremer and Yuan, 1968). However, O'Farrell and Gold (1973) have pointed out that some DE or IE genes can be transcribed from QL promoters later in infection. Transcription from these promoters does require protein synthesis. Consistent with this idea, transcription mapping shows that gene 43 is transcribed from different promoters at different times in infection (Hercules and Sauerbier, 1974).

Although the host cell RNA polymerase is used for transcription of all T4 genes, the enzyme undergoes numerous structural alterations during infection, some of which have been correlated with changes in transcription patterns and others of which have not. In the latter category are two early events, "alteration" and "modification," which involve covalent addition of new material to α subunits. The specific change in alteration has not been identified, but it is effected by an injected virion protein (Horvitz, 1974). Modification involves the attachment of ADP-ribose (Goff, 1974). Mutants defective in both of these functions are viable, so their physiological roles are unknown. Later the β and β' subunits undergo additional uncharacterized changes which are manifested in altered peptide fingerprint maps of each subunit (Schachner and Zillig, 1971).

Later in infection, RNA polymerase isolated from infected cells contains four new peptides, two of which are the products of genes 33 and 55 (Stevens, 1974; Horvitz, 1973; Ratner, 1974a). In addition, Ratner (1974b) has shown by an alternate approach that P45 is also associated with RNA polymerase late in infection. This finding provides an important clue to understanding the relationship between DNA replication and TL gene transcription. This latter problem has proven intractable because of the difficulty in developing a suitable *in vitro* system which transcribes late T4 genes. Geiduschek and colleagues have taken an alternate approach to this problem, namely attempts to uncouple late transcription from DNA replication *in vivo* by infection with appropriate multiple mutants defective in replication. Riva *et al.* (1970) found that triple mutants defective in genes 30, 46, and 43 were so uncoupled; late transcription occurred in the absence of DNA replication. This apparently occurred because single-strand interruptions in DNA, necessary for such transcription, remained unrepaired in the absence of ligase (P30) but were also not subject to further degradation by the 46/47 function. Introduction of additional mutations in genes controlling DNA replication maintained this uncoupling phenomenon, with the sole exception of gene 45 (Wu *et al.,* 1975a). Thus elucidation of the action of P45 should greatly enhance our understanding of both DNA replication and the regulation of transcription.

3.7. Late Functions

Viral assembly is discussed elsewhere in this series by King and Wood, and has also been reviewed by Casjens and King (1975), so this section will merely provide a summary. The important tools in teaching

us about T-even phage morphogenesis have been the electron microscope and the *in vitro* complementation test devised by Edgar and
Wood (1966), wherein viral subparticles produced in infection by
assembly-defective mutants can interact in appropriate mixtures of
extracts to produce infectious phage. More recently, polyacrylamide
gel electrophoresis coupled with autoradiography of labeled proteins
has become very useful (Laemmli, 1970) and has allowed, for example,
the demonstration that specific protein cleavages occur during
assembly of the T4 head but that no apparent cleavages are involved in
tail morphogenesis.

Three independent pathways generate heads, tails (baseplate plus
core plus sheath), and tail fibers. A striking feature of head assembly is
the presence in a head precursor of P22 and IPIII, which apparently
serve as an "assembly core" and are subsequently cleaved, P22 to small
peptides which remain within the completed head. In addition, P23, the
major head protein, and P24 are cleaved as the head matures, with the
help of P21. Assembly of the tail begins with the baseplate, and King's
group has recently described two distinct subpathways in baseplate
assembly (cf. Casjens and King, 1975), one of which generates a central
plug and the other of which forms a "wedge," six of these combining in
formation of one baseplate. The core is then attached to the baseplate,
followed by polymerization of sheath subunits about the core and
finally "capping" of the completed tail by P3 and P15. Attachment of
heads to tails seems to be spontaneous, whereas the final step in
assembly, the attachment of fibers to the baseplate, behaves like a
catalyzed reaction, involving P63.

The final step in the infectious cycle is lysis of the infected cell,
with concomitant release of progeny phage. This surprisingly complicated process has resisted attempts at elucidation. We do know that the
lysozyme specified by gene *e* is involved, because mutants in this gene
cannot lyse their hosts spontaneously. However, the *e* function can be
dispensed with if an additional mutation is present in *s*, the so-called
spackle gene (Emrich, 1968). Nothing is known about the biochemistry
of the *s* function, but Cornett (1974) has suggested that it may act at
points of contact between cell wall and membrane, since there is some
evidence for *s*-mediated effects at both wall and membrane.

An additional phage function controlling lysis was inferred from
the work of Mukai *et al.* (1967). They found that in cells infected with *e*
gene mutants phage production and cell metabolism stop at about the
same time as lysis would normally occur, even though the cells do not
lyse. The most reasonable interpretation is that some intracellular event

interrupts metabolism and this causes a functional disruption of the inner membrane, such that lysozyme, which by now is present in abundance, can pass through the membrane and attack the cell wall. Cronan and Wulff (1969) suggested that this event might be hydrolysis of membrane phospholipid, with subsequent uncoupling of oxidative phosphorylation by the released free fatty acids. However, Josslin (1971b) challenged this idea. It would appear that the t gene, also characterized by Josslin (1970, 1971a), controls the key step, since t mutants cannot lyse their hosts even in the presence of lysozyme. As stated earlier, t may control the synthesis or activity of a phospholipase, although the evidence for this is not conclusive. To further complicate the picture, phage particles can be released from certain bacterial mutants without lysis of the cell, including a phospholipase-deficient mutant of *E. coli* K12 (λ) (Hardaway et al., 1975) and another mutant with increased sensitivity to several antibiotics, colicins, and detergents (Sundar Raj and Wu, 1973). In the latter case, phage release occurs in the absence of phage lysozyme.

As an alternate approach to this problem, several workers have studied phage mutants unable to establish lysis inhibition—the r mutants, and, in particular, rII mutants. Lysis inhibition is a prolongation of the latent period which results when an infected cell is superinfected. This occurs whether or not lysozyme is present (Mukai et al., 1967). rII mutants have several other distinctive phenotypes, including restricted growth in host cells lysogenic for phage λ and suppression of gene 30 (DNA ligase) mutations. By use of temperature-dependent rII mutations, Heere and Karam (1975) have shown that these two expressions of the mutant rII gene are manifest at distinctly different times in the infectious cycle. The restriction in λ lysogens may be a consequence of defective membrane function, since, as we have seen, the rIIA and rIIB proteins are membrane associated, and the restriction can be overcome in the presence of high magnesium concentration or low levels of monovalent cations (Sekiguchi, 1966). Maor and Shalitin (1974) have tested the idea that faulty late T4 gene transcription results from this ionic imbalance. In a membrane–DNA system prepared from rII-infected λ lysogens, they found that the synthesis of late T4 RNA *in vitro* is sensitive to high ionic strength or low Mg^{2+} concentration, just as in the *in vivo* situation. Although this goes far to tell us why rII mutants are restricted by λ lysogens, it does not clarify the relationship between rII gene expression and lysis. It seems appropriate, perhaps, to conclude our discussion of the much studied T-even phages by discussing a still unsolved problem of some importance.

4. REPRODUCTION OF T-ODD COLIPHAGES

4.1. T1

In terms of the amount of attention it has received, T1 represents the skeleton in the T phage family closet. Like all T-odd coliphages, T1 has a "standard" base composition of A, G, C, and T. The DNA molecule is nonpermuted and linear, with an unusually long and variable terminal repetition, some 2800 base pairs long on the average, or about 6.5% of the chromosome length (MacHattie *et al.,* 1972). Apparently the molecule replicates as a circle. Nucleotides for phage DNA synthesis are derived largely from breakdown of host DNA. However, early in infection large pieces of host DNA can be packaged into T1 virions, accounting for the ability of T1 to serve as a transducing phage (Kylberg *et al.,* 1975). The sequence of T1 gene expression must be quite different from that in T4, because by the time T4 virions are being assembled the host DNA has been largely degraded. T1 can also package λ phage DNA in infection of an induced lysogen (Geiman *et al.,* 1974). Both DNAs are of similar size. Finally, with respect to effects on host cell metabolism, Male and Christensen (1970) found that T1 infection does not abolish the synthesis of host mRNA but that β-galactosidase cannot be induced in infected cells.

4.2. T3 and T7

The closely related T3 and T7 viruses are the smallest of the T phages, with DNA molecules of about 25 million molecular weight. This relatively small size renders the DNA easy to manipulate experimentally, and the DNA possesses several other features which have combined to make these phages, particularly T7, popular objects for studying gene expression at the molecular level. This field was reviewed by Studier (1972), one of those most responsible for making us aware of the advantages of T7. The close relationship between T3 and T7 can be seen both in the extensive homologies between their genetic maps (Beier and Hausmann, 1973) and in their DNA molecules (Davis and Hyman, 1971; Hyman *et al.,* 1974). However, there are some distinct differences, as reflected in the fact that either phage can exclude the growth of the other.

The T7 DNA molecule is a nonpermuted linear duplex molecule with a short (260 base pairs) region of terminal redundancy (see Fig. 9). The presence of a unique sequence has allowed detailed physical map-

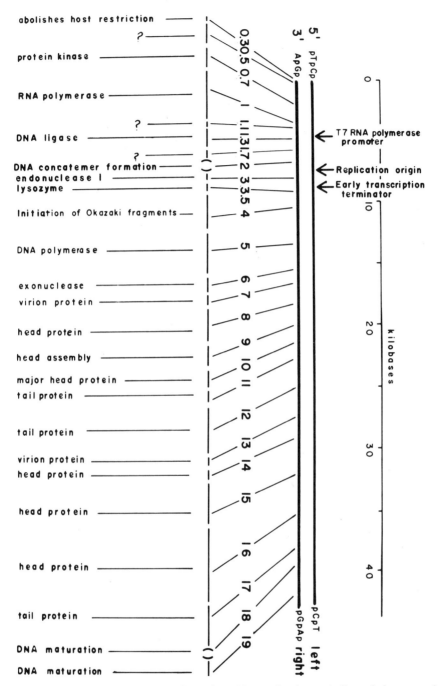

Fig. 9. The T7 phage genome. Along the DNA molecule are indicated the approximate positions of genes and other sites. The right strand is the template for all transcription. The approximate molecular weight of each gene product, where known, is indicated by each horizontal line denoting a protein (relate to the gene 1 product, with a molecular weight of approximately 100,000). Molecular weights of P2 and P18 have not been reported. The function or name of each gene product, where known, is indicated.

ping of the chromosome (Hyman, 1971; Studier, 1972; Simon and Studier, 1973), including location of the origin for the first round of DNA replication (Dressler *et al.,* 1972). This has also permitted a demonstration that injection of T7 DNA is polarized, with markers at the left end (as shown in Fig. 9) being injected first (Pao and Speyer, 1973).

Further simplifying the analysis of T7 gene expression is the historical fact that the first extensive mutant hunts (Studier and Hausmann, 1969) generated enough conditional lethal mutants to nearly saturate the map. The coding capacity of T7 DNA corresponds to some 25–30 proteins, and the *am* and *ts* mutants isolated in the early work fell into 19 complementation groups, which were numbered sequentially from left to right. Additional genes, most of which were recognized through the existence of deletions (Studier, 1973*a*), have been assigned fractional numbers corresponding to their location on the map. For example, gene 1.3 maps between genes 1 and 2. A new gene— gene 20—has recently been described (Pao and Speyer, 1975) and mapped at the right end of the genome. An additional simplifying factor is the fact that T7 gene transcription is totally asymmetrical; all genes are transcribed from the *r* strand (Summers and Szybalski, 1968). Thus all transcription, and hence translation, occurs from left to right in terms of the diagram in Fig. 9. The only exception to this pleasing symmetry is replication, which occurs bidirectionally, at least in the first two rounds (Dressler *et al.,* 1972). Moreover, T7 mRNAs are somehow stabilized in the infected cell, such that they can be identified and quantitated by gel electrophoresis (Summers, 1969, 1970; Studier, 1973*b*). From the sum of the molecular weights of all of the transcripts, one can conclude that virtually the entire *r* strand is transcribed.

Turning now to the proteins specified by the T7 genome, we see to a greater extent than with T-even phages a clustering of related functions. The genes coding for early functions—regulation and nucleic acid synthesis—map at the left, or earliest-transcribed, end of the genome, while structural proteins and those involved in assembly are controlled by genes at the right end of the map. T7 derives its DNA precursors almost exclusively from host cell DNA breakdown, and also there are no unusual nucleotides in T7 DNA. Therefore, the early functions include no enzymes of DNA precursor synthesis, but, as discussed below, they include several enzymes and proteins essential for DNA replication at the macromolecular level.

The most striking feature of the organization of the T7 genome is the fact that the earliest-expressed genes, from 0.3 through 1.3, are transcribed both *in vivo* and *in vitro* by unmodified RNA polymerase of the host (Hyman, 1971; Simon and Studier, 1973; Bräutigam and Sauerbier, 1973). A termination signal for *E. coli* RNA polymerase lies at 0.2 genome length from the left end (Simon and Studier, 1973). One of these early gene products is an RNA polymerase, coded for by gene 1 (Chamberlin *et al.,* 1970), which transcribes late genes starting from a promoter just to the left of gene 1.3 (Skare *et al.,* 1974). The T7 polymerase is quite distinct from any known cellular RNA polymerase (Chamberlin *et al.,* 1970; Niles *et al.,* 1974). It consists of a single subunit of molecular weight about 110,000, rather than four or more subunits. Moreover, both the T3 and T7 polymerases are quite species specific, to the extent that T7 polymerase transcribes T3 DNA very poorly and *vice versa.* As an approach to understanding the nature of the differences between the T3 and T7 polymerases, Beier and Hausmann (1974) have prepared a series of hybrid polymerases resulting from recombination within gene 1 in a series of T3 × T7 crosses.

Synthesis of phage-coded RNA polymerase represents a positive control mechanism. There also exist negative control mechanisms, one responsible for shutting off host transcription (Brunovskis and Summers, 1971) and one involved in the switch from early to late transcription (Ponta *et al.,* 1974). It seems likely that the protein kinase (Pai *et al.,* 1975) coded for by gene 0.7 plays the former role, possibly by phosphorylation of *E. coli* RNA polymerase (Rahmsdorf *et al.,* 1974; Ponta *et al.,* 1974; Zillig *et al.,* 1975). However, the precise role of the protein kinase is still unclear, since it also phosphorylates some ribosomal proteins (Rahmsdorf *et al.,* 1973). The enzyme is evidently required for growth only under suboptimal conditions (Hirsch-Kauffman *et al.,* 1975). Ponta *et al.* (1974) have also described the purification of a T7-specified "transcription inhibitor" which is believed to facilitate the transition from early to late transcription by inhibiting *E. coli* RNA polymerase. The same laboratory (Herrlich *et al.,* 1974) has also described a protein which interferes with host translation, at the level of polypeptide chain initiation. The gene coding for this protein lies to the left of gene 0.7 and either may represent the "gene 0.5" which appeared in one published map of T7 (Studier, 1972) but has not been mentioned since or may represent another activity of the 0.3 gene product. Studier (1975) has shown that the 0.3 protein overcomes a host restriction system. This explains the puzzling observation (Eskin *et al.,* 1973) that T7 lacking the appropriate modification grows in restricting hosts, even though DNA from such a phage is cleaved by the restriction endonuclease *in vivo.*

One other aspect of T7 gene regulation deserves comment. The entire early region of the genome is transcribed by *E. coli* RNA polymerase, from one of three promoters near the left end of the molecule to give a multicistronic RNA (the sequence of one of these promoters has been determined, Pribnow, 1975). The multicistronic RNA contains sequences encoding the products of genes 0.3, 0.7, 1, 1.1, and 1.3, but it serves as a poor template for synthesis of any of these proteins. Processing this molecule to five monocistronic messages involves cleavage by a host enzyme, ribonuclease III (Dunn and Studier, 1973; Hercules *et al.,* 1974).

Other early gene products include DNA ligase, encoded by gene 1.3 (Studier, 1972); the gene 2 product, which seems to be involved in formation of concatemeric replicative intermediates (Center, 1975); endonuclease I and exonuclease, encoded by genes 3 and 6, respectively (Center *et al.,* 1970); the gene 4 protein, which participates in initiation of Okazaki fragments as shown by its role in DNA synthesis *in vitro* (Strätling and Knippers, 1973; Scherzinger and Liftin, 1974; Hinkle and Richardson, 1975); and DNA polymerase, specified by gene 5 (Grippo and Richardson, 1971). A fascinating aspect of the function of the T7 DNA polymerase is that it requires a host protein for catalytic activity; this protein has been identified as thioredoxin, the electron transport protein in the ribonucleoside diphosphate reductase system (Modrich and Richardson, 1975).

T7 specifies at least two additional proteins of DNA metabolism whose controlling genes have not been identified: a DNA-binding protein, analogous to P32 of T4 (Reuben and Gefter, 1973, 1974), and an additional nuclease, endonuclease II (Center, 1972*a*). Like other DNA-binding proteins, the T7 protein is species specific, in that it apparently interacts only with T7 DNA polymerase *in vitro.* In this context, it is unusual that no mutants defective in this function have yet been reported. With respect to endonuclease II, the role of this enzyme is unknown. Endonuclease I and exonuclease evidently play the major roles in host DNA breakdown, for mutants in gene 3 or 6 are defective in DNA synthesis at least partly because of defective host DNA degradation (Sadowski and Kerr, 1970). Endonuclease II may be the same as an endonuclease specifically bound to DNA–membrane complexes (Pacumbaba and Center, 1974), but at present there is no strong evidence on this point.

Insofar as has been investigated, T3 induces a similar pattern of early protein synthesis. Two exceptions are the fact that T3 apparently induces no DNA ligase, using the host ligase instead, and that T3 also induces a unique enzyme ("SAMase") which cleaves *S*-adenosylmethionine to thiomethyladenosine and homoserine (Gefter *et al.,* 1966). The function of this latter enzyme appears to involve protection against host restriction systems, and in this context Studier (1975) has postulated that the 0.3 gene product of T7, which also protects against restriction, has a common evolutionary origin with the T3 SAMase, even though it contains no such catalytic activity.

As mentioned earlier, denaturation mapping of partially replicated T7 DNA indicates that replication is bidirectional from a fixed origin 17% of a genome length from the left end (Dressler *et al.*, 1972). Molecules which had initiated a second round from the same origin were also detected. Because the left-hand fork reaches the left end earlier than the right-hand fork reaches the more distant right end, many first-round replicative intermediates are Y shaped. Electron microscopic examination of both looped and branched replicative intermediates showed single-stranded regions along one strand only (Wolfson and Dressler, 1972). This suggests that DNA synthesis is discontinuous only along the lagging strand, i.e., that which grows overall in a 3′ to 5′ direction. However, one cannot rule out the possibility that synthesis is discontinuous in both directions but that leading-strand gaps are required more rapidly than lagging-strand gaps. In this context, Miller (1972*b*) has described the isolation of an RNA-linked DNA species from T7-infected cells which anneals only with *r*-strand DNA. If this species does represent an Okazaki fragment with its RNA primer still intact, one would expect it to hybridize to both strands of a bidirectionally replicating DNA molecule. Unfortunately, Miller's interesting but preliminary communication has not yet been followed up with a detailed report.

As a linear molecule which replicates without circularization, T7 DNA faces the same problem as T4 DNA, namely the completion of replication of the 5′-terminated strands. Watson (1972) has proposed a scheme analogous to that of Broker (1973), in which concatemers which are integral multiples of mature DNA are formed by recombination at redundant termini. Concatemers with the expected properties have been isolated from T7-infected cells (Schlegel and Thomas, 1972). Other fast-sedimenting and membrane-bound forms of T7 DNA have been isolated in later stages of replication (Center, 1972*b*; Strätling *et al.*, 1973; Serwer, 1974*a*), and the general picture which emerges is not unlike that already presented for T4. With respect to maturation of concatemeric intermediates, Watson (1972) proposed a mechanism involving endonucleolytic cleavage at the ends of the terminally redundant region, followed by either a strand displacement reaction involving DNA polymerase or digestion by an exonuclease followed by polymerase-catalyzed repair at the ends. He proposed the products of genes 18 and 19 as candidates for this role, but we should observe that the gene 3 and 6 nucleases may also participate in maturation (Strätling *et al.*, 1973). Further analysis of T7 DNA maturation should be greatly facilitated by two recent developments: Serwer (1974*b*) has isolated apparent intermediates in recombination, which consist of a capsid bound near the right end of either unit-length or concatemeric DNA; and Kerr and Sadowski (1974) have devised an *in vitro* system for DNA maturation and have demonstrated a role for the gene 19 protein in this process.

4.3. T5

T5 virus is intermediate between T7 and T4 in terms of size and complexity. Like T7 it has a linear, nonpermuted duplex DNA molecule with no novel nucleotides. However, the DNA molecule is about 3 times as long as that of T7, with a molecular weight of about 80 million. This represents roughly 110,000 base pairs, of which about 10,000 base pairs, or 9% of the chromosome, are repeated at each end of the molecule (Rhoades and Rhoades, 1972).

Like the T-even phages, T5 derives most of its DNA precursors from *de novo* nucleotide synthesis after infection, and to this end it induces the synthesis of several enzymes of DNA precursor synthesis, including thymidylate synthetase, dihydrofolate reductase, deoxynucleoside monophosphate kinase (Mathews, 1971*a*), and ribonucleotide reductase (Eriksson and Berglund, 1974). However, unlike the T-even phages, T5 does not utilize deoxynucleotides derived from the breakdown of bacterial DNA, even though the host cell chromosome is efficiently degraded. In fact, for reasons best known to itself, T5 induces the formation of a 5′-deoxynucleotidase, which seems to participate in the active removal from the cell of purines and pyrimidines derived from host cell DNA degradation (Warner *et al.*, 1975).

T5 contains several other unique features shared among known phages only with its close relative, phage BF23. The DNA molecule contains single-strand interruptions (repairable with DNA ligase) located at specific sites in one of the two strands. Several laboratories have studied the length of each segment and the locations of the nicks (cf. Hayward and Smith, 1972; Bujard and Hendrickson, 1973; Hayward, 1974). Although there is some disagreement over details, the model in Fig. 10 shows the essential features; the left-end fragments are the smallest; the nick within the left-hand repeat sequence is variable in position while the right-hand repeat sequence contains no such nicks; and heat-stable mutations, which involve deletion of about 6% of the

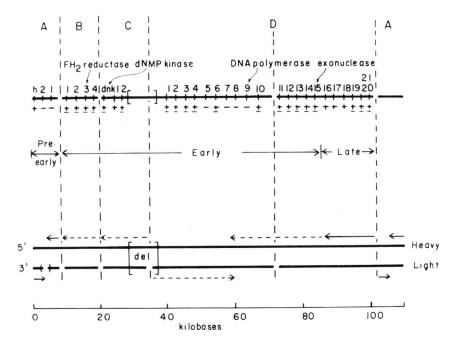

Fig. 10. The T5 phage genome. The capital letters at the top and the vertical dashed lines denote the four linkage groups. The upper heavy line denotes the genetic map, with the approximate position of each gene given, along with the identification of four gene products. Below the map is an indication of whether mutants in each gene synthesize DNA normally (+), synthesize no detectable DNA (−), or exhibit abnormal DNA synthesis (±; reduced rate, delayed or arrested synthesis, or degradation of nascent DNA). Next the time of expression of each group of genes is shown. The heavy double line represents the DNA molecule, showing the positions of single-strand interruptions (the position of the leftmost nick is variable); the DNA deleted in heat-stable mutants of T5; and the direction of transcription of each group of genes (firm assignments are indicated with solid arrows). Modified from Hendrickson and Bujard (1973).

DNA, cover the region involving the middle nick (Scheible and Rhoades, 1975). Virtually nothing is known about the biological functions of the nicks beyond the probability from their specific locations that their existence is not accidental, and the fact that the nicks are repaired early in infection (Herman and Moyer, 1974, 1975).

The other unusual aspect of T5 phage biology is its discontinuous mode of DNA transfer into the infected cell (Lanni, 1968). After the leftmost 8% of the chromosome has passed into the cell, DNA transfer stops for a while, and several genes on the "first step transfer" (FST) DNA are expressed. This is essential for transfer of the remainder of the chromosome. The head and noncontractile tail seem to play only a passive role, if any, in this latter transfer. In infected complexes which have transferred only the FST segment, one can strip off the attached heads by the shear forces involved in centrifuging the cells (Labedan and Legault-Demare, 1973). Under these conditions, the entire remaining DNA remains attached to the bacterium, waving gently in the breeze, as it were, and able to be subsequently drawn into the cell.

Development of a genetic map for T5 and its correlation with phage DNA structure have been pursued by McCorquodale and his associates (Hendrickson and McCorquodale, 1971a, 1972; Beckman et al., 1973; McCorquodale, 1975). Somewhat surprisingly, all of the mutations mapped thus far fell into four seemingly independent linkage groups, even though the entire genome consists of but one DNA molecule. One mutant of T5 exhibits abnormally low recombination frequencies, and Hendrickson and McCorquodale were able to use this to order the four fragments (Fig. 10). The basis for this apparent division of the chromosome is not known, but it may involve in some obscure way the single-strand DNA interruptions, or it may reflect a low degree of saturation of the map with mutations. Recall that many marker pairs in T4 are unlinked because of the large distance between them and the high rate of recombination of that virus. Recall also that the T4 chromosome contains about 120 known genes distributed along a DNA molecule of 170 kb, while T5 has about 30 known genes on a DNA molecule of 110 kb. Thus the density of known markers on the T5 genome is less than 40% of the corresponding value for T4.

Of the four linkage groups on the T5 chromosome, one—group A—corresponds to FST DNA, the small amount injected initially into the infected cell. Even before a T5 genetic map was available, it was possible to assign phage functions to genes on FST DNA. One could carry out infection with wild-type T5, allow FST DNA to be injected, interrupt further DNA injection by shearing the infected complexes in a blender, and ask what phage functions were expressed by the cells containing only FST DNA (Lanni, 1969). This study showed that two functions are controlled by genes on FST DNA: degradation of the host chromosome and transfer of the remaining DNA. Later Beckman et al. (1973) recognized the existence of three FST genes. Mutants in gene A2 are unable to complete transfer of the chromosome, while mutants in gene A1 show simultaneous defects in chromosome transfer, host DNA degradation, shutoff of host-specific transcription and translation, and, in some cases, ability to grow in a λ lysogen. Gene A3 controls a function which in wild-type phage is responsible for restriction of growth in host strains bearing the colicinogenic factor ColIb.

The pleiotropic effect of A1 mutations can be explained partly in terms of the existence of protein complexes involving the A1 and A2 gene products (Beckman *et al.,* 1971). The A1 and A2 proteins have subunit molecular weights of 57,000 and 15,000, respectively. Beckman and colleagues detected the presence of an oligomeric form of the A1 protein, of molecular weight 244,000, and a complex with both A1 and A2 proteins, of molecular weight 364,000. It seems reasonable to ascribe a role in DNA transfer to the A1-A2 complex, with the other functions controlled, directly or indirectly, by the A1 oligomer. Elucidation of how the A1-A2 complex interacts with the cell to drag in the 92% of T4 DNA which is non-FST should prove one of the more fascinating developments in this area of science.

Since genes of the A group are on a redundant end, one has in principle an opportunity for the existence of heterozygotes, comparable to the terminal redundancy heterozygotes of T4. However, these could never be detected in T5, because the genes on the right-hand A region cannot be expressed until after DNA transfer is complete. Once this has occurred, expression of the left-end A genes, which are classified as "pre-early" in terms of their time of expression (Hendrickson and Bujard, 1973), has ceased and been supplanted by the expression of "early" genes. These correspond to linkage groups B, C, and part of D. Relatively few of the products of these genes have been identified. Gene B3 codes for dihydrofolate reductase, gene D9 for DNA polymerase, and gene D15 for an exonuclease (Hendrickson and McCorquodale, 1972). An additional gene, *dnk,* which maps near gene C1, codes for dNMP kinase (Berget *et al.,* 1974). Since this kinase is not involved in synthesis of a unique phage DNA precursor, as in T4, *dnk* mutants are not lethal, but there is a reduction in DNA synthesis of about threefold. Surprisingly, mutants defective in dihydrofolate reductase (B3) exhibit a substantially greater reduction in DNA synthesis, about eightfold. This leads one to wonder whether some aspect of the metabolism of the T5-infected cell limits the activity of the host cell dihydrofolate reductase, since T4 mutants defective in the corresponding gene show only a two- to threefold reduction in DNA synthesis.

As expected, mutants defective in DNA polymerase (D9) exhibit a D0 phenotype, as do mutants in five other as-yet uncharacterized genes: D4, D5, D7, D8, and D11. Mutants in gene D15 show a DNA-arrest phenotype, and Frenkel and Richardson (1971) have presented evidence for a role of this enzyme in maturation of rapidly sedimenting replicative intermediates to virion DNA. The function therefore may be analogous to the 46/47 function of T4. Activity of this enzyme is also required for expression of late T5 genes (Chinnadurai and McCorquodale, 1973), even though replication is not coupled to late transcription, as it is in T4 (Hendrickson and McCorquodale, 1971*b*).

Many of the uncharacterized T5 genes show DNA-defective phenotypes as well, as summarized in Fig. 10. Of interest are mutants in genes D6 and D11, in which only a small amount of DNA is synthesized and then degraded. Controlling genes for several other T5 gene products have not yet been identified, including thymidylate synthetase, ribonucleotide reductase, and at least 14 tRNAs (Scherberg and Weiss, 1970; Chen *et al.*, 1975). Thus the correlation of genes with gene functions is still in an early stage for T5, particularly when one considers that little has yet been done in assigning genes for structural proteins (Zweig and Cummings, 1973).

The regulation of T5 gene expression is discussed more fully in the chapter by Geiduschek and Rabussay and in the review of McCorquodale (1975). Suffice it to say for our purposes that both RNA and protein species fall into three temporal classes. Class I RNA, which is transcribed from FST DNA, is synthesized from 0 to 4 min after infection. Class II transcription starts at about 4 min, and class III transcription commences at 9 min. Calcium ion, which has long been known to be essential for successful infection by T5, must be present for the transition from class I to class II transcription (Moyer and Buchanan, 1970). Syntheses of protein classes I, II, and III commence shortly after the onset of transcription of the respective RNA classes (McCorquodale and Buchanan, 1968). By means of hybridization with separated strands and specific fragments of T5 DNA, Hendrickson and Bujard (1973) have learned a great deal about regions of the chromosome and template strands corresponding to each class of transcripts (see Fig. 10).

What metabolic changes are responsible for transitions from class I to class II and from class II to class III transcription patterns? We have already seen that concurrent DNA replication is not required for normal late gene transcription. In other respects, T5 is not unlike T4 in its regulation, insofar as has been reported. T5 does use the host cell RNA polymerase for transcription of all its genes (Beckman *et al.*, 1972), and it modifies that enzyme to its own ends (Szabo *et al.*, 1975). The latter study analyzed phage proteins associated with RNA polymerase through immunoprecipitation with an antiserum against *E. coli* RNA polymerase. One class I protein and two class II proteins become associated with the enzyme. One of the latter proteins is the product of gene C2, already shown to be essential for initiation of class III transcription (Chinnadurai and McCorquodale, 1974). As stated earlier, T5 growth is restricted by the colicinogenic factor *Col*Ib. Under these abortive conditions of infection, only the single class I protein becomes bound to RNA polymerase. However, this does not pinpoint the site of action of *Col*Ib in restriction, for class II and III RNAs and proteins are not synthesized under these conditions (Moyer *et al.*, 1972).

Our picture of T5 DNA replication is still quite incomplete, although, as with other phages having linear DNA, concatemeric intermediates seem to be involved. These are very heterogeneous in size and apparently extensively nicked (cf. Carrington and Lunt, 1973). This study suggested also that mature-length DNA exists as a free intermediate between concatemers and DNA-filled heads, distinguishing this mode of DNA maturation from the corresponding process in T4.

One final aspect of T5 DNA metabolism deserves comment. Rosenkranz (1973) has reported the presence of RNA in T5 virions. T5 was labeled by growth in 5-^{3}H-labeled uridine, and deoxyribonuclease digestion of phage DNA yielded labeled material which had the density of RNA. A puzzling feature of this work is that base analysis of the total labeled nucleic acid revealed radioactivity in cytosine, uracil, and thymine. The last, however, should be nonradioactive because of removal of the 5-H by thymidylate synthetase.

5. *BACILLUS SUBTILIS* PHAGES

Next to the coliphages, the *Bacillus subtilis* phages are the most extensively studied group of bacteriophages. The list of *B. subtilis* phages which have received experimental attention is much longer than the corresponding list of coliphages, although there are fewer laboratories studying *B. subtilis* phages than those involved with coliphages. Until recent years, *B. subtilis* phages were used primarily as tools for study of host-related processes, including sporulation, transformation, and transduction, and only recently has attention focused on the biochemistry of phage reproduction. As a result, our general knowledge of this area is somewhat fragmentary, although certain aspects have received a great deal of attention. In this section, we shall concern ourselves with particularly distinctive or interesting aspects of the reproduction of these phages. The general field of *B. subtilis* phages is described in far more detail than possible here in a comprehensive review by Hemphill and Whiteley (1975).

All of the known *B. subtilis* phages have linear, nonpermuted duplex DNA molecules. These viruses include virulent and temperate phages, as do the coliphage viruses. However, there also exist a large number of defective phages, which can multiply only in the presence of a helper phage, and another class of transducing phages whose mode of infection can be described as "pseudovirulent." These phages can establish a transient state in which a lytic cycle is not established, but unlike the case in true lysogeny the viral chromosome exists in infected cells mostly as free DNA. We shall discuss some of these phages, as well as the true virulents. In general, inhibition of host cell macromolecular synthesis and degradation of the host chromosome either do not occur in infection by these phages or occur much more slowly than in T-even coliphage infection. Also, the phenomenon of superinfection exclusion is unknown. This means that one can study dominance relationships between different phages in mixed infections (cf. Whiteley *et al.*, 1974).

5.1.   Phages with Hydroxymethyluracil-Containing DNA

The several closely related phages SP01, SP82G, SP8, ϕe, and 2C all have hydroxymethyluracil-containing DNA molecules of molecular weight $1-1.3 \times 10^8$, about the same size as T-even phage genomes. Partial genetic maps for SP82G and SP01 are available, and in the case of SP82G, genes controlling DNA synthesis are clustered at one end of the map, with genes controlling tail and head formation in the middle and at the other end, respectively (Green and Laman, 1972). DNA injection is relatively slow with these phages. Two to four minutes is required, depending on temperature, and this gave McAllister (1970) an opportunity to measure the order of gene injection by shearing infected complexes in a blender at different times during injection and then carrying out marker rescue experiments with superinfecting phages. This indicated that injection is polarized, with those genes controlling DNA synthesis being injected first. Similar results were adduced from studies on partial gene transfer in ^{32}P-labeled phage, in which double-strand breaks induced by radioisotope decay had prevented injection of the distal markers (McAllister and Green, 1973).

Mechanisms for effecting the complete replacement of thymine in phage DNA by 5-hydroxymethyluracil (HMU) are comparable to those used by T-even phages to exclude cytosine from their DNA. Pathways of DNA precursor metabolism are shown in Fig. 11. dCMP deaminase provides a biosynthetic route for dUMP. Interestingly, this enzyme is unique among known dCMP deaminases in that it is not subject to feedback regulation by dNTPs (Nishihara *et al.*, 1967). The dUMP hydroxymethylase is essential for phage growth, as shown by the DNA-negative phenotype of phages unable to induce this enzyme (Price *et al.*, 1972). The same is true for HM-dUMP kinase (Kahan, 1971).

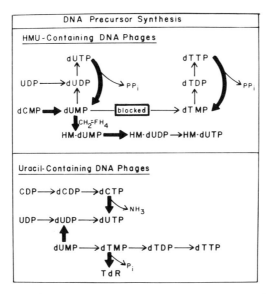

Fig. 11. Pathways of DNA precursor synthesis in phage-infected *Bacillus subtilis.*
Reactions catalyzed by phage-specified enzymes are indicated with heavy arrows.

Comparable to the mechanism used by T4 for exclusion of cytosine from its DNA is one used by HMU-containing phages for exclusion of thymine: synthesis of a new dTTPase-dUTPase. However, unlike the situation with T-even phages, this function is not essential for phage growth. Mutants unable to synthesize the enzyme are viable, despite the fact that phage DNA synthesized in infection by these mutants contains up to 20% of its HMU residues replaced by thymine (Marcus and Newlon, 1971; Dunham and Price, 1974). An additional thymine exclusion mechanism involves synthesis of a protein inhibitor of host cell thymidylate synthetase (Haslam *et al.,* 1967). This mechanism, discovered for φe, may also be operative for the other HMU-containing phages. Neither of these mechanisms seems to be involved in the phage-directed arrest of host cell DNA synthesis which is known to occur, for host shutoff occurs under conditions where a dTTP pool is maintained after infection (Marcus and Newlon, 1971). Lavi and Marcus (1972) have presented evidence for the functioning of another phage-coded protein in this process. An additional early function in SP82G inactivates a putative nuclease which had been found to inactivate phage DNA in studies on transfection, or infection of bacteria by naked DNA (McAllister and Green, 1972).

With regard to DNA replication, an extensive study of SP01 has revealed the existence of membrane-bound and concatemeric intermediates (Levner and Cozzarelli, 1972). The enzymology of phage

DNA replication is still not well understood. Replication of these phages is resistant to 6-(p-hydroxyphenylazo)uracil (HPUra), an agent which specifically blocks bacterial DNA synthesis by inhibiting DNA polymerase III (Brown, 1970; Neville and Brown, 1972). This suggests that these large phages induce their own DNA polymerases, and such an enzyme has been isolated from SP01-infected cells (Yehle and Ganesan, 1973). However, it has also been reported that host cell polymerase III is essential for φe replication, because infection at restrictive temperature of a host with a *ts* polymerase III mutation is abortive (Lavi *et al.,* 1974). These apparently contradictory findings have not yet been resolved.

Phages in this class are widely used as tools in the study of sporulation. For example, φe cannot infect cells once sporulation has begun, and RNA polymerase from sporulating cells loses its activity to transcribe φe DNA *in vitro.* This may mean that sporulation itself is controlled through changes in RNA polymerase, perhaps involving alteration of the σ subunit (Segall *et al.,* 1974). Certainly phage-induced changes in host cell RNA polymerase are involved in regulating the viral program of transcription, a complex series of events in which at least six discrete temporal classes of phage-specific mRNA can be detected. The extensive literature on this subject is capably reviewed by Hemphill and Whiteley (1975), and in Volume 8 of this series, by Rabussay and Geiduschek, and will not be further considered here.

5.2. Phages with Uracil-Containing DNA

The best-known phages in the group with uracil-containing DNA are PBS1 and its clear-plaque variant PBS2, both large viruses with DNAs of about 2×10^8 molecular weight. Of special interest are the mechanisms by which these phages synthesize DNA containing uracil instead of thymine. These include (1) replacement of the dTTP pool by dUTP through the action of phage-coded enzymes (Fig. 11) and (2) inhibition of host cell activities which degrade uracil-containing DNA. These latter activities include a nuclease which releases deoxyuridine and oligonucleotides from uracil-containing DNA (Tomita and Takahashi, 1975) and an *N*-glycosidase which releases uracil from uracil-containing DNA but apparently does not itself further degrade the DNA (Friedberg *et al.,* 1975). Of the enzymes involved in deoxyribonucleotide metabolism, there is an apparent paradox implicit in the fact that the dTMP phosphatase induced by PBS2 also cleaves dUMP, an activity which would seem to decrease the ability of the cell to synthesize dUTP (Price and Fogt, 1973a). However, the K_m for this latter activity is very high (approximately 1 mM), and it seems unlikely that the enzyme catalyzes rapid cleavage of dUMP *in vivo*.

As with the HMU-containing *B. subtilis* phages, PBS2 DNA replication is resistant to HPUra (Price and Fogt, 1973a), apparently because of the synthesis of a phage-specific DNA polymerase (Price and Cook, 1972). This enzyme utilizes either dUTP or dTTP *in vitro*, whereas cellular DNA polymerases show a distinct preference for dTTP. In parallel fashion, PBS1 reproduction was found to be insensitive to rifampicin (Rima and Takahashi, 1973), and this was followed up by the discovery that PBS2 synthesizes its own RNA polymerase, which is resistant to rifampicin (Clark *et al.*, 1974). Unlike the phage-specified RNA polymerases of T3 and T7, the PBS2 enzyme is structurally complex, containing at least four polypeptide subunits. Also, the enzyme has a marked preference for PBS2 DNA as a template, although, unlike T3 and T7 polymerases, this species specificity is not absolute.

A question of general biological interest is the teleological significance of the separate existence of thymine in DNA and uracil in RNA, when the coding properties of these two pyrimidines are identical. Phages with uracil-containing DNA present an opportunity for exploration of this question. Although it will require the development of some complex multiple mutants, it should be possible in principle to develop conditions for reinsertion of thymine into PBS2 DNA. What will be the biological consequences of this substitution?

5.3. Small *B. subtilis* Phages

Among the *B. subtilis* phages, ϕ29 can be considered as a "counterpart" to coliphage T7 in its being small enough that a complete identification of genes and their functions might possibly be affected. In fact, the task may be more approachable for ϕ29, because its genome, with a molecular weight of 11 million, is less than half the size of that of T7. Moreover, the virus is an attractive object for studies on viral morphogenesis (little studied in other *B. subtilis* phages), because of its complex structure (see Table 2).

Several laboratories have mapped conditional lethal mutations of ϕ29. The most complete map published to date shows 17 cistrons (Moreno *et al.*, 1974). Since the coding capacity of ϕ29 DNA is about 20–25 proteins, the map is approaching saturation. Analysis of proteins synthesized in UV-irradiated infected cells reveals the existence of 23 proteins, whose aggregate molecular weight accounts for about 90% of the coding capacity of the phage (Hawley *et al.*, 1973). However, some of these proteins may represent cleavage products or precursors; protein cleavage is known to occur in ϕ29 morphogenesis (Tosi *et al.*, 1975).

Infection with ϕ29 has little effect on host-specific macromolecular synthesis (cf. Schachtele *et al.*, 1972). It is for this reason that the analysis of viral proteins cited above had to utilize UV-irradiated host cells—to reduce the synthesis of bacterial proteins. For comparable studies on phage DNA replication, the reagent HPUra is useful (Ivarie and Pène, 1973), because, like larger *B. subtilis* phages, ϕ29 can replicate in the presence of this inhibitor (Schachtele *et al.*, 1973*b*). *A priori,* one might not expect so small a virus to encode its own DNA polymerase, so one must await elucidation of the mechanism of this resistance.

Because of its small size, ϕ29 represents an attractive system for studying the control of transcription. Two temporal classes of phage RNA can be detected: an early class, transcribed from the light strand of viral DNA, and a later class, synthesized without concomitant shutoff of early transcription, which is synthesized primarily from the heavy strand (Schachtele *et al.*, 1973*a*). The viral transcripts are also stabilized somehow in the infected cell, so that they can be resolved as discrete species by disc gel electrophoretic analysis; the detectable species account for about 90% of the coding capacity of this virus (Loskutoff and Pène, 1973).

In studies of ϕ29 infection of sporulating cells, Kawamura and Ito (1974) have challenged the idea that alterations in host cell RNA polymerase are primarily involved in initiating sporulation. Replication of this virus is blocked much earlier in sporulation than is that of the much larger ϕe. Under conditions of blocked viral growth, ϕ29 DNA synthesis was undetectable, whereas early phage RNA synthesis appeared normal. This would suggest that the primary alteration involves something other than bacterial RNA polymerase, although other explanations are possible.

5.4. Other *B. subtilis* Phages

Here we merely mention a few scattered points of interest with regard to other *B. subtilis* phages. Much more information is available in the previously cited reviews. Neubort and Marmur (1973) have studied the biosynthesis of the unique pyrimidine, dihydroxypentyluracil (DHPU), the existence of which in phage SP-15 was cited in Table 1. Unlike other phage DNA modifications we have discussed, this one occurs at the macromolecular level, after incorporation of uracil into DNA as dUTP. The mechanism and significance of the subsequent modifications, including attachment of a sugar phosphate to the hydroxyl positions in the modified base, are not yet known.

Another *B. subtilis* phage which has been useful for studies on replication and transcription is SPP1, because of the extraordinary ease with which its DNA strands can be separated. Spatz and Trautner (1970) carried out transfection experiments with SPP1 heteroduplexes. Each cell yielded only one of the two possible genotypes, indicating the presence of an active repair system for mismatched bases in transfecting (and presumably also transforming) DNA. Also, Klotz (1973) used transfection to determine a gradient of marker frequency in replicating SPP1 DNA. Intracellular DNA was isolated from transfected cells, and gene frequencies in this DNA were determined by marker rescue experiments in a subsequent cycle of transfection. This showed that replication of this DNA is unidirectional from an origin near one end of the molecule.

A final point relates to the existence of *B. subtilis* phages which can reproduce at high temperature, even though *B. subtilis* is not a thermophilic bacterium. LaMontagne and McDonald (1973) found that one such phage, TSP-1, can adsorb only to cells grown at temperatures above 50°C. Once adsorbed, however, phage growth still requires high temperature, because DNA replication is inhibited at temperatures below 50°C. At present, the ecological significance of these findings is quite obscure.

6. OTHER PHAGES

The coliphages and the *B. subtilis* phages are the only groups whose reproduction has been studied systematically. However, several other groups of phages have been receiving increasing attention, primarily because of their potential utility as probes for metabolic events in their hosts. These include the cyanophages, which, strictly speaking, are not bacteriophages because their hosts are blue-green algae. However, these algae are prokaryotic organisms, even though they contain a photosynthetic apparatus similar to those found in eukaryotes. As reviewed by Padan and Shilo (1973), all of the known cyanophages are tailed viruses with double-stranded DNA, morphologically quite similar to bacteriophages. Growth times are considerably longer, commonly 12–14 h for a single infectious cycle. Moreover, quantitative measurements of growth and other metabolic events are often difficult to carry out because the host grows and is infected in a filamentous form. However, we do know that growth of some cyanophages is dependent on continued photosynthetic activity of the host, while infection by other classes disrupts the photosynthetic apparatus. Further analysis of these systems should lead to new insights on the organization of photosynthetic machinery in these organisms.

The bdellovibriophages represent another intriguing class of phages, because the hosts, bdellovibrios, are cellular parasites which can only grow and divide within another bacterial cell, such as *E. coli* (Varon and Levisohn, 1972; Kessel and Varon, 1973). Thus one has a three-component parasitic system, in which a phage can only replicate in a bdellovibrio which is in turn parasitizing another bacterium. There do exist host-independent mutants of bdellovibrio in which phage replication can occur in the absence of a cellular host for the parasite. Little is known as yet about the biochemistry of these phages, although they do appear to contain double-stranded DNA, and nucleotides for their DNA synthesis seem to be derived from both the host bdellovibrio and its own host.

Taylor and Guha (1975) have initiated a study of the molecular biology of phages with anaerobic bacterial hosts. Initial studies have focused on transcription in *Clostridium sporogenes* infected with phage F1. Individual transcripts were analyzed by polyacrylamide gel electrophoresis. Five early species were derived from the heavy DNA strand, as were five more late species. Even later in infection, two other mRNA species were synthesized from the light strand, and host-specific ribosomal RNA synthesis continued throughout infection.

We close this chapter with a topic close to that with which we began it: the biosynthesis of unique bases. Of the known base substitutions that were listed in Table 1, we have discussed all those known to occur in the coliphages and the *B. subtilis* phages. The other two include the biosynthesis of α-putrescinylthymine in *Pseudomonas acidovorans* infected by phage ϕW14 (Kelln and Warren, 1973) and the biosynthesis of 5-methylcytosine, which replaces cytosine in phage XP-12 of *Xanthomonas oryzae,* originally isolated from a Chinese rice paddy (Ehrlich *et al.,* 1975). The former substitution has been found to occur at the mononucleotide level. Infection by ϕW14 induces the synthesis of at least two new enzymes, thymidylate synthetase and dUMP hydroxymethylase. The latter enzyme generates 5-hydroxymethyl-dUMP, which is apparently an intermediate in putrescinylthymidylate biosynthesis. Since this nucleotide does not completely substitute for thymine in the DNA of this phage, one is left with the question of whether there is any specificity regarding the location within DNA sequences of the modified base, and, if so, how it is generated. Regarding 5-methylcytosine biosynthesis, this base normally arises in nucleic acids, where it exists as a minor constitutent, by an S-adenosylmethionine-dependent methyl transfer to a preformed polynucleotide chain. In the case of phage XP-12, the methyl group of methylcytosine is derived from the β-carbon of serine, suggesting the involvement of 5,10-methylenetetrahydrofolate as a single-carbon donor. Whether this one-carbon transfer occurs at the mononucleotide level or after completion of a polynucleotide chain is not known at the time of this writing.

7. REFERENCES

Abelson, J. N., and Thomas, C. A., Jr., 1966, The anatomy of the T5 bacteriophage DNA molecule, *J. Mol. Biol.* **18**:262.

Abelson, J., Fukada, K., Johnson, P., Lamfrom, H., Nierlich, D. P., Otsuka, A., Paddock, G. V., Pinkerton, T. C., Sarabhai, A., Stahl, S., Wilson, J. H., and Yesian, H., 1975, Bacteriophage T4 tRNA's: Structure, genetics, and biosynthesis, in: *Processing of RNA*, Brookhaven Symposia in Biology, No. 26, p. 8.

Adams, M. H., 1959, *Bacteriophages*, Interscience, New York.

Alberts, B. M., and Frey, L., 1970, T4 bacteriophage gene 32: A structural protein in the replication and recombination of DNA, *Nature (London)* **227**:1313.

Alberts, B. M., Morris, F., Sinha, N., Mace, D., Bittner, M., and Moran, L., 1975, *In vitro* DNA synthesis catalyzed by purified T4 bacteriophage replication proteins, in: *DNA Synthesis and Its Regulation* (M. Goulian and P. Hanawalt, eds.), ICN-UCLA Symposium, Benjamin, Menlo Park, Calif.

Altman, S., and Meselson, M., 1970, A T4-induced endonuclease which attacks T4 DNA, *Proc. Natl. Acad. Sci. USA* **66**:716.

Ames, B. N., and Dubin, D. T., 1960, Polyamines in the neutralization of bacteriophage DNA, *J. Biol. Chem.* **235**:769.

Anderson, C. W., and Eigner, J., 1971, Breakdown and exclusion of superinfecting T-even bacteriophage in *Escherichia coli*, *J. Virol.* **8**:869.

Anderson, C. W., Williamson, J. R., and Eigner, J., 1971, Localization of parental DNA from superinfecting T4 bacteriophage in *Escherichia coli*, *J. Virol.* **8**:887.

Anderson, T. F., 1945, The role of tryptophane in the adsorption of two bacterial viruses on their host, *E. coli*, *J. Cell. Comp. Physiol.* **25**:17.

Ando, T., Takagi, J., Kojawa, T., and Ikeda, Y., 1970, Substrate specificity of the nicking enzymes isolated from phage T4-infected *Escherichia coli*, *J. Biochem.* **67**:497.

Arscott, P. G., and Goldberg, E. B., 1975, Cooperative action of the T4 tail fibers and baseplate in triggering conformational change and in determining host range, *Virology* **69**:15.

Astrachan, L., and Miller, J. F., 1973, Cadaverine in bacteriophage T4, *J. Virol.* **11**:792.

Bachrach, U., Friedmann, A., Levin, R., and Nygaard, A. P., 1974, Transfer of internal proteins from phage to host and their association with bacterial membranes, *J. Gen. Virol.* **23**:117.

Baker, J. O., and Hattman, S., 1970, Interference by bacteriophage T4 in the reproduction of the single-stranded DNA phage M13, *Virology* **42**:28.

Baldy, M., 1968, Repair and recombination in phage T4. II. Genes affecting UV sensitivity, *Cold Spring Harbor Symp. Quant. Biol.* **33**:333.

Baltz, R. H., and Drake, J. W., 1972, Bacteriophage T4 transformation: An assay for mutations induced *in vitro, Virology* **49**:462.

Barry, J., and Alberts, B. M., 1972, *In vitro* complementation as an assay for new proteins required for bacteriophage DNA replication, *Proc. Natl. Acad. Sci. USA* **69**:2717.

Bayer, M. E., 1968, Adsorption of bacteriophage to adhesions between cell wall and membrane of *Escherichia coli, J. Virol.* **2**:346.

Beckendorf, S., 1973, Structure of the distal half of the bacteriophage T4 tail fiber, *J. Mol. Biol.* **73**:37.

Becker, A., and Hurwitz, J., 1967, The enzymatic cleavage of phosphate termini from polynucleotides, *J. Biol. Chem.* **242**:936.

Beckey, A. D., Wulff, J. L., and Earhart, C. F., 1974, Early synthesis of membrane protein after bacteriophage T4 infection, *J. Virol.* **14**:886.

Beckman, L. D., Hoffman, M. S., and McCorquodale, D. J., 1971, Pre-early proteins of bacteriophage T5: Structure and function, *J. Mol. Biol.* **62**:551.

Beckman, L. D., Witonsky, P., and McCorquodale, D. J., 1972, Effect of rifampicin on the growth of bacteriophage T5, *J. Virol.* **10**:179.

Beckman, L. D., Anderson, G. C., and McCorquodale, D. J., 1973, Arrangement on the chromosome of the known pre-early genes of bacteriophage T5 and BF23, *J. Virol.* **12**:1191.

Behme, M. T., and Ebisuzaki, K., 1975, Characterization of a bacteriophage T4 mutant lacking DNA-dependent ATPase, *J. Virol.* **15**:50.

Beier, H., and Hausmann, R., 1973, Genetic map of bacteriophage T3, *J. Virol.* **12**:417.

Beier, H., and Hausmann, R., 1974, T3 × T7 phage crosses leading to recombinant RNA polymerases, *Nature (London)* **251**:538.

Bello, L. J., and Bessman, M. J., 1963, The enzymology of virus-infected bacteria. V. Phosphorylation of hydroxymethyl-dCDP and dTDP in normal and bacteriophage-infected *Escherichia coli, Biochim. Biophys. Acta* **72**:647.

Benz, W. C., and Goldberg, E. B., 1973, Interactions between modified phage T4 particles and spheroplasts, *Virology* **53**:225.

Berget, P. B., and Warner, H. R., 1975, Identification of P48 and P54 as components of phage T4 baseplates, *J. Virol.* **16**:1669.

Berget, S. M., Warner, H. R., and McCorquodale, D. J., 1974, Isolation and partial characterization of bacteriophage T5 mutants deficient in the ability to induce deoxynucleoside monophosphate kinase. *J. Virol.* **13**:78.

Berglund, O., 1972, Ribonucleoside diphosphate reductase induced by bacteriophage T4. II. Allosteric regulation of substrate specificity and catalytic activity, *J. Biol. Chem.* **247**:7276.

Berglund, O., and Holmgren, A., 1975, Thioredoxin reductase-mediated hydrogen transfer from *Escherichia coli* thioredoxin-$(SH)_2$ to phage T4 thioredoxin-S_2, *J. Biol. Chem.* **250**:2778.

Bernstein, C., and Bernstein, H., 1974, Coiled rings of DNA released from cells infected with bacteriophages T7 or T4 or from uninfected *Escherichia coli, J. Virol.* **13**:1346.

Bernstein, H., and Bernstein, C., 1973, Circular and branched circular concatenates as possible intermediates in bacteriophage T4 DNA replication, *J. Mol. Biol.* **77**:355.

Black, L. W., 1974, Bacteriophage T4 internal protein mutants: Isolation and properties, *Virology* **60**:166.

Black, L. W., and Abremski, K., 1974, Restriction of phage T4 internal protein I mutants by a strain of *Escherichia coli, Virology* **60**:180.

Black, L. W., and Ahmad-Zadeh, C., 1971, Internal proteins of bacteriophage T4D: Their characterization and relation to head structure and assembly, *J. Mol. Biol.* **57**:71.

Boikov, P. Y., and Gumanov, L. L., 1972, Modification of cell membrane structures of *Escherichia coli* B infected with various *r*II mutants in phage T4B, *Biokhimiya* **37**:142.

Bolle, A., Epstein, R. H., Salser, W., and Geiduschek, E. P., 1968, Transcription during bacteriophage T4 development: Requirements for late messenger synthesis, *J. Mol. Biol.* **33**:339.

Bradley, D. E., 1967, Ultrastructure of bacteriophages and bacteriocins, *Bacteriol. Rev.* **31**:230.

Brandon, C. Gallop, P. M., Marmur, J., Hayashi, H., and Nakanishi, K., 1972, Structure of a new pyrimidine from *Bacillus subtilis* phage SP-15 nucleic acid, *Nature (London) New Biol.* **239**:70.

Bräutigam, A. R., and Sauerbier, W., 1973, Transcription unit mapping in bacteriophage T7, *J. Virol.* **12**:882.

Bremer, H., and Yuan, D., 1968, Chain growth rate of messenger RNA in *Escherichia coli* infected with bacteriophage T4, *J. Mol. Biol.* **34**:527.

Broker, T. R., 1973, An electron microscopic analysis of pathways for bacteriophage T4 DNA recombination, *J. Mol. Biol.* **81**:1.

Brooks, J., and Hattman, S., 1973, Location of the DNA-adenine methylase gene on the genetic map of phage T2, *Virology* **55**:285.

Brown, N. C., 1970, 6-(*p*-Hydroxyphenylazo)-uracil: A selective inhibitor of host DNA replication in phage-infected *Bacillus subtilis, Proc. Natl. Acad. Sci. USA* **67**:1454.

Brunovskis, I., and Summers, W. C., 1971, The process of infection with coliphage T7. V. Shutoff of host RNA synthesis by an early phage function, *Virology* **45**:224.

Buckley, P. J., Kosturko, L. D., and Kozinski, A. W., 1972, *In vivo* production of an RNA-DNA copolymer after infection of *Escherichia coli* by bacteriophage T4, *Proc. Natl. Acad. Sci. USA* **69**:3165.

Bujard, H., and Hendrickson, H. E., 1973, Structure and function of the genome of coliphage T5. I. The physical structure of the chromosome of T5$^+$, *Eur. J. Biochem.* **33**:517.

Bujard, H., Mazaitis, A. J., and Bautz, E. K. F., 1970, The size of the *r*II region of bacteriophage T4, *Virology* **42**:717.

Buller, C. S., and Astrachan, L., 1968, Replication of T4 *r*II bacteriophage in *Escherichia coli* K12(λ), *J. Virol.* **2**:298.

Buller, C. S., Vander Maten, M., Faurot, D., and Nelson, E. T., 1975, Phospholipase activity in bacteriophage-infected *Escherichia coli*. II. Activation of phospholipase by T4 ghost infection, *J. Virol.* **15**:1141.

Cairns, J., Stent, G. S., and Watson, J. D. (eds.), 1966, *Phage and the Origins of Molecular Biology,* Cold Spring Harbor Laboratory, Cold Spring Harbor, N.Y.

Campbell, A., 1961, Sensitive mutants of bacteriophage λ, *Virology* **14**:22.

Capco, G. R., and Mathews, C. K., 1973, Bacteriophage-coded thymidylate synthetase: Evidence that the T4 enzyme is a capsid protein, *Arch. Biochem. Biophys.* **158**:736.

Carlson, K., 1973, Multiple initiation of bacteriophage T4 DNA replication: Delaying effect of bromodeoxyuridine, *J. Virol.* **12**:349.

Carrington, J. M., and Lunt, M., 1973, Studies on the replication of bacteriophage T5, *J. Gen. Virol.* **18**:91.

Carroll, R. B., Neet, K., and Goldthwait, D. A., 1973, Self-association of gene-32 protein of bacteriophage T4, *Proc. Natl. Acad. Sci. USA* **69**:2741.

Carroll, R. B., Neet, K., and Goldthwait, D. A., 1975, Studies of the self-association of bacteriophage T4 gene 32 protein by equilibrium sedimentation, *J. Mol. Biol.* **91**:275.

Casjens, S., and King, J., 1975, Virus assembly, *Annu. Rev. Biochem.* **44**:555.

Celis, J. E., Smith, J. D., and Brenner, S., 1973, Correlation between genetic and translational maps of gene 23 in bacteriophage T4, *Nature (London)* **241**:130.

Center, M. S., 1972a, Bacteriophage T7-induced endonuclease II, *J. Biol. Chem.* **247**:146.

Center, M. S., 1972b, Replicative intermediates of bacteriophage T7 DNA, *J. Virol.* **10**:115.

Center, M. S., 1975, Role of gene 2 in bacteriophage T7 DNA synthesis, *J. Virol.* **16**:94.

Center, M. S., Studier, F. W., and Richardson, C. C., 1970, The structural gene for a T7 endonuclease essential for phage DNA synthesis, *Proc. Natl. Acad. Sci. USA* **65**:242.

Chace, K. V., and Hall, D. H., 1975a, Characterization of new regulatory mutants of bacteriophage T4. II. New class of mutants, *J. Virol.* **15**:929.

Chace, K. V., and Hall, D. H., 1975b, Isolation of mutants of bacteriophage T4 unable to induce thymidine kinase activity. II. Location of the structural gene for thymidine kinase, *J. Virol.* **15**:855.

Chamberlin, M., McGrath, J., and Waskell, L., 1970, New RNA polymerase from *Escherichia coli* infected with bacteriophage T7, *Nature (London)* **228**:227.

Chan, V. L., and Ebisuzaki, K., 1970, Polynucleotide kinase mutant of bacteriophage T4, *Mol. Gen. Genet.* **109**:162.

Chan, V. L., and Ebisuzaki, K., 1973, Intergenic suppression of amber polynucleotide ligase mutation in bacteriophage T4, *Virology* **53**:60.

Chao, J., Chao, L., and Speyer, J. F., 1974, Bacteriophage T4 head morphogenesis: Host DNA enzymes affect frequency of petite forms, *J. Mol. Biol.* **85**:41.

Chen, M., Shiau, R. P., Hwang, L., Vaughan, J., and Weiss, S. B., 1975, Methionine and formylmethionine specific tRNA's coded by bacteriophage T5, *Proc. Natl. Acad. Sci. USA* **72**:558.

Chiang, T., and Harm, W., 1974, Evidence against phenotypic mixing between bacteriophage T4 wild type and T4v⁻, *J. Virol.* **14**:592.

Childs, J. D., 1971, A map of molecular distances between mutations of bacteriophage T4D, *Genetics* **67**:455.

Childs, J. D., 1973, Superinfection exclusion by incomplete genomes of bacteriophage T4, *J. Virol.* **11**:1.

Chinnadurai, G., and McCorquodale, D. J., 1973, Requirement of a phage-induced 5′exonuclease for the expression of late genes of bacteriophage T5, *Proc. Natl. Acad. Sci. USA* **70**:3502.

Chinnadurai, G., and McCorquodale, D. J., 1974, Regulation of expression of late genes of bacteriophage T5, *J. Virol.* **13**:85.

Chiu, C. S., and Greenberg, G. R., 1968, Evidence for a possible direct role of dCMP hydroxymethylase in T4 phage DNA synthesis, *Cold Spring Harbor Symp. Quant. Biol.* **33**:351.

Chrispeels, M. J., Boyd, R. F., Williams, L. S., and Neidhardt, F. C., 1968, Modification of valyl tRNA synthetase by bacteriophage in *Escherichia coli, J. Mol. Biol.* **31**:463.

Clark, S., Losick, R., and Pero, J., 1974, New RNA polymerase from *Bacillus subtilis* infected with phage PBS2, *Nature (London)* **252**:21.

Cohen, S. S., 1968, *Virus-Induced Enzymes,* Columbia University Press, New York.

Collinsworth, W. L., and Mathews, C. K., 1974, Biochemistry of DNA-defective mutants of bacteriophage T4. IV. DNA synthesis in plasmolyzed cells, *J. Virol.* **13**:908.

Conley, M. P., and Wood, W. B., 1975, Bacteriophage T4 whiskers: a rudimentary environment-sensing device, *Proc. Natl. Acad. Sci. USA* **72**:3701.

Coppo, A., Manzi, A., Pulitzer, J. F., and Takahashi, H., 1973, Abortive bacteriophage T4 head assembly in mutants of *Escherichia coli, J. Mol. Biol.* **76**:61.

Cornett, J. B., 1974, Spackle and immunity functions of bacteriophage T4, *J. Virol.* **13**:312.

Cowie, D. B., Avery, R. J., and Champe, S. P., 1971, DNA homology among the T-even bacteriophages, *Virology* **45**:30.

Cranston, J. W., Silber, R., Malathi, V. G., and Hurwitz, J., 1974, Studies on RNA ligase, *J. Biol. Chem.* **249**:7447.

Cronan, J. E., Jr., and Vagelos, P. R., 1971, Abortive infection by phage T4 under conditions of defective host membrane lipid biosynthesis, *Virology* **43**:412.

Cronan, J. E., Jr., and Wulff, D. L., 1969, A role for phospholipid hydrolysis in the lysis of *Escherichia coli* infected with bacteriophage T4, *Virology* **38**:241.

Cummings, D. J., 1964, Sedimentation and biological properties of T-even phages of *Escherichia coli, Virology* **23**:408.

Curtis, M. J., and Alberts, B., 1976, Studies on the structure of intracellular bacteriophage T4 DNA, *J. Mol. Biol.* **102**:793.

Davis, R. W., and Hyman, R. W., 1971, A study in evolution: The DNA base sequence homology between coliphages T7 and T3, *J. Mol. Biol.* **62**:287.

Dawes, J., 1975, Characterization of the bacteriophage T4 receptor site, *Nature (London)* **256**:127.

Dawes, J., and Goldberg, E. B., 1973a, Functions of baseplate components in bacteriophage T4 infection. I. Dihydrofolate reductase and dihydropteroylhexaglutamate, *Virology* **55**:380.

Dawes, J., and Goldberg, E. B., 1973b, Functions of baseplate components in bacteriophage T4 infection. II. Products of genes 5, 6, 7, 8, and 10, *Virology* **55**:391.

Delius, H., Howe, C., and Kozinski, A. W., 1971, Structure of the replicating DNA from bacteriophage T4, *Proc. Natl. Acad. Sci. USA* **68**:3049.

Demerec, M., and Fano, U., 1945, Bacteriophage-resistant mutants in *Escherichia coli, Genetics* **30**:119.

DePamphilis, M. L., 1971, Isolation of bacteriophages T2 and T4 attached to the outer membrane of *Escherichia coli, J. Virol.* **7**:683.

Depew, R. E., and Cozzarelli, N. R., 1974, Genetics and physiology of bacteriophage T4 3′ phosphatase: Evidence for involvement of the enzyme in T4 DNA metabolism, *J. Virol.* **13**:888.

Depew, R. E., Snopek, T. J., and Cozzarelli, N. R., 1975, Characterization of a new class of deletions of the D region of the bacteriophage T4 genome. *Virology* **64**:144.

deWaard, A., Ubbink, T., and Beukman, W., 1967, On the specificity of bacteriophage-induced hydroxymethylcytosine glucosyl transferases, *Eur. J. Biochem.* **2**:303.

Dewey, J. J., Wiberg, J. S., and Frankel, F. R., 1974, Genetic control of whisker antigen of bacteriophage T4D, *J. Mol. Biol.* **84**:625.

Dicou, L., and Cozzarelli, N. R., 1973, Bacteriophage T4-directed DNA synthesis in toluene-treated cells, *J. Virol.* **12**:1293.

Doermann, A. H., 1948, Intracellular growth of bacteriophage, *Carnegie Institution Yearbook* **47**:176.

Doermann, A. H., 1974, T4 and the rolling circle model of replication, *Annu. Rev. Genet.* **7**:325.

Doermann, A. H., Eiserling, F. A., and Boehner, L., 1973, Capsid length in bacteriophage T4 and its genetic control, in: *Virus Research* (C. F. Fox and W. S. Robinson, eds.), p. 243, Academic Press, New York.

Drake, J. W., 1974, The role of mutation in microbial evolution, *Symp. Soc. Gen. Microbiol.* **24**:41.

Drake, J. W., and Greening, E. D., 1970, Suppression of chemical mutagenesis in bacteriophage T4 by genetically modified DNA polymerases, *Proc. Natl. Acad. Sci. USA* **66**:823.

Dressler, D., Wolfson, J., and Magazin, M., 1972, Initiation and reinitiation of DNA synthesis during replication of bacteriophage T7, *Proc. Natl. Acad. Sci. USA* **69**:998.

Drexler, H., 1973, Transduction of *gal*+ by coliphage T1. III. Requirement for transcription and translation in recipient cells, *J. Virol.* **12**:1072.

Dube, S. K., and Rudland, P. S., 1970, Control of translation by T4 phage: Altered binding of disfavoured messengers, *Nature (London)* **226**:820.

Duckworth, D. H., 1970*a*, Biological activity of bacteriophage ghosts and "take-over" of host functions by bacteriophage, *Bacteriol. Rev.* **34**:344.

Duckworth, D. H., 1970*b*, The metabolism of T4 phage ghost infected cells. I. Macromolecular syntheses and transport of nucleic acid and protein precursors, *Virology* **40**:673.

Duckworth, D. H., 1971*a*, Inhibition of T4 bacteriophage multiplication by superinfecting ghosts and the development of tolerance after bacteriophage infection, *J. Virol.* **7**:8.

Duckworth, D. H., 1971*b*, Inhibition of host DNA synthesis by T4 bacteriophage in the absence of protein synthesis, *J. Virol.* **8**:754.

Duckworth, D. H., and Winkler, H. H., 1972, Metabolism of T4 bacteriophage ghost-infected cells. II. Do ghosts cause a generalized permeability change? *J. Virol.* **9**:917.

Dukes, P. P., and Kozloff, L. M., 1959, Phosphatases in bacteriophages T2, T4, and T5, *J. Biol. Chem.* **234**:534.

Dunham, L. F., and Price, A. R., 1974, Mutants of *Bacillus subtilis* bacteriophage φe defective in dTTP-dUTP nucleotidohydrolase, *J. Virol.* **14**:709.

Dunn, J. J., and Studier, F. W., 1973, T7 early RNA's and *Escherichia coli* ribosomal RNA's are cut from a large precursor RNA's in *vivo* by ribonuclease III, *Proc. Natl. Acad. Sci. USA* **70**:3296.

Earhart, C. F., 1970, The association of host and phage DNA with the membrane of *Escherichia coli*, *Virology* **42**:429.

Earhart, C. F., Sauri, C. J., Fletcher, G., and Wulff, J. L., 1973, Effect of inhibition of macromolecule synthesis on the association of bacteriophage T4 DNA with membrane, *J. Virol.* **11**:527.

Ebisuzaki, K., Behme, M. J., Senior, C., Shannon, D., and Dunn, D., 1972, An alternative approach to the study of new enzymatic reactions involving DNA, *Proc. Natl. Acad. Sci. USA* **69**:515.

Edgar, R. S., and Wood, W. B., 1966, Morphogenesis of bacteriophage T4 in extracts of mutant-infected cells, *Proc. Natl. Acad. Sci. USA* **55**:498.

Ehrlich, M., Ehrlich, K., and Mayo, J., 1975, Unusual properties of the DNA from *Xanthomonas* phage in which 5-methylcytosine completely replaces cytosine, *Biochim. Biophys. Acta* **395**:109.

Ellis, E. L., and Delbrück, M., 1939, The growth of bacteriophage, *J. Gen. Physiol.* **22**:365.

Emanuel, B. S., 1973, Replicative hybrid of T4 bacteriophage DNA, *J. Virol.* **12**:408.

Emrich, J., 1968, Lysis of T4-infected bacteria in the absence of lysozyme, *Virology* **35**:158.

Emrich, J., and Streisinger, G., 1968, The role of phage lysozyme in the life cycle of phage T4, *Virology* **36**:387.

Ennis, H. L., and Kievitt, K. D., 1973, Association of the *r*IIA protein with the bacterial membrane, *Proc. Natl. Acad. Sci. USA* **70**:1468.

Epstein, R. H., Bolle, A., Steinberg, C. M., Kellenberger, E., Boy de la Tour, E., Chevalley, R., Edgar, R. S., Sussman, M., Denhardt, G. H., and Lielausis, A., 1963, Physiological studies of conditional lethal mutants of bacteriophage T4D, *Cold Spring Harbor Symp. Quant. Biol.* **28**:375.

Erickson, J. S., and Mathews, C. K., 1973, Dihydrofolate reductases of *Escherichia coli* and bacteriophage T4: A spectrofluorometric study, *Biochemistry* **12**:372.

Erikson, R. L., and Szybalski, W., 1964, The Cs_2SO_4 equilibrium density gradient and its application for the study of T-even phage DNA: Glucosylation and replication, *Virology* **22**:111.

Eriksson, S., and Berglund, O., 1974, Bacteriophage-induced ribonucleotide reductase systems, *Eur. J. Biochem.* **46**:271.

Eskin, B., Lautenberger, J. A., and Linn, S., 1973, Host-controlled modification and restriction of bacteriophage T7 by *Escherichia coli* B, *J. Virol.* **11**:1020.

Espejo, R. T., Canelo, E. S., Sinsheimer, R. L., 1969, DNA of bacteriophage PM2: A closed circular double-stranded molecule, *Proc. Natl. Acad. Sci. USA* **63**:1164.

Fabricant, R., and Kennell, D., 1970, Inhibition of host protein synthesis during infection of *Escherichia coli* by bacteriophage T4. III. Inhibition by ghosts, *J. Virol.* **6**:772.

Fleischman, R. A., and Richardson, C. C., 1971, Analysis of host range restriction in *Escherichia coli* treated with toluene, *Proc. Natl. Acad. Sci. USA* **68**:2527.

Fleischman, R. A., Campbell, J. L., and Richardson, C. C., 1975, *In vitro* restriction of DNA containing 5-hydroxymethyldeoxycytidine, *Fed. Proc.* **34**:554.

Fletcher, G., and Earhart, C. F., 1975, Alterations in host envelope which result from bacteriophage T4 late protein synthesis, Abstracts of the Annual Meeting of the American Society for Microbiology, p. 258.

Fletcher, G., Wulff, J. L., and Earhart, C. F., 1974, Localization of membrane protein synthesized after infection with bacteriophage T4, *J. Virol.* **13**:73.

Follansbee, S., Vanderslice, R. W., Chavez, L. G., and Yegian, C. D., 1974, A set of adsorption mutants of bacteriophage T4D: Identification of a new gene, *Virology* **58**:180.

Frankel, F. R., 1966, Studies on the nature of DNA in T4 infected *Escherichia coli, J. Mol. Biol.* **18**:127.

Frankel, F. R., 1968, Evidence for long DNA strands in the replicating pool after T4 infection, *Proc. Natl. Acad. Sci. USA* **59**:131.

Frankel, F. R., Majumdar, C., Weintraub, S., and Frankel, D. M., 1968, DNA polymerase and the cell membrane after T4 infection, *Cold Spring Harbor Symp. Quant. Biol.* **33**:495.

Frankel, F., Batcheler, M., and Clark, C., 1971, The role of gene 49 in DNA replication and head morphogenesis in bacteriophage T4, *J. Mol. Biol.* **62**:439.

Freedman, M. L., and Krisch, R. E., 1971a, Enlargement of *Escherichia coli* after bacteriophage infection. I. Description of the phenomenon, *J. Virol.* **8**:87.

Freedman, M. L., and Krisch, R. E., 1971b, Enlargement of *Escherichia coli* after bacteriophage infection. II. Proposed mechanism, *J. Virol.* **8**:95.

Frenkel, G. D., and Richardson, C. C., 1971, The deoxyribonuclease induced after infection of *Escherichia coli* by bacteriophage T5, *J. Biol. Chem.* **246**:4848.

Friedberg, E. C., Minton, K., Pawl, G., and Verzola, P., 1974, Excision of thymine dimers *in vitro* by extracts of bacteriophage infected *Escherichia coli, J. Virol.* **13**:953.

Friedberg, E. C., Ganesan, A. K., and Minton, K., 1975, *N*-Glycosidase activity in extracts of *Bacillus subtilis* and its inhibition after infection with bacteriophage PBS2, *J. Virol.* **16**:315.

Furrow, M., and Pizer, L. I., 1968, Phospholipid synthesis in *Escherichia coli* infected with T4 bacteriophages, *J. Virol.* **2**:594.

Gamow, R. I., and Kozloff, L. M., 1968, Chemically induced cofactor requirement for bacteriophage T4D, *J. Virol.* **2**:480.

Gefter, M., Hausmann, R., Gold, M., and Hurwitz, J., 1966, The enzymatic methylation of RNA and DNA. X. Bacteriophage T3-induced *S*-adenosylmethionine cleavage, *J. Biol. Chem.* **241**:1995.

Geiman, J. M., Christensen, J. R., and Drexler, H., 1974, Interactions between the vegetative states of phages λ and T1, *J. Virol.* **14**:1430.

Georgopoulos, C. P., and Revel, H. R., 1971, Studies with glucosyl transferase mutants of the T-even bacteriophages, *Virology* **44**:271.

Georgopoulos, C. P., Hendrix, R. W., Kaiser, A. D., and Wood, W. B., 1972, Role of the host cell in bacteriophage morphogenesis: Effects of a bacterial mutation on T4 head assembly, *Nature (London)* **239**:38.

Gillin, F. D., and Nossal, N. G., 1975, T4 DNA polymerase has a lower apparent K_m for deoxynucleoside triphosphates complementary rather than noncomplementary to the template, *Biochem. Biophys. Res. Commun.* **64**:457.

Goff, C. G., 1974, Chemical structure of a modification of the *Escherichia coli* RNA polymerase α polypeptides induced by bacteriophage T4 infection, *J. Biol. Chem.* **249**:6181.

Goldberg, E. B., 1966, The amount of DNA between genetic markers in phage T4, *Proc. Natl. Acad. Sci. USA* **56**:1457.

Goldman, E., and Lodish, H. F., 1971, Inhibition of replication of RNA bacteriophage f2 by superinfection with bacteriophage T4, *J. Virol.* **8**:417.

Goldman, E., and Lodish, H. F., 1973, T4 phage and T4 ghosts inhibit f2 phage replication by different mechanisms, *J. Mol. Biol.* **74**:151.

Goodman, M. F., Gore, W. C., Muzyczka, N., and Bessman, M. J., 1974, Studies on the biochemical basis of spontaneous mutation. III. Rate model for DNA polymerase-effected nucleotide misincorporation, *J. Mol. Biol.* **88**:423.

Goscin, L. A., and Hall, D. H., 1972, Hydroxyurea-sensitive mutants of bacteriophage T4, *Virology* **50**:84.

Goscin, L. A., Hall, D. H., and Kutter, E. M., 1973, Hydroxyurea-sensitive mutants of T4. II. Degradation and utilization of bacterial DNA, *Virology* **56**:207.

Green, D. M., and Laman, D., 1972, Organization of gene functions in *Bacillus subtilis* bacteriophage SP82G, *J. Virol.* **9**:1033.

Grippo, P., and Richardson, C. C., 1971, DNA polymerase of bacteriophage T7, *J. Biol. Chem.* **246**:6867.

Guha, A., Szybalski, W., Salser, W., Bolle, A., Geiduschek, E. P., and Pulitzer, J. F., 1971, Controls and polarity of transcription during bacteriophage T4 development, *J. Mol. Biol.* **59**:329.

Guthrie, C. D., and McClain, W. H., 1973, Conditionally lethal mutants of bacteriophage T4 defective in production of a transfer RNA, *J. Mol. Biol.* **81**:137.

Hall, D. H., 1967, Mutants of bacteriophage T4 unable to induce dihydrofolate reductase activity, *Proc. Natl. Acad. Sci. USA* **58**:584.

Hamlett, N. V., and Berger, H., 1975, Mutations altering genetic recombination and repair of DNA in bacteriophage T4, *Virology* **63**:539.

Hardaway, K. L., Vander Maten, M., and Buller, C. S., 1975, Phospholipase activity in bacteriophage-infected *Escherichia coli*. III. Phospholipase A involvement in lysis of T4-infected cells, *J. Virol.* **16**:867.

Haslam, E. A., Roscoe, D. H., and Tucker, R. G., 1967, Inhibition of thymidylate synthetase in bacteriophage-infected *Bacillus subtilis, Biochim. Biophys. Acta* **134**:312.

Hattman, S., 1970*a*, Influence of T4 superinfection on the formation of RNA bacteriophage coat protein, *J. Mol. Biol.* **47**:599.

Hattman, S., 1970*b*, DNA methylation of T-even bacteriophages and of their nonglucosylated mutants: Its role in P1-directed restriction, *Virology* **42**:359.

Hausmann, R., and Gold, M., 1966, The enzymatic methylation of RNA and DNA. IX. DNA methylase in bacteriophage-infected *Escherichia coli, J. Biol. Chem.* **241**:1985.

Hawley, L. A., Reilly, B. E., Hagen, E. W., and Anderson, D. L., 1973, Viral protein synthesis in bacteriophage ϕ29-infected *Bacillus subtilis, J. Virol.* **12**:1149.

Hayward, G. S., 1974, Unique double-stranded fragments of bacteriophage T5 DNA resulting from preferential shear-induced breakage at nicks, *Proc. Natl. Acad. Sci. USA* **71**:2108.

Hayward, G. S., and Smith, M. G., 1972, The chromosome of bacteriophage T5. II. Arrangement of the single-stranded DNA fragments in the T5$^+$ and T5*st*(0) chromosome, *J. Mol. Biol.* **63**:397.

Heere, L. J., and Karam, J. D., 1975, Analysis of expressions of the *r*II gene function of bacteriophage T4, *J. Virol.* **16**:974.

Hemphill, H. E., and Whiteley, H. R., 1975, Bacteriophages of *Bacillus subtilis, Bacteriol. Rev.* **39**:257.

Hendrickson, H. E., and Bujard, H., 1973, Structure and function of the genome of coliphage T5, *Eur. J. Biochem.* **33**:529.

Hendrickson, H. E., and McCorquodale, D. J., 1971*a*, Genetic and physiological studies of bacteriophage T5. I. An expanded genetic map of T5, *J. Virol.* **7**:612.

Hendrickson, H., and McCorquodale, D. J., 1971*b*, Genetic and physiological studies of bacteriophage T5. 2. The relationship between phage DNA synthesis and protein synthesis in T5-infected cells, *Biochem. Biophys. Res. Commun.* **43**:735.

Hendrickson, H. E., and McCorquodale, D. J., 1972, Genetic and physiological studies of bacteriophage T5. III. Patterns of DNA synthesis induced by mutants of T5, *J. Virol.* **9**:981.

Hercules, K., and Sauerbier, W., 1973, Transcription units in bacteriophage T4, *J. Virol.* **12**:872.

Hercules, K., and Sauerbier, W., 1974, Two modes of *in vivo* transcription for genes 43 and 45 of phage T4, *J. Virol.* **14**:341.

Hercules, K., and Wiberg, J. S., 1971, Specific suppression of mutations in genes 46 and 47 by *das*, a new class of mutations in bacteriophage T4D, *J. Virol.* **8**:603.

Hercules, K., Schweiger, M., and Sauerbier, W., 1974, Cleavage by RNase III converts T3 and T7 early precursor RNA into translatable message, *Proc. Natl. Acad. Sci. USA* **71**:8400.

Herman, R. C., and Moyer, R. W., 1974, *In vivo* repair of the single-strand interruptions contained in bacteriophage T5 DNA, *Proc. Natl. Acad. Sci. USA* **71**:680.

Herman, R. C., and Moyer, R. W., 1975, *In vivo* repair of bacteriophage T5 DNA: An assay for viral growth control, *Virology* **66**:393.

Herrlich, P., Rahmsdorf, H. J., Pai, S. H., and Schweiger, M., 1974, Translational control induced by bacteriophage T7, *Proc. Natl. Acad. Sci. USA* **71**:1088.

Hershfield, M. S., and Nossal, N. G., 1972, Hydrolysis of template and newly synthesized DNA by the 3′ to 5′ exonuclease activity of T4 DNA polymerase, *J. Biol. Chem.* **247**:3393.

Hewlett, M. J., and Mathews, C. K., 1975, Bacteriophage–host interaction and restriction of nonglucosylated T6, *J. Virol.* **15**:776.

Hinkle, D. C., and Richardson, C. C., 1975, Bacteriophage T7 DNA replication *in vitro*, *J. Biol. Chem.* **250**:5523.

Hirsch-Kauffman, M., Herrlich, P., Ponta, H., and Schweiger, M., 1975, Helper function of T7 protein kinase in virus propagation, *Nature (London)* **255**:508.

Homyk, T., Jr., and Weil, J., 1974, Deletion analysis of two nonessential regions of the T4 genome, *Virology* **61**:505.

Hopfield, J. J., 1974, Kinetic proofreading: A new mechanism for reducing errors in biosynthetic processes requiring high specificity, *Proc. Natl. Acad. Sci. USA* **71**:4135.

Horvitz, H. R., 1973, Polypeptide bound to the host RNA polymerase is specified by T4 control gene 33, *Nature (London)* **244**:138.

Horvitz, H. R., 1974, Bacteriophage T4 mutants deficient in alteration and modification of the *Escherichia coli* RNA polymerase, *J. Mol. Biol.* **90**:739.

Hosoda, J., and Levinthal, C., 1968, Protein synthesis by *Escherichia coli* infected with bacteriophage T4D, *Virology* **34**:709.

Hosoda, J., Mathews, E., and Jansen, B., 1971, Role of genes 46 and 47 in bacteriophage T4 reproduction. I. *In vivo* DNA replication, *J. Virol.* **8**:372.

Hosoda, J., Takacs, B., and Brack, C., 1974, Denaturation of T4 DNA by an *in vitro* processed gene 32-protein, *FEBS Lett.* **47**:338.

Howe, C. C., Buckley, P. J., Carlson, K. M., and Kozinski, A. W., 1973, Multiple and specific initiation of T4 DNA replication, *J. Virol.* **12**:130.

Hsu, W.-T., 1973, Nondiscrimination of RNA viral message in binding to 30S ribosomes derived from T4 phage infected *Escherichia coli*, *Biochem. Biophys. Res. Commun.* **52**:974.

Huang, W. M., 1975, Membrane-associated proteins of T4-infected *Escherichia coli*, *Virology* **66**:508.

Huang, W. M., and Buchanan, J. M., 1974, Synergistic interactions of T4 early proteins concerned with their binding to DNA, *Proc. Natl. Acad. Sci. USA* **71**:2226.

Huberman, J. A., 1968, Visualization of replicating mammalian and T4 bacteriophage DNA, *Cold Spring Harbor Symp. Quant. Biol.* **33**:509.

Huberman, J. A., Kornberg, A., and Alberts, B. M., 1971, Stimulation of bacteriophage T4 DNA polymerase by the protein product of T4 gene 32, *J. Mol. Biol.* **62**:39.

Hulick-Bursch, C. J., and Snustad, D. P., 1975, Packaging of DNA into T4 bacteriophage: Exclusion of host DNA despite the absence of both host DNA degradation and nuclear disruption, *Virology* **65**:276.

Hyman, R. W., 1971, Physical mapping of T7 messenger RNA, *J. Mol. Biol.* **61**:369.

Hyman, R. W., Brunovskis, I., and Summers, W. C., 1974, A biochemical comparison of the related bacteriophages T7, φI, φII, W31, H, and T3, *Virology* **57**:189.

Iida, S., and Sekiguchi, M., 1971, Infection of actinomycin-permeable mutants of *Escherichia coli* with urea-disrupted bacteriophage, *J. Virol.* **7**:121.

Israeli, M., and Artman, M., 1970, Leakage of β-galactosidase from phage-infected *Escherichia coli*: A re-evaluation, *J. Gen. Virol.* **7**:137.

Ivarie, R. D., and Pène, J. J., 1973, DNA replication in bacteriophage φ29, *Virology* **52**:351.

Jacob, F., Brenner, S., and Cuzin, F., 1963, On the regulation of DNA replication in bacteria, *Cold Spring Harbor Symp. Quant. Biol.* **28**:329.

Jesaitis, M. A., 1956, Differences in the chemical composition of the phage nucleic acids, *Nature (London)* **178**:637.

Josslin, R., 1970, The lysis mechanism of phage T4: Mutants affecting lysis, *Virology* **40**:719.

Josslin, R., 1971a, Physiological studies on the *t* gene defect in T4-infected *Escherichia coli, Virology* **44**:101.

Josslin, R., 1971b, The effect of phage T4 infection on phospholipid hydrolysis in *Escherichia coli, Virology* **44**:94.

Kahan, E., 1971, Early and late gene functions in bacteriophage SP82, *Virology* **46**:634.

Kallen, R. G., Simon, M., and Marmur, J., 1962, The occurrence of a new pyrimidine base replacing thymine in a bacteriophage DNA: 5-Hydroxymethyl uracil, *J. Mol. Biol.* **5**:248.

Kammen, H. O., and Strand, M., 1967, Thymine metabolism in *Escherichia coli*. II. Altered uptake of thymine after bacteriophage infection, *J. Biol. Chem.* **242**:1854.

Kano-Sueoka, T., and Sueoka, N., 1969, Leucine tRNA and cessation of *Escherichia coli* protein synthesis upon phage T2 infection, *Proc. Natl. Acad. Sci. USA* **62**:1229.

Kaplan, D. A., and Nierlich, D. P., 1975, Cleavage of nonglucosylated bacteriophage T4 DNA by restriction endonuclease Eco RI, *J. Biol. Chem.* **250**:2395.

Karam, J. D., and Barker, B., 1971, Properties of bacteriophage T4 mutants defective in gene 30 and the *r*II gene, *J. Virol.* **7**:260.

Karam, J. D., and Bowles, M. G., 1974, Mutation to overproduction of bacteriophage T4 gene products, *J. Virol.* **13**:428.

Karam, J. D., and Chao, J., 1975, On the possible interaction between DNA polymerase and dCMP hydroxymethylase of T4, Abstracts of Phage Meetings, p. 57, Cold Spring Harbor, N.Y.

Kasai, T., and Bautz, E. K. F., 1969, Regulation of gene-specific RNA synthesis in bacteriophage T4, *J. Mol. Biol.* **41**:401.

Kawamura, F., and Ito, J., 1974, Bacteriophage gene expression in sporulating cells of *Bacillus subtilis* 168, *Virology* **62**:414.

Kellenberger, E., 1960, The physical state of the bacterial nucleus, in: *Microbial Genetics,* p. 39, Tenth Symposium of the Society for General Microbiology, Cambridge University Press, London.

Kelln, R. A., and Warren, R. A. J., 1973, Studies on the biosynthesis of M-putre-scinylthymine in bacteriophage φW-14-infected *Pseudomonas acidovorans, J. Virol.* **12**:1427.

Kells, S. S., and Haselkorn, R., 1974, Bacteriophage T4 short tail fibers are the product of gene 12, *J. Mol. Biol.* **83**:473.

Kemper, B., and Hurwitz, J., 1973, Studies on T4-induced nucleases: Isolation and characterization of a manganese-activated T4-induced endonuclease, *J. Biol. Chem.* **248**:91.

Kennell, D., 1968, Inhibition of host protein synthesis during infection of *Escherichia coli* by bacteriophage T4. I. Continued synthesis of host RNA, *J. Virol.* **2**:1262.

Kennell, D., 1970, Inhibition of host protein synthesis during infection of *Escherichia coli* by bacteriophage T4. II. Induction of host mRNA and its exclusiom from polysomes, *J. Virol.* **6**:208.

Kerr, C., and Sadowski, P. D., 1974, Packaging and maturation of DNA of bac-teriophage T7 *in vitro, Proc. Natl. Acad. Sci. USA* **71**:3545.

Kessel, M., and Varon, M., 1973, Development of bdellophage VL-1 in parasitic and saprophytic bdellovibrios, *J. Virol.* **12**:1522.

Kim, J.-S., and Davidson, N., 1974, Electron microscope heteroduplex study of sequence relations of T2, T4, and T6 bacteriophage DNA's, *Virology* **57**:93.

King, J., and Laemmli, U., 1971, Polypeptides of the tail fibres of bacteriophage T4, *J. Mol. Biol.* **62**:465.

King, J., and Mykolajewycz, N., 1973, Bacteriophage T4 tail assembly: Proteins of the sheath, core, and baseplate, *J. Mol. Biol.* **75**:339.

Klem, E. B., Hsu, W., and Weiss, S. B., 1970, The selective inhibition of protein initia-tion by T4 phage-induced factors, *Proc. Natl. Acad. Sci. USA* **67**:696.

Klotz, G., 1973, Direction of SPP1 DNA replication in transfected *B. subtilis* cells, *Mol. Gen. Genet.* **120**:95.

Knight, C. A., 1975, *Chemistry of Viruses,* 2nd ed., Springer-Verlag, New York.

Koch, R. E., 1973, Ligase-defective bacteriophage T4. II. Physiological studies, *J. Virol.* **11**:41.

Kornberg, A., 1974, *DNA Synthesis,* Freeman, San Francisco.

Kozinski, A. W., and Doermann, A. H., 1975, Repetitive DNA replication of the incomplete genomes of phage T4 petite particles, *Proc. Natl. Acad. Sci. USA* **72**:1734.

Kozloff, L. M., 1968, Biochemistry of the T-even bacteriophages of *Escherichia coli,* in: *Molecular Basis of Virology* (H. Fraenkel-Conrat, ed.), p. 435, Reinhold, New York.

Kozloff, L. M., and Lute, M., 1965, Folic acid, a structural component of T4 bac-teriophage, *J. Mol. Biol.* **12**:780.

Kozloff, L., and Lute, M., 1973, Bacteriophage tail components. IV. Pteroyl polyglutamate synthesis in T4D-infected *Escherichia coli* B, *J. Virol.* **11**:630.

Kozloff, L. M., Lute, M., and Crosby, L. K., 1970a, Bacteriophage tail components. III. Use of synthetic pteroyl hexaglutamate for T4D tail plate assembly, *J. Virol.* **6**:754.

Kozloff, L. M., Lute, M., Crosby, L. K., Rao, N., Chapman, V. A., and DeLong, S. S., 1970b, Bacteriophage tail components. I. Pteroyl polyglutamates in T-even bac-teriophages, *J. Virol.* **5**:726.

Kozloff, L. M., Verses, C., Lute, M., and Crosby, L. K., 1970c, Bacteriophage tail components. II. Dihydrofolate reductase in T4D bacteriophage, *J. Virol.* **5**:740.

Kozloff, L. M., Lute, M., and Baugh, C. M., 1973, Bacteriophage tail components. V.

Complementation of T4D gene 28-infected bacterial extracts with pteroyl hexa-glutamate, *J. Virol.* **11**:637.

Kozloff, L. M., Crosby, L. K., and Lute, M., 1975a, Bacteriophage baseplate components. III. Location and properties of the phage structural thymidylate synthetase, *J. Virol.* **16**:1409.

Kozloff, L. M., Crosby, L. K., Lute, M., and Hall, D. H., 1975b, Bacteriophage base-plate components. II. Binding and location of phage-induced dihydrofolate reductase, *J. Virol.* **16**:1401.

Kozloff, L. M., Lute, M., and Crosby, L. K., 1975c, Bacteriophage baseplate components. I. Binding and location of the folic acid, *J. Virol.* (in press).

Krauss, S. W., Stollar, B. D., and Friedkin, M., 1973, Genetic and immunologic studies of bacteriophage T4 thymidylate synthetase, *J. Virol.* **11**:783.

Krisch, H. M., Shah, D. B., and Berger, H., 1971, Replication and recombination in ligase-deficient rII bacteriophage T4D, *J. Virol.* **7**:491.

Krisch, H. M., Bolle, A., and Epstein, R. H., 1974, Regulation of the synthesis of bac-teriophage T4 gene 32 protein, *J. Mol. Biol.* **88**:89.

Kropinski, A. M. B., Bose, R. J., and Warren, R. A. J., 1973, 5-(4-Aminobutyl-aminomethyl)uracil, an unusual pyrimidine from the DNA of bacteriophage ϕW-14, *Biochemistry* **12**:151.

Krylov, V. N., 1972, A mutation of T4B phage, which enhances suppression of ligase mutants with rII mutations, *Virology* **50**:291.

Krylov, V. N., and Plotnikova, T. G., 1971, A suppressor in the genome of phage T4 inhibiting phenotypic expression of mutations in genes 46 and 47, *Genetics* **67**:319.

Krylov, V. N., and Yankofsky, N. K., 1975, Mutations in the new gene st III of bac-teriophage T4B suppressing the lysis defect of gene st II and gene e mutants, *J. Virol.* **15**:22.

Kuo, T.-T., Huang, T.-C., and Teng, M.-H., 1968, 5-Methylcytosine replacing cytosine in the DNA of a bacteriophage for *Xanthomonas oryzae*, *J. Mol. Biol.* **34**:373.

Kutter, E. M., and Wiberg, J. S., 1968, Degradation of cytosine-containing bacterial and bacteriophage DNA after infection of *Escherichia coli* B with bacteriophage T4D wild type and with mutants defective in genes 46, 47, and 56, *J. Mol. Biol.* **38**:395.

Kutter, E. M., and Wiberg, J. S., 1969, Biological effects of substituting cytosine for 5-hydroxymethylcytosine in the DNA of bacteriophage T4, *J. Virol.* **4**:439.

Kutter, E., Beug, A., Sluss, R., Jensen, L., and Bradley, D., 1975, The production of undegraded cytosine-containing DNA by bacteriophage T4 in the absence of dCTPase and endonucleases II and IV, and its effects on T4-directed protein syn-thesis, *J. Mol. Biol.* **99**:591.

Kylberg, K. J., Bendig, M. M., and Drexler, H., 1975, Characterization of transduction by bacteriophage T1: Time of production and density of transducing particles, *J. Virol.* **16**:854.

Labedan, B., and Legault-Demare, J., 1973, Penetration into host cells of naked, partially injected (post-FST) DNA of bacteriophage T5, *J. Virol.* **12**:226.

Laemmli, U. K., 1970, Cleavage of structural proteins during the assembly of the head of bacteriophage T4, *Nature (London)* **227**:680.

Laemmli, U. K., and Favre, M., 1973, Maturation of the head of bacteriophage T4. I. DNA packaging events, *J. Mol. Biol.* **80**:575.

Laemmli, U. K., Paulson, J. R., and Hitchins, V., 1974, Maturation of the head of bac-teriophage T4. V. A possible DNA packaging mechanism: *in vitro* cleavage of the head proteins and the structure of the core of the polyhead, *J. Supramol. Struct.* **2**:276.

LaMontagne, J. R., and McDonald, W. C., 1973, A bacteriophage of *Bacillus subtilis* which forms plaques only at temperatures above 50°C, *J. Virol.* **9**:659.

Lanni, Y. T., 1968, First-step-transfer DNA of bacteriophage T5, *Bacteriol. Rev.* **32**:227.

Lanni, Y. T., 1969, Function of two genes in the first-step-transfer DNA of bacteriophage T5, *J. Mol. Biol.* **44**:173.

Lavi, U., and Marcus, M., 1972, Arrest of host DNA synthesis in *Bacillus subtilis* infected with phage φe, *Virology* **49**:668.

Lavi, U., Nattenberg, A., Ronen, A., and Marcus, M., 1974, *Bacillus subtilis* DNA polymerase III is required for the replication of the virulent bacteriophage φe, *J. Virol.* **14**:1337.

Lehman, I. R., 1974, DNA ligase: Structure, mechanism, and function, *Science* **186**:790.

Lehman, I. R., and Pratt, E. A., 1960, On the structure of the glucosylated hydroxymethylcytosine nucleotides of coliphages T2, T4, and T6, *J. Biol. Chem.* **235**:3254.

Levner, M. H., and Cozzarelli, N. R., 1972, Replication of viral DNA in SP01-infected *Bacillus subtilis, Virology* **48**:402.

Lichtenstein, J., and Cohen, S. S., 1960, Nucleotides derived from enzymatic digests of nucleic acids of T2, T4, and T6 bacteriophages, *J. Biol. Chem.* **235**:1134.

Lillehaug, J. R., and Kleppe, K., 1975, Kinetics and specificity of T4 polynucleotide kinase, *Biochemistry* **14**:1221.

Linné, T., Oberg, B., and Philipson, L., 1974, RNA ligase activity in phage-infected bacteria and animal cells, *Eur. J. Biochem.* **42**:157.

Little, J. W., 1973, Mutants of bacteriophage T4 which allow amber mutants of gene 32 to grow in ochre-suppressing hosts, *Virology* **53**:47.

Lo, K., and Bessman, M. J., 1976, An antimutator DNA polymerase. II. *In vitro* and *in vivo* studies of its temperature sensitivity, *J. Biol. Chem.* **251**:2480.

Loeb, M. R., 1974, Bacteriophage T4-mediated release of envelope components from *Escherichia coli, J. Virol.* **13**:631.

Loskutoff, D. J., and Pène, J. J., 1973, Gene expression during the development of *Bacillus subtilis* bacteriophage φ29, *J. Virol.* **11**:87.

Luckey, M., Wayne, R., and Neilands, J. B., 1975, *In vitro* competition between ferrichrome and phage for the outer membrane T5 receptor complex of *Escherichia coli, Biochem. Biophys. Res. Commun.* **64**:687.

Luftig, R. B., and Lundh, N. P., 1973, Bacteriophage T4 head morphogenesis. V. The role of DNA synthesis in maturation of an intermediate in head assembly, *Virology* **51**:432.

MacHattie, L. A., Rhoades, M., and Thomas, C. A., Jr., 1972, Large repetition in the non-permuted nucleotide sequence of bacteriophage T1 DNA, *J. Mol. Biol.* **72**:645.

Mahmood, N., and Lunt, M. R., 1972, Biochemical changes during mixed infections with bacteriophages T2 and T4, *J. Gen. Virol.* **16**:185.

Majumdar, C., Dewey, M., and Frankel, F. R., 1972, Bacteriophage-directed association of DNA polymerase I with host membrane: A dispensable function, *Virology* **49**:134.

Male, C. J., and Christensen, J. R., 1970, Synthesis of messenger RNA after bacteriophage T1 infection, *J. Virol.* **6**:727.

Male, C. J., and Kozloff, L. M., 1973, Function of T4D structural dihydrofolate reductase in bacteriophage infection, *J. Virol.* **11**:840.

Maley, G. F., Guarino, D. U., and Maley, F., 1972, T2r$^+$ Bacteriophage-induced enzymes. I. The purification and properties of deoxycytidylate deaminase, *J. Biol. Chem.* **247**:931.

Maor, G., and Shalitin, C., 1974, Competence of membrane-bound T4rII DNA for *in vitro* "late" mRNA transcription, *Virology* **62**:500.

Marcus, M., and Newlon, M. C., 1971, Control of DNA synthesis in *Bacillus subtilis* by phage ϕe, *Virology* **44**:83.

Marsh, R. C., Breschkin, A. M., and Mosig, G., 1971, Origin and direction of bacteriophage T4 DNA replication. II. A gradient of marker frequencies in partially replicated T4 DNA as assayed by transformation, *J. Mol. Biol.* **60**:213.

Mathews, C. K., 1966, on the metabolic role of T6 phage-induced dihydrofolate reductase: Intracellular reduced pyridine nucleotides, *J. Biol. Chem.* **241**:5008.

Mathews, C. K., 1967, Evidence that bacteriophage-induced dihydrofolate reductase is coded by the viral genome, *J. Biol. Chem.* **242**:4083.

Mathews, C. K., 1968, Biochemistry of DNA-defective amber mutants of bacteriophage T4. I. RNA metabolism, *J. Biol. Chem.* **243**:5610.

Mathews, C. K., 1971*a*, *Bacteriophage Biochemistry*, Van Nostrand Reinhold, New York.

Mathews, C. K., 1971*b*, Identity of genes coding for soluble and structural dihydrofolate reductases in bacteriophage T4, *J. Virol.* **7**:531.

Mathews, C. K., 1972, Biochemistry of DNA-defective mutants of bacteriophage T4. III. Nucleotide pools, *J. Biol. Chem.* **247**:7430.

Mathews, C. K., 1976, Biochemistry of DNA-defective mutants of bacteriophage T4. V. Thymine nucleotide pool dynamics, *Arch. Biochem. Biophys.* **172**:178.

Mathews, C. K., Crosby, L. K., and Kozloff, L. M., 1973, Inactivation of T4D bacteriophage by antiserum against bacteriophage dihydrofolate reductase, *J. Virol.* **12**:74.

Mattson, T., Richardson, J., and Goodin, D., 1974, Mutant of bacteriophage T4D affecting expression of many early genes, *Nature (London)* **250**:48.

Maynard-Smith, S., and Symonds, N., 1973, The unexpected location of a gene conferring abnormal radiation sensitivity on phage T4, *Nature (London)* **241**:395.

McAllister, W. T., 1970, Bacteriophage infection: Which end of the SP82G genome goes in first? *J. Virol.* **5**:194.

McAllister, W. T., and Green, D. M., 1972, Bacteriophage SP82G inhibition of an intracellular DNA inactivation process in *Bacillus subtilis*, *J. Virol.* **10**:51.

McAllister, W. T., and Green, D. M., 1973, Effects of the decay of incorporated ^{32}P on the transfer of the bacteriophage SP82G genome, *J. Virol.* **12**:300.

McClain, W. H., Guthrie, C. D., and Barrell, B. G., 1972, Eight transfer RNA's induced by infection of *Escherichia coli* with bacteriophage T4, *Proc. Natl. Acad. Sci. USA* **69**:3703.

McCorquodale, D. J., 1975, The T-odd bacteriophages, *CRC Crit. Rev. Microbiol.* **4**:101.

McCorquodale, D. J., and Buchanan, J. M., 1968, Patterns of protein synthesis in T5-infected *Escherichia coli*, *J. Biol. Chem.* **243**:2550.

Mekshenkov, M. I., and Guseinov, R. D., 1970, Cyclic gene arrangement in phage T4r$^+$ chromosomes, *Dokl. Akad. Nauk SSSR* **191**:457.

Miller, R. C., Jr., 1972a, Association of replicative T4 DNA and bacterial membranes, *J. Virol.* **10**:920.

Miller, R. C., Jr., 1972b, Assymetric [*sic*] annealing of an RNA linked DNA molecule isolated during the initiation of bacteriophage T7 DNA replication, *Biochem. Biophys. Res. Commun.* **49**:1082.

Miller, R. C., Jr., 1975, T4 DNA polymerase is required *in vivo* for repair of gaps in recombinants, *J. Virol.* **15**:316.

Miller, R. C., Jr., and Buckley, P., 1970, Early intracellular events in the replication of bacteriophage T4 DNA. VI. Newly synthesized proteins in the T4 protein–DNA complex, *J. Virol.* **5**:502.

Miller, R. C., Jr., Kozinski, A. W., and Litwin, S., 1970, Molecular recombination in T4 bacteriophage DNA. III. Formation of long single strands during recombination, *J. Virol.* **5**:368.

Minton, K., Dunphy, M., Taylor, R., and Friedberg, E. C., 1975, The ultraviolet endo-nuclease of bacteriophage T4: Further characterization, *J. Biol. Chem.* **250**:2823.

Modrich, P., and Richardson, C. C., 1975, Bacteriophage T7 DNA replication *in vitro*, *J. Biol. Chem.* **250**:5508.

Moise, H., and Hosoda, J., 1976, T4 gene 32 protein model for control of activity at replication fork, *Nature* **259**:455.

Montgomery, D. L., and Snyder, L. R. 1973, A negative effect of β-glucosylation on T4 growth in certain RNA polymerase mutants of *Escherichia coli, Virology* **53**:349.

Moreno, F., Camacho, E., Viñuela, E., and Salas, M., 1974, Suppressor-sensitive mutants and genetic map of *Bacillus subtilis* bacteriophage ϕ29, *Virology* **62**:1.

Morse, J. W., and Cohen, P. S., 1975, Synthesis of functional bacteriophage T4 delayed early mRNA in the absence of protein synthesis, *J. Mol. Biol.* **16**:330.

Mortelmans, K., and Friedberg, E. C., 1972, DNA repair in bacteriophage T4: Observations on the roles of the *x* and *v* genes and of host factors, *J. Virol.* **10**:730.

Mosig, G., 1968, A map of distances along the DNA molecule of phage T4, *Genetics* **59**:137.

Mosig, G., 1970, A preferred origin and direction of bacteriophage T4 DNA replica-tion. I. A gradient of allele frequencies in crosses between normal and small T4 parti-cles, *J. Mol. Biol.* **53**:503.

Mosig, G., and Breschkin, A. M., 1975, Genetic evidence for an additional function of phage T4 gene 32 protein: Interaction with ligase, *Proc. Natl. Acad. Sci. USA* **72**:1226.

Mosig, G., and Werner, R., 1969, On the replication of incomplete chromosomes of phage T4, *Proc. Natl. Acad. Sci. USA* **64**:747.

Mosig, G., Bowden, D. W., and Bock, S., 1972, *E. coli* DNA polymerase I and other host functions participate in T4 DNA replication and recombination, *Nature (London)* **240**:12.

Moyer, R. W., and Buchanan, J. M., 1970, Effect of calcium ions on synthesis of T4-specific RNA, *J. Biol. Chem.* **245**:5904.

Moyer, R. W., Fu, A. S., and Szabo, C., 1972, Regulation of bacteriophage T5 development by *Col* I factors, *J. Virol.* **9**:804.

Mufti, S., 1972, A bacteriophage T4 mutant defective in protection against superinfect-ing phage, *J. Gen. Virol.* **17**:119.

Mufti, S., and Bernstein, H., 1974, The DNA-delay mutants of bacteriophage T4, *J. Virol.* **14**:860.

Mukai, F., Streisinger, G., and Miller, B., 1967, The mechanism of lysis in phage T4-infected cells, *Virology* **33**:398.

Müller, U. R., and Marchin, G. L., 1975, Temporal appearance of bacteriophage T4-modified valyl tRNA synthetase in *Escherichia coli, J. Virol.* **15**:238.

Munch-Petersen, A., and Schwartz, M., 1972, Inhibition of the catabolism of deoxyribonucleosides in *Escherichia coli* after infection by T4 phage, *Eur. J. Biochem.* **27**:443.

Muzyczka, N., Poland, R. L., and Bessman, M. J., 1972, Studies on the biochemical basis of spontaneous mutation. I. A study of DNA polymerases of mutator, antimutator and wild type strains of bacteriophage T4, *J. Biol. Chem.* **247**:7116.

Naot, Y., and Shalitin, C., 1973, Role of gene 52 in bacteriophage T4 DNA synthesis, *J. Virol.* **11**:862.

Nashimoto, H., and Uchida, H., 1969, Indole as an activator for *in vitro* attachment of tail fibers in the assembly of bacteriophage T4D, *Virology* **37**:1.

Nelson, E. T., and Buller, C. S., 1974, Phospholipase activity in bacteriophage-infected *Escherichia coli*. I. Demonstration of a T4 bacteriophage-associated phospholipase, *J. Virol.* **14**:479.

Neubort, S., and Marmur, J., 1973, Synthesis of the unusual DNA of *Bacillus subtilis* bacteriophage SP-15, *J. Virol.* **12**:1078.

Neville, M. M., and Brown, N. C., 1972, Inhibition of a discrete bacterial DNA polymerase by 6-(*p*-hydroxyphenylazo)-uracil and 6-(*p*-hydroxyphenylazo)-isocytosine, *Nature (London)* **240**:80.

Niles, E. G., Conlon, S. W., and Summers, W. C., 1974, Purification and physical characterization of T7 RNA polymerase from T7-infected *Escherichia coli* B, *Biochemistry* **13**:3904.

Nishihara, M., Chrambach, A., and Aposhian, H. V., 1967, The deoxycytidylate deaminase found in *Bacillus subtilis* infected with phage SP8, *Biochemistry* **6**:1877.

Nomura, M., Matsubara, K., Okamoto, K., and Fujimura, R., 1962, Inhibition of host nucleic acid and protein synthesis by bacteriophage T4: Its relation to the physical and functional integrity of host chromosome, *J. Mol. Biol.* **5**:535.

North, T. W., Stafford, M. E., and Mathews, C. K., 1976, Biochemistry of DNA-defective mutants of bacteriophage T4. VI. Biological functions of gene 42, *J. Virol.* **17**:973.

Nossal, N. G., 1969, A T4 bacteriophage mutant which lacks DNA polymerase but retains the polymerase-associated nuclease, *J. Biol. Chem.* **244**:218.

Nossal, N. G., 1974, DNA synthesis on a double-stranded DNA template by the T4 bacteriophage DNA polymerase and the T4 gene 32 DNA unwinding protein, *J. Biol. Chem.* **249**:5668.

O'Donnell, P. V., and Karam, J. D., 1972, On the direction of reading of bacteriophage T4 gene 43, *J. Virol.* **9**:990.

O'Farrell, P. Z., and Gold, L. M., 1973, Bacteriophage T4 gene expression: Evidence for two classes of prereplicative cistrons, *J. Biol. Chem.* **248**:5502.

O'Farrell, P. Z., Gold, L. M., and Huang, W. M., 1973, The identification of prereplicative bacteriophage T4 proteins, *J. Biol. Chem.* **248**:5499.

Ohshima, S., and Sekiguchi, M., 1972, Induction of a new enzyme activity to excise pyrimidine dimers in *Escherichia coli* infected with bacteriophage T4, *Biochem. Biophys. Res. Commun.* **47**:1126.

Onorato, L., and Showe, M. K., 1975, Gene 21 protein-dependent proteolysis *in vitro* of purified gene 22 product of bacteriophage T4, *J. Mol. Biol.* **92**:395.

Okazaki, R., Okazaki, T., Sakabe, K., Sugimoto, K., and Sugino, A., 1968, Mechanism of DNA chain growth. I. Possible discontinuity and unusual secondary structure of newly synthesized chains, *Proc. Natl. Acad. Sci. USA* **59**:598.

Okker, R. J. H., 1974, The fate of parental DNA of bacteriophage T2 in crosses with bacteriophage T4, *Biochim. Biophys. Acta* **353**:36.

Pacumbaba, R. P., and Center, M. S., 1974, Studies on an endonuclease activity associated with the bacteriophage T7 DNA–membrane complex, *J. Virol.* **14**:1380.

Padan, E., and Shilo, M., 1973, Cyanophages—Viruses attacking blue-green algae, *Bacteriol. Rev.* **37**:343.

Pai, S., Rahmsdorf, H., Ponta, H., Hirsch-Kauffmann, M., Herrlich, P., and Schweiger, M., 1975, Protein kinase of bacteriophage T7, *Eur. J. Biochem.* **55**:305.

Panet, A., Van de Sande, J. H., Loewen, P. C., Khorana, H. G., Raae, A. J., Lillehaug, J. R., and Kleppe, K., 9173, Physical characterization and simultaneous purification of bacteriophage T4 induced polynucleotide kinase, polynucleotide ligase, and DNA polymerase, *Biochemistry* **12**:5045.

Pao, C., and Speyer, J. F., 1973, Order of injection of T7 bacteriophage DNA, *J. Virol.* **11**:1024.

Pao, C. C., and Speyer, J. F., 1975, Mutants of T7 bacteriophage inhibited by lambda prophage, *Proc. Natl. Acad. Sci. USA* **72**:3642.

Parson, K. A., and Snustad, D. P., 1975, Host DNA degradation after infection of *Escherichia coli* with bacteriophage T4: Dependence of the alternate pathway of degradation which occurs in the absence of both T4 endonuclease II and nuclear disruption on T4 endonuclease IV, *J. Virol.* **15**:221.

Parson, K. A., Warner, H. R., Anderson, D. L., and Snustad, D. P., 1973, Analysis of nuclear disruption and binding of intermediates in host DNA breakdown to membranes after infection of *Escherichia coli* with bacteriophages T4 and T7, *J. Virol.* **11**:806.

Pees, M., and deGroot, B., 1975, Mutants of bacteriophage T4 unable to exclude T2 from the progeny of crosses, *Virology* **67**:94.

Peterson, R. H. F., and Buller, C. S., 1969, Phospholipid metabolism in T4 bacteriophage-infected *Escherichia coli* K12 (λ), *J. Virol.* **3**:463.

Plate, C. A., Suit, J. L., Jetton, A. M., and Luria, S. E., 1974, Effects of colicin K on a mutant of *Escherichia coli* deficient in Ca^{+2}, Mg^{+2}-activated adenosine triphosphatase, *J. Biol. Chem.* **249**:6138.

Pollock, P. N., and Duckworth, D. H., 1973, Outer-membrane proteins induced by T4 bacteriophage, *Biochim. Biophys. Acta* **322**:321.

Ponta, H., Rahmsdorf, H. J., Pai, S. H., Hirsch-Kauffman, M., Herrlich, P., and Schweiger, M., 1974, Control of gene expression in bacteriophage T7: Transcriptional controls, *Mol. Gen. Genet.* **134**:281.

Pribnow, D., 1975, Nucleotide sequence of an RNA polymerase binding site at an early T7 promoter, *Proc. Natl. Acad. Sci. USA* **72**:784.

Price, A. R., and Cook, S. J., 1972, New DNA polymerase induced by *Bacillus subtilis* phage PBS2, *J. Virol.* **9**:602.

Price, A. R., and Fogt, S. M., 1973a, dTMP phosphohydrolase induced by bacteriophage PBS2 during infection of *Bacillus subtilis*, *J. Biol. Chem.* **248**:1372.

Price, A. R., and Fogt, S., 1973b, Resistance of bacteriophage PBS2 infection to 6-(*p*-hydroxyphenylazo)-uracil, an inhibitor of *Bacillus subtilis* DNA synthesis, *J. Virol.* **11**:338.

Price, A. R., and Warner, H. R., 1969, Bacteriophage T4-induced dCTP-dUTP nucleotidohydrolase: Its properties and its role during phage infection of *Escherichia coli*, *Virology* **37**:882.

Price, A. R., Dunham, L. F., and Walker, R. L., 1972, dTTP nucleotidohydrolase and dUMP hydroxymethylase induced by mutants of *Bacillus subtilis* bacteriophage SP82G, *J. Virol.* **10**:1240.

Puck, T. T., and Lee, H. H., 1955, Mechanism of cell wall penetration by viruses. II. Demonstration of cyclic permeability changes accompanying virus infection of *Escherichia coli* B cells, *J. Exp. Med.* **101**:151.

Rahmsdorf, H. J., Herrlich, P., Pai, S. H., Schweiger, M., and Wittmann, H. G., 1973, Ribosomes after infection with bacteriophage T4 and T7, *Mol. Gen. Genet.* **127**:259.

Rahmsdorf, H. J., Pai, S. H., Ponta, H., Herrlich, P., Roskosi, R., Jr., Schweiger, M., and Studier, F. W., 1974, Protein kinase induction in *Escherichia coli* by bacteriophage T7, *Proc. Natl. Acad. Sci. USA* **71**:586.

Ratner, D., 1974a, Bacteriophage T4 transcriptional control gene 55 codes for a protein bound to *Escherichia coli* RNA polymerase, *J. Mol. Biol.* **89**:803.

Ratner, D., 1974b, The interaction of bacterial and phage proteins with immobilized *Escherichia coli* RNA polymerase, *J. Mol. Biol.* **88**:373.

Reuben, R. C., and Gefter, M. L., 1973, A DNA-binding protein induced by bacteriophage T7, *J. Biol. Chem.* **249**:3843 (*Proc. Natl. Acad. Sci. USA* **70**:1846, 1974).

Revel, H. R., and Georgopoulos, C. P., 1969, Restriction of nonglucosylated T-even bacteriophages by prophage P1, *Virology* **39**:1.

Revel, H. R., and Hattman, S., 1971, Mutants of T2gt with altered DNA methylase activity: Relation to restriction by prophage P1, *Virology* **45**:484.

Revel, H. R., and Luria, S. E., 1970, DNA glucosylation in T-even phages: Genetic determination and role in phage-host interaction, *Annu. Rev. Genet.* **4**:177.

Reznikoff, W. S., and Thomas, C. A., Jr., 1969, The anatomy of the SP50 bacteriophage DNA molecule, *Virology* **37**:309.

Rhoades, M., and Rhoades, E. A., 1972, Terminal repetition in the DNA of bacteriophage T5, *J. Mol. Biol.* **69**:187.

Richardson, C. C., 1965, Phosphorylation of nucleic acid by an enzyme from bacteriophage-infected *Escherichia coli*, *Proc. Natl. Acad. Sci. USA* **54**:158.

Rima, B. K., and Takahashi, I., 1973, The synthesis of nucleic acids in *Bacillus subtilis* infected with phage PBS1, *Can. J. Biochem.* **51**:1219.

Ritchie, D. A., Jamieson, A. T., and White, F. E., 1974, The induction of deoxythymidine kinase by bacteriophage T4, *J. Gen. Virol.* **24**:115.

Riva, S., Cascino, A., and Geiduschek, E. P., 1970, Coupling of late transcription to viral replication in bacteriophage T4 development, *J. Mol. Biol.* **54**:85.

Rosenthal, D., and Reid, P., 1973, Rifampicin resistant DNA synthesis in phage T4-infected *Escherichia coli*, *Biochem. Biophys. Res. Commun.* **55**:993.

Rosenkranz, H. S., 1973, RNA in coliphage T5, *Nature (London)* **242**:327.

Russel, M., 1973, Control of bacteriophage T4 DNA polymerase synthesis, *J. Mol. Biol.* **79**:83.

Russell, R. L., 1974, Comparative genetics of the T-even bacteriophages, *Genetics* **78**:967.

Russell, R. L., and Huskey, R. J., 1974, Partial exclusion between T-even bacteriophages: An incipient genetic isolation mechanism, *Genetics* **78**:989.

Sadowski, P. D., and Bakyta, I., 1972, T4 endonuclease IV. Improved purification procedure and resolution from T4 endonuclease III, *J. Biol. Chem.* **247**:405.

Sadowski, P., and Hurwitz, J., 1969, Enzymatic breakage of DNA. I. Purification and properties of endonuclease II from T4 phage-infected *Escherichia coli*, *J. Biol. Chem.* **244**:6182.

Sadowski, P. D., and Kerr, C., 1970, Degradation of *E. coli* B DNA after infection with DNA-defective amber mutants of bacteriophage T7, *J. Virol.* **6**:149.

Sakaki, Y., 1974, Inactivation of the ATP-dependent DNase of *Escherichia coli* after infection with double-stranded DNA phages, *J. Virol.* **14**:1611.

Salser, W., Bolle, A., and Epstein, R., 1970, Transcription during bacteriophage T4 development, *J. Mol. Biol.* **49**:271.

Sano, H., and Feix, G., 1974, RNA ligase activity of DNA ligase from phage T4 infected *Escherichia coli, Biochemistry* **13**:5110.

Sauri, C. J., and Earhart, C. F., 1971, Superinfection with bacteriophage T4: Inverse relationship between genetic exclusion and membrane association of DNA of secondary bacteriophage, *J. Virol.* **8**:856.

Schachner, M., and Zillig, W., 1971, Fingerprint maps of tryptic peptides from subunits of *Escherichia coli* and T4-modified DNA-dependent RNA polymerases, *Eur. J. Biochem.* **22**:513.

Schachtele, C. F., deSain, C. V., Hawley, L. A., and Anderson, D. L., 1972, Transcription during the development of bacteriophage ϕ29: Production of host- and ϕ29-specific RNA, *J. Virol.* **10**:1170.

Schachtele, C. F., deSain, C. V., and Anderson, D. L., 1973*a*, Transcription during the development of bacteriophage ϕ29: Definition of "early" and "late" RNA, *J. Virol.* **11**:9.

Schachtele, C. F., Reilly, B. E., deSain, C. V., Whittington, M. O., and Anderson, D. L., 1973*b*, Selective replication of bacteriophage ϕ29 DNA in 6-(*p*-hydroxyphenylazo)-uracil-treated *Bacillus subtilis, J. Virol.* **11**:153.

Schedl, P. D., Singer, R. E., and Conway, T. W., 1970, A factor required for the translation of bacteriophage f2 RNA in extracts of T4-infected cells, *Biochem. Biophys. Res. Commun.* **38**:631.

Scheible, P. P., and Rhoades, M., 1975, Heteroduplex mapping of heat-resistant deletion mutants of bacteriophage T5, *J. Virol.* **15**:1276.

Scherberg, N. H., and Weiss, S. B., 1970, Detection of bacteriophage T4-and T5-coded transfer RNA's, *Proc. Natl. Acad. Sci. USA* **67**:1164.

Scherzinger, E., and Liftin, F., 1974, *In vitro* studies on the role of phage T7 gene 4 product in DNA replication, *Mol. Gen. Genet.* **135**:73.

Schiff, N., Miller, M. J., and Wahba, A. J., 1974, Purification and properties of chain initiation factor 3 from T4-infected and uninfected *Escherichia coli* MRE 600, *J. Biol. Chem.* **249**:3797.

Schlegel, R. A., and Thomas, C. A., Jr., 1972, Some special structural features of intracellular bacteriophage T7 concatemers, *J. Mol. Biol.* **68**:319.

Schnitzlein, C. F., Albrecht, I., and Drake, J. W., 1974, Is bacteriophage T4 DNA polymerase involved in the repair of ultraviolet damage? *Virology* **59**:580.

Schnös, M., and Inman, R. B., 1970, Position of branch points in replicating λ DNA, *J. Mol. Biol.* **51**:61.

Schweiger, M., and Herrlich, P., 1974, DNA-directed enzyme synthesis *in vitro, Curr. Top. Microbiol. Immunol.* **65**:58.

Scocca, J. J., Panny, S. R., and Bessman, M. J., 1969, Studies of deoxycytidylate deaminase from T4-infected *Escherichia coli, J. Biol. Chem.* **244**:3698.

Scofield, M. S., Collinsworth, W. L., and Mathews, C. K., 1974, Continued synthesis of bacterial DNA after infection by bacteriophage T4, *J. Virol.* **13**:847.

Segal, J., Tjian, R., Pero, J., and Losick, R., 1974, Chloramphenicol restores sigma factor activity to sporulating *Bacillus subtilis, Proc. Natl. Acad. Sci. USA* **71**:4860.

Sekiguchi, M., 1966, Studies on the physiological defect in *r*II mutants of bacteriophage T4, *J. Mol. Biol.* **16**:503.

Serwer, P., 1974*a*, Fast sedimenting bacteriophage T7 DNA from T7-infected *Escherichia coli, Virology* **59**:70.

Serwer, P., 1974*b*, Complexes between bacteriophage T7 capsids and T7 *DNA, Virology* **59**:89.

Shah, D. B., and Berger, H. D., 1971, Replication of gene 46–47 amber mutants of bacteriophage T4D, *J. Mol. Biol.* **57**:17.

Shalitin, C., and Naot, Y., 1971, Role of gene 46 in bacteriophage T4 DNA synthesis, *J. Virol.* **8**:142.

Shames, R. B., Lorkiewicz, Z. K., and Kozinski, A. W., 1973, Injection of ultraviolet-damage-specific enzyme by T4 bacteriophage, *J. Virol.* **12**:1.

Shapira, A., Giberman, E., and Kohn, A., 1974, Recoverable potassium fluxes variations following adsorption of T4 phage and their ghosts on *Escherichia coli* B, *J. Gen. Virol.* **23**:159.

Short, E. C., Jr., and Koerner, J. F., 1969, Separation and characterization of deoxyribonucleases of *Escherichia coli* B. II. Further purification and properties of an exonuclease induced by infection with bacteriophage T2, *J. Biol. Chem.* **244**:1487.

Siegel, P. J., and Schaechter, M., 1973, Bacteriophage T4 head maturation: Release of progeny DNA from the host cell membrane, *J. Virol.* **11**:359.

Silber, R., Malathi, V. G., and Hurwitz, J., 1972, Purification and properties of bacteriophage T4-induced RNA ligase, *Proc. Natl. Acad. Sci. USA* **69**:3009.

Silver, S., 1965, Acriflavine resistance: A bacteriophage mutation affecting the uptake of dye by the infected bacterial cells, *Proc. Natl. Acad. Sci. USA* **53**:24.

Silver, S., 1967, Acridine sensitivity of bacteriophage T2: A virus gene affecting cell permeability, *J. Mol. Biol.* **29**:191.

Silver, S., Levine, E., and Spielman, P. M., 1968, Cation fluxes and permeability changes accompanying bacteriophage infection of *Escherichia coli, J. Virol.* **2**:763.

Simon, L. D., 1969, The infection of *Escherichia coli* by T2 and T4 bacteriophages as seen in the electron microscope. III. Membrane-associated intracellular bacteriophages, *Virology* **38**:285.

Simon, L. D., 1972, Infection of *Escherichia coli* by T2 and T4 bacteriophages as seen in the electron microscope. IV. T4 head morphogenesis, *Proc. Natl. Acad. Sci. USA* **69**:907.

Simon, L. D., and Anderson, T. F., 1967*a*, The infection of *Escherichia coli* by T2 and T4 bacteriophages as seen in the electron microscope. I. Attachment and penetration, *Virology* **32**:279.

Simon, L. D., and Anderson, T. F., 1967*b*, The infection of *Escherichia coli* by T2 and T4 bacteriophages as seen in the electron microscope. II. Structure and function of the base plate, *Virology* **32**:298.

Simon, L. D., Swan, J. G., and Flatgaard, J. E., 1970, Functional defects in T4 bacteriophages lacking the gene 11 and gene 12 products, *Virology* **41**:77.

Simon, L. D., Snover, D., and Doermann, A. H., 1974, Bacterial mutation affecting T4 phage DNA synthesis and tail production, *Nature (London)* **252**:451.

Simon, L. D., McLaughlin, T. J. M., Snover, D., Ou, J., Grisham, C., and Loeb, M. R., 1975, *E. coli* membrane lipid alteration affecting T4 capsid morphogenesis, *Nature (London)* **256**:379.

Simon, M. N., and Studier, F. W., 1973, Physical mapping of the early region of bacteriophage T4 DNA, *J. Mol. Biol.* **79**:249.

Singer, R. E., and Conway, T. W., 1975, Comparison of the effects of bacteriophage T4 infection and N-ethylmaleimide on the translational specificity of *Escherichia coli* ribosomes, *Arch. Biochem. Biophys.* **166**:549.

Sinha, N. K., and Snustad, D. P., 1971, DNA synthesis in bacteriophage T4-infected *Escherichia coli*: Evidence supporting a stoichiometric role for gene 32-product, *J. Mol. Biol.* **62**:267.

Skalka, A., Poonian, M., and Bartl, P., 1972, Concatemers in DNA replication: Electron microscopic studies of partially denatured intracellular λ DNA, *J. Mol. Biol.* **64**:541.

Skare, J., Niles, E. G., and Summers, W. C., 1974, Localization of the leftmost initiation site for T7 late transcription *in vivo* and *in vitro, Biochemistry* **13**:3912.

Smith, F. A., and Haselkorn, R., 1969, Proteins associated with ribosomes in T4-infected *E. coli, Cold Spring Harbor Symp. Quant. Biol.* **34**:91.

Snustad, D. P., and Conroy, L. M., 1974, Mutants of bacteriophage T4 deficient in the ability to induce nuclear disruption. I. Isolation and genetic characterization, *J. Mol. Biol.* **89**:663.

Snustad, D. P., Warner, H. R., Parson, K. A., and Anderson, D. L., 1972, Nuclear disruption after infection of *Escherichia coli* with a bacteriophage T4 mutant unable to induce endonuclease II, *J. Virol.* **10**:124.

Snustad, D. P., Parson, K. A., Warner, H. R., Tutas, D. J., Wehner, J. M., and Koerner, J. F., 1974, Mutants of bacteriophage T4 deficient in the ability to induce nuclear disruption. II. Physiological state of the host nucleoid in infected cells, *J. Mol. Biol.* **89**:675.

Snustad, D. P., Bursch, C. J. H., Parson, K. A., and Hefeneider, S. H., 1976a, Mutants of bacteriophage T4 deficient in the ability to induce nuclear disruption: shutoff of host DNA and protein synthesis, gene dosage experiments, identification of a restrictive host, and possible biological significance, *J. Virol.* **18**:268.

Snustad, D. P., Tigges, M. A., Parson, K. A., Bursch, C. J. H., Caron, F. M., Koerner, J. F., and Tutas, D. J., 1976b, Identification and preliminary characterization of a mutant defective in the bacteriophage T4-induced unfolding of the *Escherichia coli* nucleoid, *J. Virol.* **17**:622.

Snyder, L., 1973, Change in RNA polymerase associated with the shutoff of host transcription by T4, *Nature (London)* **243**:131.

Spatz, H. C., and Trautner, T. A., 1970, One way to do experiments on gene conversion? *Mol. Gen. Genet.* **109**:84.

Speyer, J. F., and Rosenberg, D., 1968, The function of T4 DNA polymerase, *Cold Spring Harbor Symp. Quant. Biol.* **33**:345.

Speyer, J. F., Chao, J., and Chao, L., 1972, Ribonucleotides covalently linked to DNA in T4 bacteriophage, *J. Virol.* **10**:902.

Stent, G. S., 1963, *Molecular Biology of Bacterial Viruses,* Freeman, San Francisco.

Stevens, A., 1974, DNA-dependent RNA polymerase from two T4 phage-infected systems, *Biochemistry* **13**:493.

Strätling, W., and Knippers, R., 1973, Function and purification of gene 4 protein of phage T7, *Nature (London)* **245**:195.

Strätling, W., Krause, E., and Knippers, R., 1973, Fast sedimenting DNA in bacteriophage T7-infected cells, *Virology* **51**:109.

Streisinger, G., Emrich, J., and Stahl, M. M., 1967, Chromosome structure in phage T4. III. Terminal redundancy and length determination, *Proc. Natl. Acad. Sci. USA* **57**:292.

Studier, F. W., 1972, Bacteriophage T7, *Science* **176**:367.

Studier, F. W., 1973*a*, Genetic analysis of non-essential bacteriophage T7 genes, *J. Mol. Biol.* **79**:227.

Studier, F. W., 1973*b*, Analysis of bacteriophage T7 early RNA's and proteins on slab gels, *J. Mol. Biol.* **79**:237.

Studier, F. W., 1975, Gene 0.3 of bacteriophage T7 acts to overcome the DNA restriction system of the host, *J. Mol. Biol.* **94**:283.

Studier, F. W., and Hausmann, R., 1969, Integration of two sets of T7 mutants, *Virology* **39**:587.

Sugino, A., and Okazaki, R., 1972, Mechanism of DNA chain growth. VII. Direction and rate of growth of T4 nascent short DNA chains, *J. Mol. Biol.* **64**:61.

Summers, W. C., 1969, The process of infection with coliphage T7. I. Characterization of T7 RNA by polyacrylamide gel electrophoretic analysis, *Virology* **39**:175.

Summers, W. C., 1970, The process of infection with coliphage T7. IV. Stability of RNA in bacteriophage-infected cells, *J. Mol. Biol.* **51**:671.

Summers, W. C., and Szybalski, W., 1968, Size, number, and distribution of poly G binding sites on the separated strands of coliphage T7, *Biochim. Biophys. Acta* **166**:371.

Sundar Raj, C. V., and Wu, H. C., 1973, *Escherichia coli* mutants permissive for T4 bacteriophage with deletion in *e* gene, *J. Bacteriol.* **114**:656.

Swift, R. L., and Wiberg, J. S., 1971, Bacteriophage T4 inhibits colicin E2-induced degradation of *Escherichia coli* DNA. I. Protein synthesis-dependent inhibition, *J. Virol.* **8**:303.

Swift, R. L., and Wiberg, J. S., 1973*a*, II. Inhibition by T4 ghosts and by T4 in the absence of protein synthesis, *J. Virol.* **11**:386.

Swift, R. L., and Wiberg, J. S., 1973*b*, III. Zone sedimentation analyses of the DNA degradation products, *J. Mol. Biol.* **80**:743.

Symonds, N., Heindl, H., and White, P., 1973, Radiation sensitive mutants of phage T4: A comparative study, *Mol. Gen. Genet.* **120**:253.

Szabo, C., Dharmgrongartama, B., and Moyer, R. W., 1975, The regulation of transcription in bacteriophage T5-infected *Escherichia coli, Biochemistry* **14**:989.

Takahashi, I., and Marmur, J., 1963, Replacement of thymidylic acid by deoxyuridylic acid of a transducing phage for *Bacillus subtilis, Nature* (*London*) **197**:794.

Takano, T., and Kakefuda, T., 1972, Involvement of a bacterial factor in morphogenesis of bacteriophage capsid, *Nature* (*London*) **239**:34.

Takeishi, K., and Kaji, A., 1975, Presence of active polyribosomes in bacterial cells infected with T4 bacteriophage ghosts, *J. Virol.* **16**:62.

Taketo, A., Yasuda, S., and Sekiguchi, M., 1972, Initial step of excision repair in *Escherichia coli*: Replacement of defective function of *uvr* mutants by T4 endonuclease V, *J. Mol. Biol.* **70**:1.

Tanner, D., and Oishi, M., 1971, The effect of bacteriophage T4 infection on an ATP-dependent deoxyribonuclease in *Escherichia coli, Biochim. Biophys. Acta* **228**:767.

Taylor, D. E., and Guha, A., 1975, Development of bacteriophage F1 in *Clostridium sporogenes*: Characterization of RNA transcripts, *J. Virol.* **16**:107.

Thomas, C. A., Jr., and MacHattie, L. A., 1967, The anatomy of viral DNA molecules, *Annu. Rev. Biochem.* **36**:485.

Tikhonenko, A. S., and Poglazov, B. F., 1963, Localization of ATPase activity in the structural elements of bacteriophage T2, *Biokhimiya* **28**:274.

Tomich, P. K., and Greenberg, G. R., 1973, On the defect of a dCMP hydroxymethylase mutant of bacteriophage T4 showing enzyme activity in extracts, *Biochem. Biophys. Res. Commun.* **50**:1032.

Tomich, P. K., Chiu, C.-S., Wovcha, M. G., and Greenberg, G. R., 1974, Evidence for a complex regulating the *in vivo* activities of early enzymes induced by bacteriophage T4, *J. Biol. Chem.* **249**:7613.

Tomita, F., and Takahashi, I., 1975, DNase specific for uracil-containing bacteriophage DNA, *J. Virol.* **15**:1081.

Tosi, M. E., Reilly, B. E., and Anderson, D. L., 1975, Morphogenesis of bacteriophage φ29 of *Bacillus subtilis*: Cleavage and assembly of the neck appendage protein, *J. Virol.* **16**:1282.

Tutas, D. J., Wehner, J. M., and Koerner, J. F., 1974, Unfolding of the host genome after infection of *Escherichia coli* with bacteriophage T4, *J. Virol.* **13**:548.

Vallée, M., and Cornett, J. B., 1972, A new gene of bacteriophage T4 determining immunity against superinfecting ghosts and phage in T4-infected *Escherichia coli, Virology* **48**:777.

Vallée, M., and Cornett, J. B., 1973, The immunity reaction of bacteriophage T4: A noncatalytic reaction, *Virology* **53**:441.

Vander Maten, M., Nelson, E. T., and Buller, C. S., 1974, Does phospholipase have a role in killing and SDS lysis of T4 ghost-infected *Escherichia coli? J. Virol.* **14**:1617.

Varon, M., and Levisohn, R., 1972, Three-membered parasitic system: A bacteriophage, *Bdellovibrio bacteriovorus*, and *Escherichia coli, J. Virol.* **9**:519.

Vetter, D., and Sadowski, P. D., 1974, Point mutants in the D2a region of bacteriophage T4 fail to induce T4 endonuclease IV, *J. Virol.* **14**:207.

Wais, A. C., and Goldberg, E. B., 1969, Growth and transformation of phage T4 in *Escherichia coli* B/4, *Salmonella, Aerobacter, Proteus*, and *Serratia, Virology* **39**:153.

Warner, H. R., and Hobbs, M. D., 1967, Incorporation of uracil-^{14}C into nucleic acids in *Escherichia coli* infected with bacteriophage T4 and T4 amber mutants, *Virology* **33**:376.

Warner, H. R., Snustad, D. P., Jorgenson, S. E., and Koerner, J. G., 1970, Isolation of bacteriophage T4 mutants defective in the ability to degrade host DNA, *J. Virol.* **5**:700.

Warner, H. R., Snustad, D. P., Koerner, J. F., and Childs, J. D., 1972, Identification and genetic characterization of mutants of bacteriophage T4 defective in the ability to induce exonuclease A, *J. Virol.* **9**:399.

Warner, H. R., Drong, R. F., and Berget, S. M., 1975, Early events after infection of *Escherichia coli* by bacteriophage T5, *J. Virol.* **15**:273.

Watson, J. D., 1972, Origin of concatemeric DNA, *Nature (London)* **239**:197.

Weintraub, S. B., and Frankel, F. R., 1972, Identification of the T4 *r*IIB gene product as a membrane protein, *J. Mol. Biol.* **70**:589.

Werner, R., 1968, Distribution of growing points in DNA of bacteriophage T4, *J. Mol. Biol.* **33**:679.

Whiteley, H. R., Kolenbrander, P. E., and Hemphill, H. E., 1974, Mixed infections of *Bacillus subtilis* involving bacteriophages SP82 and β22, *J. Virol.* **14**:1463.

Wiberg, J. S., Mendelsohn, S., Warner, V., Hercules, K., Aldrich, C., and Munro, J. L., 1973, SP62, a viable mutant of T4D defective in regulation of phage enzyme synthesis, *J. Virol.* **12**:775.

Wilson, J. H., 1973, Function of the bacteriophage T4 transfer RNA's, *J. Mol. Biol.* **74**:753.

Wilson, J. H., and Abelson, J. N., 1972, Bacteriophage T4 transfer RNA. II. Mutants of T4 defective in the formation of functional suppressor transfer RNA, *J. Mol. Biol.* **69**:57.

Wilson, J. H., Kim, J. S., and Abelson, J. N., 1972, Bacteriophage T4 transfer RNA. III. Clustering of the genes for the T4 transfer RNA's, *J. Mol. Biol.* **71**:547.

Witmer, H. J., 1974, Regulation of bacteriophage T4 gene expression, *Progr. Mol. Submol. Biol.* **4**:65.

Witmer, H. J., Baros, A., and Forbes, J., 1975, Effect of chloramphenicol and starvation for an essential amino acid on polypeptide and polyribonucleotide synthesis in *Escherichia coli* infected with bacteriophage T4, *Arch. Biochem. Biophys.* **169**:406.

Wolfson, J., and Dressler, D., 1972, Regions of single-stranded DNA in the growing points of replicating bacteriophage T7 chromosomes, *Proc. Natl. Acad. Sci. USA* **69**:2682.

Wood, W. B., 1974, Genetic map of bacteriophage T4, In *Handbook of Genetics,* Vol. 1 (R. C. King, ed.), pp. 327–331, Plenum, New York.

Wovcha, M. G., Tomich, P. K., Chiu, C.-S., and Greenberg, G. R., 1973, Direct participation of dCMP hydroxymethylase in T4 phage DNA replication, *Proc. Natl. Acad. Sci. USA* **70**:2196.

Wu, R., and Geiduschek, E. P., 1975, The role of replication proteins in the regulation of bacteriophage T4 transcription. I. Gene 45 and hydroxymethyl-C-containing DNA, *J. Mol. Biol.* **96**:513.

Wu, R., and Yeh, Y.-C., 1974, DNA arrested mutants of gene 59 of bacteriophage T4. II. Replicative intermediates, *Virology* **59**:108.

Wu, R., Geiduschek, E. P., and Cascino, A., 1975a, The role of replication proteins in the regulation of bacteriophage T4 transcription. II. Gene 45 and late transcription uncoupled from replication, *J. Mol. Biol.* **96**:539.

Wu, R., Wu, J.-L., and Yeh, Y.-C., 1975b, Role of gene 59 of bacteriophage T4 in repair of UV-irradiated and alkylated DNA *in vivo, J. Virol.* **16**:5.

Wyatt, G. R., and Cohen, S. S., 1953, The base of the nucleic acids of some bacterial and animal viruses: The occurrence of 5-hydroxymethylcytosine, *Biochem. J.* **55**:774.

Yamamoto, M., and Uchida, H., 1975, Organization and function of the tail of bacteriophage T4. II. Structural control of the tail contraction, *J. Mol. Biol.* **92**:207.

Yamazaki, Y., 1969, Enzymatic activities on cell walls in bacteriophage T4, *Biochim. Biophys. Acta* **178**:542.

Yanagida, M., and Ahmad-Zadeh, C., 1970, Determination of gene product positions in bacteriophage T4 by specific antibody association, *J. Mol. Biol.* **51**:411.

Yasuda, S., and Sekiguchi, M., 1970, T4 endonuclease involved in repair of DNA, *Proc. Natl. Acad. Sci. USA* **67**:1839.

Yegian, C. D., Mueller, M., Selzer, G., Russo, V., and Stahl, F. W., 1971, Properties of DNA-delay mutants of bacteriophage T4, *Virology* **46**:900.

Yeh, Y.-C., and Tessman, I., 1972, Control by bacteriophage T4 of the reduction of adenoside nucleotide to deoxyadenosine nucleotide, *J. Biol. Chem.* **247**:3252.

Yehle, C. O., and Ganesan, A. T., 1973, DNA synthesis in bacteriophage SPO1-infected *Bacillus subtilis, J. Biol. Chem.* **248**:7456.

Yudelevich, H., 1971, Specific cleavage of an *Escherichia coli* leucine transfer RNA following bacteriophage T4 infection, *J. Mol. Biol.* **60**:21.

Zetter, B. R., and Cohen, P. S., 1974, Post-transcriptional regulation of T4 enzyme synthesis, *Arch. Biochem. Biophys.* **162**:560.

Zillig, W., Fujiki, H., Blum, W., Janekovic, D., Schweiger, M., Rahmsdorf, H., Ponta, H., and Hirsch-Kauffman, M., 1975, *In vivo* and *in vitro* phosphorylation of DNA-dependent RNA polymerase of *Escherichia coli* by bacteriophage T7-induced protein kinase, *Proc. Natl. Acad. Sci. USA* **72**:2506.

Zweig, M., and Cummings, D. J., 1973, Structural proteins of bacteriophage T5, *Virology* **51**:443.

Index